BLUEPRINTS
SURGERY

Fifth Edition

BLUEPRINTS
SURGERY

Fifth Edition

Seth J. Karp, MD
Attending Surgeon
Beth Israel Deaconess Medical Center
Assistant Professor of Surgery
Harvard Medical School
Boston, Massachusetts

James P.G. Morris, MD, FACS
Thoracic and General Surgeon
The Permanente Medical Group
Chief of Surgery
South San Francisco Kaiser Hospital
South San Francisco, California

Questions and answers provided by

Stanley Zaslau, MD, MBA, FACS
Associate Professor
Division of Urology
West Virginia University
School of Medicine
Morgantown, West Virginia

 Wolters Kluwer | Lippincott Williams & Wilkins
Health
Philadelphia • Baltimore • New York • London
Buenos Aires • Hong Kong • Sydney • Tokyo

Acquisitions Editor: Charles W. Mitchell
Senior Managing Editor: Stacey Sebring
Editorial Assistant: Catherine Noonan
Marketing Manager: Jennifer Kuklinski
Creative Director: Doug Smock
Associate Production Manager: Kevin P. Johnson
Compositor: International Typesetting and Composition

Fifth Edition

351 West Camden Street   530 Walnut Street
Baltimore, MD 21201   Philadelphia, PA 19106

Printed in China

15 14
9 8 7 6 5 4

Library of Congress Cataloging-in-Publication Data

Karp, Seth J.
  Surgery / Seth J. Karp, James P.G. Morris ; questions and answers provided by Stanley Zaslau.—5th ed.
      p. ; cm.—(Blueprints)
  Rev. ed. of: Blueprints surgery / Seth J. Karp, James P.G. Morris. 4th ed. c2006.
  Includes bibliographical references and index.
  ISBN-13: 978-0-7817-8868-7
  ISBN-10: 0-7817-8868-4
  1. Surgery—Outlines, syllabi, etc.   I. Morris, James, 1964-   II. Zaslau, Stanley.   III. Karp, Seth J. Blueprints surgery.   IV. Title.   V. Series.
  [DNLM: 1. Surgical Procedures, Operative—Examination Questions. WO 18.2 K18s 2009]
    RD37.3.K37 2009
    617'.910076—dc22

                                             2008035981

To purchase additional copies of this book, call our customer service department at **(800) 638-3030** or fax orders to **(301) 223-2320**. International customers should call **(301) 223-2300**.

Visit Lippincott Williams & Wilkins on the Internet: http://www.lww.com. Lippincott Williams & Wilkins customer service representatives are available from 8:30 am to 6:00 pm, EST.

To Lauren, Sarah, and Jay. S.J.K.

To Caroline, Isabel, Grant, and Cameron. J.P.G.M.

Preface

It has been 12 years since the first five books in the *Blueprints* series were published. Originally intended as board review for medical students, interns, and residents who wanted high-yield, accurate clinical content for U.S. Medical Licensing Examination (USMLE) Steps 2 and 3, the series now also serves as a guide to students during third-year and senior rotations. We are extremely proud that the original books and the entire *Blueprints* brand of review materials have far exceeded our expectations and have been dependable reference sources for so many students.

The fifth edition of *Blueprints Surgery* has been significantly revised. Reorganization of the Table of Contents creates a more logical flow to the chapters. Every chapter includes updates to reflect current practices in the field. A new chapter in the gastrointestinal section explores bariatric surgery. Similar to the previous edition, sample operative reports are included in an appendix. As *Blueprints* is used in a wider range of clinical settings, students have had the opportunity to review and comment on what additional material would be useful. In response, an increased number of figures, including radiographic studies, photographs, and drawings, integrate with the text. This fifth edition is the first to include a color insert, showing detailed depictions of surgical techniques. The Questions and Answers sections include 25% more material for USMLE Board review. Finally, suggestions for additional reading are available online, along with an additional 50 USMLE-format questions and answers for further self-study.

We sincerely hope this edition preserves the original vision of *Blueprints* to provide concise, useful information for students and that the additional material enhances this vision.

Seth J. Karp, MD
James P.G. Morris, MD

Contributors

Ramzi Alami, MD
Bariatric & General Surgeon
Department of Surgery
The Permanente Medical Group
South San Francisco Kaiser Hospital
South San Francisco, CA
Chapter 10

Rona L.T. Chen, MD, FACS
General Surgeon
Department of Surgery
The Permanente Medical Group
South San Francisco Kaiser Hospital
South San Francisco, CA
Chapter 14

Grant Cooper, MD
Fellow
Spine, Sports and Musculoskeletal Medicine
Orthopedics and Rehabilitation Medicine
Beth Israel Medical Center
New York, NY
Chapter 25

Jason Cooper, MD
Plastic Surgery Resident
Department of Surgery
Brigham and Women's Hospital
Harvard Plastic Surgery
Boston, MA
Chapter 24

David Le, MD
Bariatric & General Surgeon
Department of Surgery
The Permanente Medical Group
South San Francisco Kaiser Hospital
South San Francisco, CA
Chapter 10

Alice Yeh, MD, FACS
Surgical Oncologist
Department of Surgery
The Permanente Medical Group
South San Francisco Kaiser Hospital
South San Francisco, CA
Chapter 12 and 13

Stanley Zaslau, MD, MBA, FACS
Program Director, Associate Professor
Division of Urology
West Virginia University
Morgantown, WV
Questions and Answers

Contents

xii • Contents

Abbreviations

ABGs	arterial blood gases	CN	cranial nerve
ACAS	Asymptomatic Carotid Atherosclerosis Study	CNS	central nervous system
		COPD	chronic obstructive pulmonary disease
ACE	angiotensin-converting enzyme	CPAP	continuous positive airway pressure
ACTH	adrenocorticotropic hormone	CRF	corticotropin-releasing factor
ADH	antidiuretic hormone	CRH	corticotropin-releasing hormone
AFP	alpha-fetoprotein	CSF	cerebrospinal fluid
AI	aortic insufficiency	CT	computed tomography
ALT	alanine transaminase	CXR	chest x-ray
ANA	antinuclear antibody	DCIS	ductal carcinoma in situ
AP	anteroposterior	DEXA	dual-energy x-ray absorptiometry
APKD	adult polycystic kidney disease	DHT	dihydrotestosterone
ARDS	adult respiratory distress syndrome	DIC	disseminated intravascular coagulation
AS	aortic stenosis	DIP	distal interphalangeal
ASD	atrial septal defect	DNA	deoxyribonucleic acid
AST	aspartate transaminase	DTRs	deep tendon reflexes
ATLS	Advanced Trauma Life Support	ECG	electrocardiography
AUA-IPSS	American Urological Association Symptom Score	EEG	electroencephalogram
		EGD	esophagogastroduodenoscopy
AV	arteriovenous	EMG	electromyography
BCC	basal cell carcinoma	ERCP	endoscopic retrograde cholangiopancreatography
BCG	bacill (bacillus) Calmette-Guérin		
BE	barium enema	ESR	erythrocyte sedimentation rate
β-hCG	beta-human chorionic gonadotropin	EUS	endoscopic esophageal ultrasound
		ESWL	extracorporeal shock wave lithotripsy
BP	blood pressure	FDG-PET	fluorodeoxyglucose positron emission tomography
BPH	benign prostatic hypertrophy		
BRCA	breast cancer gene	FNA	fine-needle aspiration
BUN	blood urea nitrogen	FSH	follicle-stimulating hormone
CABG	coronary artery bypass graft	G-6-PD	glucose-6-phosphate dehydrogenase
CAD	coronary artery disease	GBM	glioblastoma multiforme
CBC	complete blood count	GCS	Glasgow Coma Scale
CCK	cholecystokinin	GERD	gastroesophageal reflux disease
CDC	Centers for Disease Control and Prevention	GGT	gamma-glutamyl transferase
		GH	growth hormone
CEA	carcinoembryonic antigen	GI	gastrointestinal
CES	cauda equina syndrome	GU	genitourinary
CHF	congestive heart failure	Hb	hemoglobin
CIS	carcinoma in situ	hCG	human chorionic gonadotropin
CMF	cyclophosphamide, methotrexate, and 5-fluorouracil	HIDA	hepatobiliary iminodiacetic acid
		HIV	human immunodeficiency virus
CMV	cytomegalovirus	HLA	human leukocyte antigen

HPF	high-power field	PBS	peripheral blood smear
HPI	history of present illness	PCNL	percutaneous nephrolithotomy
HPV	human papilloma virus	PDA	posterior descending coronary artery
HR	heart rate	PDS	polydioxanone
ICP	intracranial pressure	PE	physical examination
ID/CC	identification and chief complaint	PEEP	positive end-expiratory pressure
IgA	immunoglobulin A	PET	positron-emission tomography
IL-2	interleukin-2	PFTs	pulmonary function tests
IMA	inferior mesenteric artery	PIP	proximal interphalangeal
IMV	inferior mesenteric vein	PMI	point of maximal impulse
INR	international normalized ratio	PP	pancreatic polypeptide
ITP	immune thrombocytopenic purpura	PPI	proton-pump inhibitors
IVP	intravenous pyelography	PSA	prostate-specific antigen
JVD	jugular venous distention	PT	prothrombin time
KUB	kidneys/ureter/bladder	PTC	percutaneous transhepatic cholangiography
LAD	left anterior descending coronary artery	PTH	parathyroid hormone
LCA	left coronary artery	PTU	propylthiouracil
LCIS	lobular carcinoma in situ	RA	right atrium
LCX	left circumflex	RBC	red blood cell
LDH	lactate dehydrogenase	RCA	right coronary artery
LES	lower esophageal sphincter	REM	rapid eye movement
LFTs	liver function tests	RPLND	retroperitoneal lymph node dissection
LH	luteinizing hormone	RR	respiratory rate
LH-RH	luteinizing hormone-releasing hormone	RV	right ventricular
LM	left main coronary artery	RVH	right ventricular hypertrophy
LVH	left ventricular hypertrophy	SAH	subarachnoid hemorrhage
Lytes	electrolytes	SBFT	small bowel follow-through
MCP	metacarpophalangeal	SBO	small bowel obstruction
MCV	mean corpuscular volume	SCC	squamous cell carcinoma
MELD	Model for End-Stage Liver Disease	SIADH	syndrome of inappropriate secretion of ADH
MEN	multiple endocrine neoplasia		
MHC	major histocompatibility complex	SLNB	sentinel lymph node biopsy
MI	myocardial infarction	SMA	superior mesenteric artery
MMF	mycophenolate mofetil	SMV	superior mesenteric vein
MPA	mycophenolic acid	SSI	surgical site infection
MR	mitral regurgitation	STD	sexually transmitted disease
MRCP	magnetic resonance cholangiopancreatography	STSG	split-thickness skin graft
		TCC	transitional cell carcinoma
MRI	magnetic resonance imaging	TIA	transient ischemic attack
MS	mitral stenosis	TIBC	total iron-binding capacity
MTC	medullary thyroid carcinoma	TIPS	transjugular intrahepatic portosystemic shunt
MVA	motor vehicle accident		
NASCET	North American Symptomatic Carotid Endarterectomy Trial	TNM	tumors, nodes, metastases classification
		TPN	total parenteral nutrition
NG	nasogastric	TRAM	transverse rectus abdominis myocutaneous
NPO	nil per os (nothing by mouth)		
NSAID	nonsteroidal anti-inflammatory drug	TRH	thyrotropin-releasing hormone
NSGCT	nonseminomatous germ cell tumor	TSH	thyroid-stimulating hormone
Nuc	nuclear medicine	TUBD	transurethral balloon dilatation
OPSS	overwhelming postsplenectomy sepsis	TUNA	transurethral needle ablation
PA	posteroanterior		

TURP	transurethral resection of the prostate	VMA	vanillylmandelic acid
UA	urinalysis	VS	vital signs
UGI	upper gastrointestinal	VSD	ventricular septal defect
US	ultrasound	WBC	white blood cell
UTI	urinary tract infection	XR	x-ray
UV	ultraviolet		

Part I

Introduction

Surgical Techniques

INTRODUCTION

As with most endeavors in life, the healing arts are divided into both the theoretical and the practical spheres. Surgeons are fortunate to practice equally in both spheres by applying their intellect and technical skill to the diagnosis and treatment of sickness. The practice of surgery is unique in the realm of medicine and correspondingly carries added responsibilities. Patients literally place their trust in the hands of surgeons. The profound nature of cutting into another human being, and artfully manipulating his or her physical being to achieve wellness, requires reverence, skill, and judgment.

Technologic advances in modern medicine have led to the rise and establishment of procedure-related specialties, including invasive cardiology and radiology, dermatology, intensive care medicine, and emergency medicine, to name a few. Manipulative skills are now required not only in the operating room but also in procedure rooms and emergency rooms for invasive treatments and repairing traumatic injuries. Therefore, medical students and residents should master the basics of surgical technique so they are well prepared for the challenges ahead.

PREOPERATIVE ISSUES

For well-trained and experienced surgeons, performing an operation is usually a routine affair and is relatively simple. One of the difficulties in taking care of surgical patients, however, is actually making the decision to operate. Operating is simple; deciding not to operate is the more difficult decision. Ultimately, the surgeon and patient must assess the risk-to-benefit

ratio and decide whether the potential benefits of surgery outweigh the potential risks. Once the decision has been made to proceed with surgery, the surgeon must formulate a clear operative plan, taking into account and preparing for any potential deviations that may be required based on the intraoperative findings.

The relationship between patient and doctor is based on a special trust. In the surgical sphere, individuals grant their surgeon permission to render them unconscious, invade their body cavities, and remove or manipulate their internal structures to a degree that the latter deems appropriate. Physicians must never minimize the importance of this special trust that underlies the surgical relationship. A surgeon gains a patient's trust by engaging in a thorough discussion before the decision to operate is reached, outlining the clinical situation and indications for surgery. All reasonable management options should be reviewed and the risks and potential complications of each presented. This process of decision making is known as informed consent. Appropriate written documentation must be obtained—usually a "request" for operation, rather than a more passive "consent"—and signed by the patient or guardian, the person performing the procedure, and a witness.

Adequate preparation of a patient for surgery depends on examining the magnitude and nature of the intended operation in light of the patient's general medical condition. The surgical patient must be able to endure the potential insults of surgery (hypotension, hypoxemia, hypothermia, anemia, and postoperative pain) without being exposed to unacceptable risks of morbidity and mortality. All patients, particularly older adult patients with multiple medical problems, should undergo an appropriate preoperative evaluation to identify and thoroughly evaluate medical illnesses and thereby more accurately establish the degree of

■ TABLE 1-1 Preoperative Diagnostic Testing

Body System/Specialty	Tests Used	Disorders Identified
Cardiac*	Electrocardiography	Ischemic heart disease
	Echocardiography	Cardiac arrhythmias
	Radionuclide ventriculography	Congestive heart failure
	Thallium scintigraphy	Valvular heart disease
	Pathophysiologic limitations of testing	Hypertension
Respiratory	Chest x-ray	Chronic obstructive pulmonary disease
	Arterial blood gas	Obstructive sleep apnea
	Peak expiratory flow rate	
	Pulmonary function test	
	Sleep study	
Endocrine	Blood test	Diabetes mellitus
		Adrenal disorder
		Thyroid disorder
Hematology	Blood test	Thromboembolic disease
		Bleeding disorder
Gastrointestinal	Blood test	Liver disease
	Radiographic imaging	Intestinal obstruction
	Endoscopy	Malnutrition

*Scoring systems include Goldman Index, Eagle Criteria, Detsky Score, and Revised Cardiac Risk Index.

perioperative risk that the proposed surgery entails. The two main goals of preoperative evaluation are to assess and maximize the patient's health, as well as to anticipate and avoid possible perioperative complications. Consultation with a cardiologist, pulmonologist, endocrinologist, or internist may involve specific diagnostic tests and laboratory studies (Table 1-1).

Preoperative assessment is also made by an anesthesiologist before surgery to determine the patient's fitness for anesthesia, which is evaluated according to the American Society of Anesthesiologists Physical Status Classification System. Class I indicates a fit and healthy patient, whereas class V indicates a moribund patient not expected to survive 24 hours with or without an operation (Table 1-2).

Routine preoperative screening tests are ordered only when indicated by rational guidelines. Gone are the days when asymptomatic, low-risk, minor surgery patients were subjected to an extensive and expensive battery of tests (blood tests, chest x-ray, urinalysis, and electrocardiogram). The belief was that a thorough array of tests would systematically detect occult conditions, thereby avoiding potential morbidity and mortality. Over time, such an approach has been devalued, as published studies have shown that routine medical testing has not measurably increased

■ TABLE 1-2 American Society of Anesthesiologists Physical Status Classification System

Class	Description
Class I	A fit and healthy patient
Class II	A patient with mild systemic disease (e.g., hypertension)
Class III	A patient with severe systemic disease that limits activity but is not incapacitating
Class IV	A patient with an incapacitating systemic disease that is a constant threat to life
Class V	A moribund patient not expected to survive 24 hours with or without an operation

Note: If the procedure is performed as an emergency, an "E" is added to the physical status classification. Example: A healthy 70-year-old male with mild hypertension undergoing emergent appendectomy is considered class II E.

surgical safety. Therefore, modern preoperative testing relies on defined guidelines that focus on evaluating the risk arising from patient-specific comorbidities and conditions.

A foundational principle of the medical tradition is to do no harm: primum non nocere. In 2000, a widely publicized report from the Institute of Medicine, *To Err is Human*, estimated that 98,000 people die each year in U.S. hospitals as a result of medical injuries. This report, among others already in the literature, led to the creation of a number of national quality improvement projects that were specifically designed to improve surgical care in hospitals. One of the best known is the Surgical Care Improvement Project (SCIP), part of a national campaign aimed at reducing surgical complications by 25% by 2010. The multiyear project is sponsored by the Centers for Medicare and Medicaid Services in partnership with the U.S. Centers for Disease Control and Prevention (CDC), the Joint Commission, Institute for Healthcare Improvement, and the American Hospital Association. With a goal of saving lives and reducing patient injuries, SCIP examines the process and outcome measures related to infectious, cardiac, venous thromboembolic, and respiratory care. As hospitals incorporate these measures into their provision of care, it is expected that the rates of postoperative wound infection, perioperative myocardial infarction, deep venous thrombosis and pulmonary embolism, and ventilator-related pneumonia will decrease (Table 1-3).

Regarding antibiotic prophylaxis for the prevention of surgical site infections, broad implementation of the measures outlined by SCIP could decrease the overall incidence significantly. In essence, selecting the appropriate antibiotic, administering it within 60 minutes of incision, and discontinuing it within 24 hours postoperatively is the goal.

Regarding preoperative hair removal, minimal or no hair removal is preferred. The CDC guidelines for hair removal state that only the interfering hair around the incision site should be removed, if necessary. Removal should be done immediately before the operation, preferably with electric clippers. Using electric clippers minimizes microscopic skin cuts, which are more common from traditional blade razors and serve as foci for bacterial multiplication.

Category	Outcome Measure
■ TABLE 1-3 SCIP Measures	
Infectious	Prophylactic antibiotic received within 1 hour before surgical incision.
	Appropriate prophylactic antibiotic selection.
	Prophylactic antibiotics discontinued within 24 hours after surgery end time.
	Appropriate method of hair removal.
	Normothermia maintained in colorectal surgery patients postoperatively.
	Cardiac surgery patients have controlled 6 AM postoperative serum glucose.
	Postoperative wound infection diagnosed during index hospitalization.
Cardiac	Patients on a beta-blocker before operation receive continued beta-blockade during the perioperative period.
	Patients with evidence of coronary artery disease receive beta-blockers during perioperative period.
	Postoperative myocardial infarction diagnosed during index hospitalization or within 30 days of surgery.
Venous thromboembolic	Recommended venous thromboembolic prophylaxis ordered.
	Appropriate venous thromboembolic prophylaxis received within 24 hours before surgery to 24 hours after surgery.
	Pulmonary embolism diagnosed during index hospitalization and within 30 days of surgery.
	Deep venous thrombosis diagnosed during index hospitalization and within 30 days of surgery.
Respiratory	Several process and outcome measures related to ventilated surgery patients.

Maintaining patient core body temperature to avoid hypothermia should be standard practice. Both passive and active warming measures should be used when indicated (e.g., blankets, fluid warmer, forced-air warmer).

Traditional practice for colon surgery has included preoperative mechanical and chemical cleansing of the large intestine in an attempt to decrease intraluminal bacterial counts and thereby minimize anastomotic leakage and postoperative infectious complications. This established practice is based on observational studies and animal experiments and is not supported by prospective randomized trial data. Interestingly, recent prospective randomized trials call the routine use of mechanical bowel preparation into question, and a Cochrane Review (2005) concludes, "Mechanical bowel preparation before colorectal surgery cannot be recommended as routine." Given the present data, mechanical bowel preparation should be used selectively depending on the clinical situation.

Regarding active infections at the time of elective surgery, CDC guidelines advise diagnosis and treatment of "all infections remote to the surgical site before elective operation and postpone elective operations on patients with remote site infections until the infection has resolved."

The publication of the Institute of Medicine report in 2000 brought into focus, and set as a national priority, an issue that had been steadily growing since the mid-1990s: improving medical and surgical safety. Before the report, large medical organizations had begun to apply a systems approach to examining medical errors. Pioneering efforts by the Veterans Health Administration to decrease medical errors led to the establishment of the National Surgical Quality Improvement Program in 1994. The core concept of such programs is to create systems of safety similar to the aviation and nuclear power industries. Highly visible aviation accidents have been found to involve human error 70% of the time, as shown by National Aeronautics and Space Administration research. This statistic parallels the less visible medical experience, as analysis of Joint Commission data on sentinel events shows that communication failures were the primary root cause in more than 70% of events. Additional oft-cited studies indicate that surgical errors result from communication failure, fatigue, and lack of surgical proficiency. In an effort to inculcate a culture of safety and minimize surgical misadventure through miscommunication, many hospitals have instituted Highly Reliable Surgical Team (HRST) training. This training is modeled on Crew Resources Management training from the aviation industry, which has been shown to enhance error reduction. Some of the HRST training goals are creating an open and free communication environment, minimizing disruptions to patient care, improving coordination among departments, and conducting quality preoperative briefings and verifications.

INTRAOPERATIVE ISSUES

After completing the HRST preoperative briefing communication with the anesthesiologist and operating room team, ensure that the overall operating room environment is to your satisfaction. The operating table and overhead lights should be correctly positioned. Room temperature and ambient noise should be adjusted as necessary. Play music if appropriate. Ensure adequate positioning and prepping of the patient. Communicate again with the team to confirm readiness. Then scrub, gown, and drape. Before incision, again to minimize surgical errors, many hospitals call for a final check or "time out" to ensure that the correct patient is undergoing the correct procedure.

Deciding where to make the skin incision is usually straightforward. Thought should be taken to consider possible need for extending the incision or possibly converting from a laparoscopic approach to open surgery. Before incising the skin, consider the skin's intrinsic tension lines to maximize wound healing and cosmesis of the healed scar. Incisions made parallel to the natural lines of tension usually heal with thinner scars because the static and dynamic forces on the wound are minimized. When making elective facial skin excisions or repairs of traumatic facial lacerations, keep in mind that incisions perpendicular to these tension lines will result in wider, less cosmetically acceptable scars (Fig. 1-1).

Although general anesthetic techniques are usually the anesthesiologist's job, all invasive practitioners should have a working knowledge of local anesthetics. Depending on the procedure being performed, the choice of local anesthetic must be tailored to each patient. Local anesthetics diffuse across nerve membranes and interfere with neural depolarization and transmission. Each local anesthetic agent has a different onset of action, duration of activity, and toxicity. Epinephrine is often administered concurrently with the local anesthetic agent to induce vasoconstriction, thereby prolonging the duration of action and decreasing bleeding. The two most commonly used local anesthetics are the shorter-acting lidocaine (Xylocaine) and

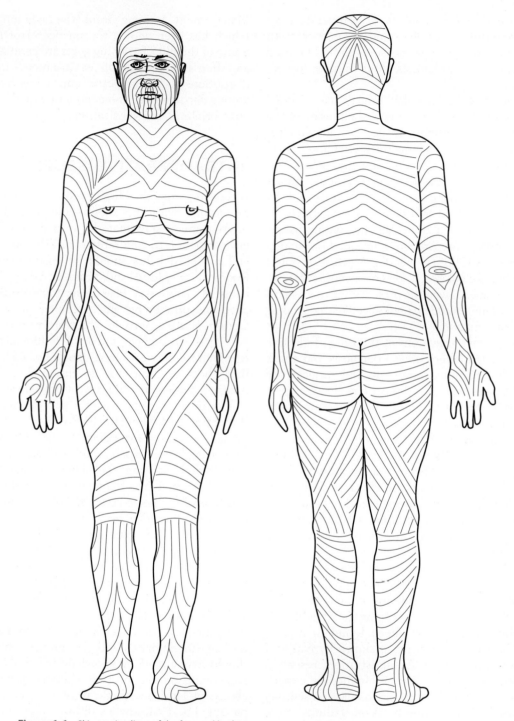

Figure 1-1 • Skin tension lines of the face and body.
Adapted from Simon R, Brenner B. *Procedures and Techniques in Emergency Medicine.* Baltimore, MD: Williams & Wilkins; 1982.

■ **TABLE 1-4** Pharmacologic Properties of Local Anesthetic Agents

Onset of Action

Agent	Concentration	Infiltration	Block	Duration of Action	Maximum Allowable Dose One Time
Lidocaine (Xylocaine)	1.0%	Immediate	4–10 min	60–120 min (for blocks)	4.5 mg/kg of 1% (30 mL per average adult)
Bupivacaine (Marcaine)	0.25%	Slower	8–12 min	240–480 min (for blocks)	3 mg/kg of 0.25% (50 mL per average adult)

Adapted from Trott A. *Wounds and Lacerations: Emergency Care and Closure.* 2nd ed. St. Louis, MO: Mosby–Year Book; 1997:31.

the longer-acting bupivacaine (Marcaine), the properties of which are outlined in Table 1-4.

Lidocaine (1% and 2%, with and without epinephrine) has a rapid onset of action, achieving sensory block in 4 to 10 minutes. The duration of action is approximately 75 minutes (range, 60 to 120 minutes). The maximum allowable dosage is 4.5 mg/kg per dose without epinephrine or 7 mg/kg per dose with epinephrine.

Bupivacaine (0.25%, 0.5%, and 0.75%, with and without epinephrine) has a slower onset of action, taking 8 to 12 minutes for a simple block. Duration of action is approximately four times longer than that of lidocaine, lasting 2 to 8 hours, making bupivacaine the preferred agent for longer procedures and for prolonged action. The maximum allowable dosage is 3 mg/kg per dose.

INSTRUMENTS

The basic tools of a surgeon are a knife for cutting and a needle with suture for restoring tissues to their appropriate position and function. Additional tools and instrumentation simply allow operations to be performed with greater finesse.

The most commonly used knife blades are illustrated in Figure 1-2 and are made functional by attachment to a standard no. 3 Bard-Parker knife handle. Choose the size and shape of the blade based on the intended indication. Abdominal or thoracic skin incisions are typically made with no. 10, 20, or 22 blades, whereas more delicate incisions could require the smaller no. 15 blade. The sharp-tipped no. 11 blade is ideal for entering and draining an abscess or for making an arteriotomy by incising a blood vessel in preparation for vascular procedures.

Scissors are mainly used for dissecting and cutting tissues. All scissors are designed for right-handed use. Each pair of scissors should only be used for the indication for which it was designed (Fig. 1-3). Most scissors have either straight or curved tips. Fine iris scissors are used for delicate dissection and cutting. Metzenbaum scissors are versatile, general-use instruments. Sturdy Mayo scissors are used for cutting thick or dense tissues, such as fascia, scar, or tendons.

Various forceps have been developed to facilitate manipulation of objects within the operative field, as well as to stabilize tissues and assist in dissection. All forceps perform essentially the same function but differ in the design of their tips and their intrinsic delicacy of form (Fig. 1-4). Toothed forceps are useful for stabilizing and moving tissues, whereas smooth atraumatic forceps are more appropriate for delicate vascular manipulation. DeBakey forceps are good general-use instruments with

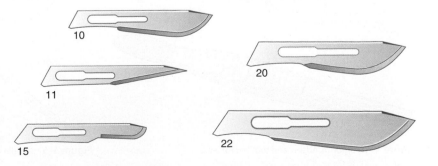

Figure 1-2 • General surgery knife blades. Shown here are Bard-Parker knife blades nos. 10, 11, 15, 20, and 22.

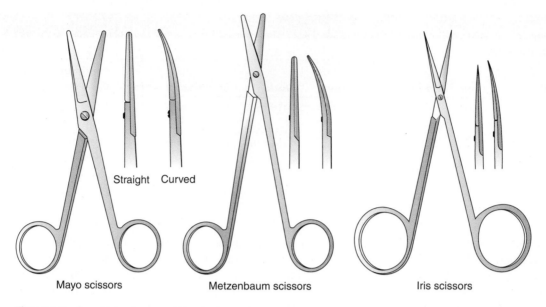

Figure 1-3 • Mayo, Metzenbaum, and iris scissors.

atraumatic flat tips and tiny fine serrations. Fine-toothed Adson forceps are ideal for skin closure, and stout-toothed Bonney forceps are excellent for facial closure.

Needle and suture are used to maintain tissue apposition until healing has occurred. The array of needles and suture material is vast; therefore, the surgeon's choice is based on the specific indication at hand.

Needles come either straight or curved. Curved needles are usually half circle or three-eighths circle. Sewing in a deep hole may require a five-eighths circle

needle, whereas microsurgery often requires quarter circle needles.

Needles can have an eye for threading the suture (French eye) or an already attached suture (swaged). Most needles today are swaged, meaning they are a needle-suture combination. Etymologically, a swage is a blacksmithing tool used to shape metal. Thus a swaged needle is manufactured by placing the suture into the hollow shank of a needle and then compressing the needle around the suture, holding it firm. Some sutures are swaged to needles in such a manner that they pop off if excess tension is applied between suture and needle.

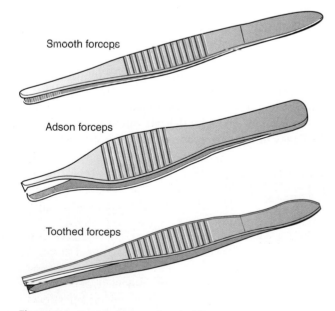

Figure 1-4 • Smooth, Adson, and toothed forceps.

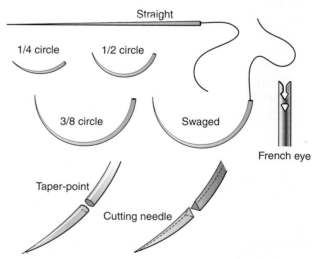

Figure 1-5 • Needle characteristics.

■ TABLE 1-5 Common Suture Material

	Material	Loss of Tensile Strength	Inflammatory Reaction	Absorbed	Common Uses
Absorbable					
Gut					
Plain	Sheep intestine	7-10 days	Moderate	2 months	Supcrficial vessels; closure of tissues that heal rapidly (buccal mucosa) and require minimal support
Chromic	Treated with chromium salt	10-14 days	Moderate but less	3 months	
Polyglactic acid (Vicryl); polyglycolic acid (Dexon)	Synthetic polyfilament	4-5 wk	Minimal	3 months	Dermis; fat muscle
Polyglyconate (Maxon, Monocryl)	Synthetic monofilament	3-4 wk	Minimal	3-4 months	Subcuticular close and soft tissue approximation
Polydioxanone (PDS)	Synthetic monofilament	8 wk	Minimal	6 months	Muscle; fascia
Nonabsorbable					
Polypropylene (Prolene)	Polymer of propylene	Years[a]	Minimal	—	Fascia; muscle; vessels
Nylon (Surgilon, Nurolon)	Polyamide	Years[a]	Minimal	—	Skin; drains; microsurgical anastomoses
Silk	Raw silk spun by silk worm	1 yr	Intense	—	Tie off vessels; bowel
Staples	Iron-chromium-nickel	—	Minimal	—	Skin

[a]With reoperation, polypropylene and nylon remain present but decompose slightly.
From Taylor JA. *Blueprints Plastic Surgery*. Malden, MA: Blackwell Science; 2005.

Needle tips are either tapered or cutting. Tapered needles are circumferentially smooth and slide between the elements of tissues, whereas cutting needles are triangular in cross section and cut through tissues like a tiny knife (Fig. 1-5).

Suture material is categorized according to its permanence (absorbable or nonabsorbable), its structure (braided or monofilament), and its caliber (Table 1-5). Absorbable suture material is made from either naturally derived, collagen-based materials or synthetic polymers. Examples of absorbable suture material are gut (plain and chromic), polyglactic acid (Vicryl), polyglycolic acid (Dexon), polyglyconate (Maxon), and polydioxanone (PDS). The suture is either hydrolyzed by water or undergoes enzymatic digestion, thereby losing tensile strength over time.

Permanent nonabsorbable sutures are made from materials impervious to significant chemical degradation and are useful for maintaining long-term tissue apposition. Examples of permanent nonabsorbable suture material are nylon, polypropylene, stainless steel, and silk.

CLOSURE TECHNIQUES

There are many techniques for closing wounds (Fig. 1-6). Wounds can be closed using a continuous stitch that is quick to perform and results in tension distributed along the length of the suture. Simple interrupted stitching allows for precise tissue approximation (skin or fascia). Mattress stitches can be placed either vertically or horizontally, allowing excellent skin apposition and eversion while minimizing tension. Subcuticular stitching using an absorbable suture at the dermal-epidermal junction is a convenient skin-closure technique, allowing epidermal apposition so that postoperative suture removal is unnecessary. Regardless of the closure technique used, certain basic principles must be considered to avoid wound breakdown and to achieve a well-healed, cosmetically satisfactory scar:

- skin incision along intrinsic tension lines
- gentle handling of intraoperative tissue
- meticulous hemostasis
- tension-free closure
- eversion of skin edges

An alternative to sutured skin closure of wounds is skin apposition using metal staples. Many elective surgical wounds are closed with skin staples, because the technique allows for rapid skin closure, minimal wound inflammatory response, and near-equivalent cosmetic results. This technique usually works best with two operators: one to evert and align the skin edges with forceps and another to fire the stapler (Fig. 1-7).

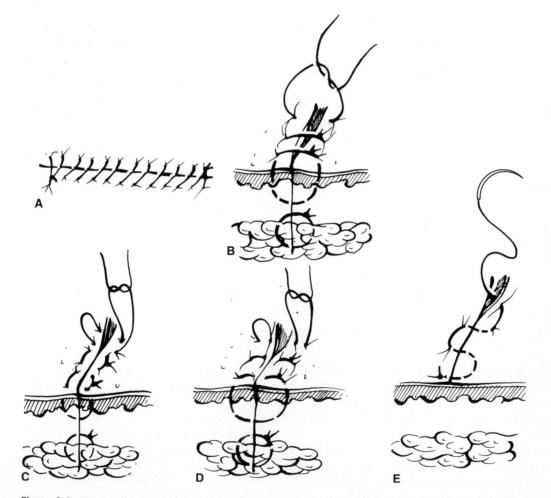

Figure 1-6 • Suturing techniques: **(A)** Continuous, **(B)** simple interrupted, **(C)** horizontal mattress, **(D)** vertical mattress, and **(E)** subcuticular.
(From Taylor JA. *Blueprints Plastic Surgery*. Malden, MA: Blackwell Publishing; 2005:7.)

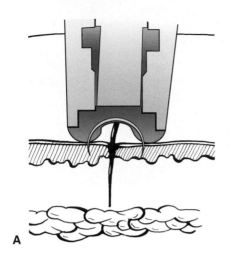

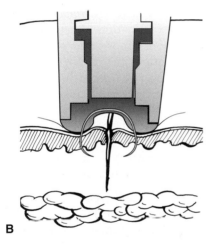

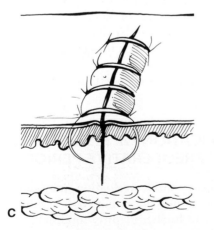

Figure 1-7 • Wound closure using metal staples.

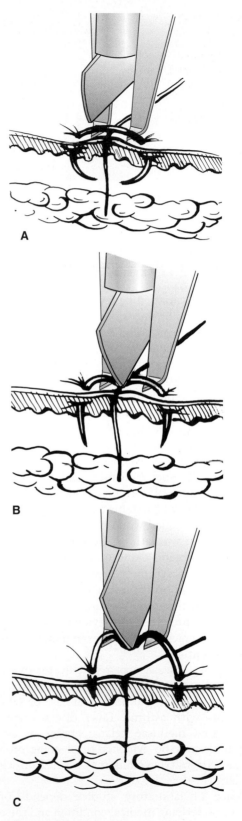

Removal of staples is performed using a simple handheld device that deforms the staple and reconfigures the staple shape, allowing for smooth, easy withdrawal (Fig. 1-8).

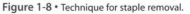

Figure 1-8 • Technique for staple removal.

Care of the Surgical Patient

PREOPERATIVE EVALUATION

Preoperative evaluation has two main purposes: identification of modifiable risk factors and risk assessment. Unless the situation is emergent, every patient should have a detailed history and physical examination. In all patients, attention should be given to a history of cerebrovascular accident, heart disease of any kind, pulmonary disease, renal disease, liver disease and other gastrointestinal disorders, diabetes, prior surgeries, bleeding problems, clotting problems, difficulty with anesthesia, poor nutrition, alcohol use, and illicit drug use. Allergies, current medications, family history, social history, and a careful and complete review of systems should be conducted. Often, the review of systems will reveal problems that require more detailed workup.

Physical examination should be focused on identifying problems that require further workup. For example, facial asymmetry, speech problems, weakness, or a carotid bruit may suggest prior cerebrovascular incident that requires further workup. Cardiac disease may present with evidence of congestive heart failure, crackles on lung examination, or jugular venous distention.

Pulmonary disease may result in, for example, a barrel chest with poor air movement in patients with chronic obstructive pulmonary disease or wheezing in patients with asthma. Liver disease may cause ascites, caput medusae, telangiectasias, or asterixis. Ecchymosis may be evidence of bleeding problems, whereas extremity swelling may result from clotting disorders.

Choice of laboratory studies depends on the patient's underlying medical condition and the extent of the surgery. There has been a trend toward less routine testing and increased reliance on the history and physical examination. In otherwise healthy patients undergoing minor surgery, laboratory studies, including coagulation studies, are probably not indicated. Similarly, in patients with no history of pulmonary or cardiac disease and no significant risk factors undergoing minor or moderate surgery, electrocardiogram (ECG) and chest x-ray (CXR) are also probably not indicated.

General guidelines for preoperative testing in patients without risk factors are as follows:

ECG: Male older than 40 years or female older than 50 years undergoing cardiovascular procedures

CXR: All patients older than 60 years or undergoing thoracic procedures

Hematocrit: All patients if the procedure is expected to cause >500 mL of blood loss

Creatinine: Patients older than 50 years or if the procedure has a high risk for generating renal failure

Pregnancy test: All women of childbearing age if pregnancy status is uncertain

MODIFICATION OF RISK FACTORS IN THE PREOPERATIVE PERIOD

Initial preoperative evaluation may suggest additional testing needed, either to determine the surgical risk or to further identify modifiable factors. For example, chest pain or shortness of breath with mild exertion should prompt a more thorough cardiac evaluation, including an ECG and stress test. If these tests show cardiac disease, a decision will need to be made regarding whether the patient requires an intervention before surgery. If preoperative assessment demonstrates carotid artery disease, it may be best to perform an endarterectomy before the originally planned surgery. Other issues, such as poorly controlled diabetes, obesity, and malnutrition, should also be addressed before surgery. This may involve modifications of diet and insulin dose, weight loss, or inpatient admission for total parenteral nutrition. Good glucose control in diabetics as measured by hemoglobin A1c levels is associated with improved outcomes after surgery. In patients suffering from malnutrition scheduled for surgery, preoperative total parenteral nutrition has been shown to improve outcomes.

TIMING OF SURGERY

Once the risk factors for surgery have been identified, a frank discussion should be held with the patient explaining the potential risks and benefits of the surgery and which risk factors should be addressed before the surgery. This discussion should be the basis for the informed consent for surgery. The outcome of this discussion may be that the surgery should proceed without delay, that the procedure is too risky and should not be attempted, or somewhere in between. For example, in a young healthy person with a symptomatic inguinal hernia, surgery without delay is indicated. On the other hand, if the hernia is small and asymptomatic and the patient has advanced liver disease with uncontrolled ascites, the risk of the surgery probably outweighs the benefits. In a patient with end-stage renal disease undergoing workup for a kidney transplant who is found to have unstable angina and coronary disease amenable to intervention, the coronary intervention should proceed before transplantation. When operation occurs within 3 months of a myocardial infarction, the risk of a subsequent one is approximately 30% in the perioperative period and decreases to less than 5% after 6 months, so that surgery should be delayed in these patients if at all possible. The Goldman criteria, although offered in 1977, are still widely used to evaluate surgical risk (Table 2-1). More recent criteria from the American College of Cardiology and the American Heart Association provide algorithms for assessing risk. Outcomes, especially for class IV risk patients, are much better with improvements in medical and surgical care, but the classification is a useful one to help stratify surgical risk.

■ TABLE 2-1 Goldman Criteria for Cardiac Risk

Factor	Point Value
Age >70 years	5
Myocardial infarction within 6 months	10
S3 gallop or JVP >12 cm	11
Significant valvular stenosis	3
Rhythm other than sinus, or atrial ectopy	7
Ventricular premature beats >5/min at any time	7
$PO_2 < 60$ or $PCO_2 > 50$ mm Hg, or Potassium < 3 mEq/L or $HCO_3 < 20$, or BUN >50 mg/dL or creatinine >3.0 mg/dL, or chronic liver disease or debilitation	3
Intraperitoneal, intrathoracic, or aortic surgery	3
Emergency surgery	4

Risk assessed as follows: 0–5 points, class I, 1% complication risk; 6–12 points, class II, 7% complication risk; 13–25 points, class III, 14% complication risk; >25 points, class IV, 78% complication risk. JVP, jugular venous pressure; PO_2, partial pressure of oxygen; PCO_2, partial pressure of carbon dioxide; HCO_3, bicarbonate; BUN, blood urea nitrogen.

DIABETES MANAGEMENT BEFORE SURGERY

There are a number of ways to manage glucose levels before and during surgery in patients with diabetes. If possible, patients with diabetes should be scheduled as the first case of the day to simplify glucose control, as patients will not be eating. For day surgery, in patients with type I diabetes or those with type II diabetes requiring multiple injections, patients should take one half of their usual dose of intermediate-acting or long-acting insulin the morning of surgery. When these patients undergo major surgery, they can hold their insulin entirely in preparation for intravenous therapy during the operation.

For patients with type II diabetes taking once-daily or twice-daily insulin, or for patients on oral medications undergoing day surgery, oral hypoglycemics should be held, and one half dose of intermediate-acting insulin should be given in the morning. Patients undergoing major surgery can be managed intraoperatively with intravenous insulin. Glucose levels should be checked on arrival for surgery and every 2 hours while waiting.

PERIOPERATIVE MANAGEMENT

FLUIDS AND ELECTROLYTES

Fluids and electrolytes must be provided in adequate amounts to replace intraoperative losses. This will maintain blood pressure and ensure optimal cardiac function. Choice of fluids depends on the underlying medical problems. For example, the use of potassium-containing fluids should be avoided in patients with renal failure. For longer and more complicated cases, consideration of loss of other electrolytes, including calcium and magnesium, must be addressed.

BLOOD PRODUCTS

Administration of blood products depends on the underlying health of the patient and the type of operation. Whereas in a healthy patient with a limited intraoperative event in which 500 mL of blood is lost, resulting in a hematocrit of 24%, a transfusion may not be indicated. However, for a patient undergoing liver transplantation with expected ongoing blood loss, transfusion may be indicated at a level of 28%. Transfusion of fresh-frozen plasma and platelets should be considered for patients with coagulopathy or thrombocytopenia.

CARDIAC RISK FACTORS

In patients with known cardiac disease, aggressive intraoperative lowering of myocardial oxygen demand with beta-blockers has been shown in randomized trials to improve outcomes and should be used.

ANTIBIOTICS

Antibiotics are of benefit in all procedures in which a body cavity is opened and are probably useful in clean procedures. Guidelines for the use of antibiotics include administration before the incision (within 1 hour) and redosing after 4 hours. Specific recommendations are shown in Table 2-2.

DIABETES MANAGEMENT

A large randomized controlled trial published in 2001 by Van den Berge et al demonstrated improved

■ TABLE 2-2 Antibiotic Recommendations

Type of Procedure	Antibiotic Choice
Clean	Cefazolin or none
Cardiovascular	Cefazolin
Colorectal	Oral: Neomycin/erythromycin base plus mechanical cleansing before surgery Parenteral: cefazolin/metronidazole or cefotetan
Prosthetic joint	Cefazolin

outcomes in surgical intensive care patients maintained with strict blood sugar control between 80 and 110 mg/dL. Since then, there has been tremendous activity in defining which patients benefit from this therapy and evaluating the complications. Many patients, including those undergoing general or cardiac surgery, benefit from improved outcomes and decreased infectious complications, including reduced septicemia. Patients using these regimens must be monitored carefully to prevent the development of hypoglycemia.

PREVENTION OF DEEP VENOUS THROMBOSIS

Prevention of deep venous thrombosis is of major importance. Although rare, this complication is potentially life-threatening. Randomized clinical trials are abundantly clear. When heparin is given, it should be done so in the preoperative area, before the incision. Administration of any anticoagulation in the perioperative period must carefully consider the risk of bleeding, and therapy should be individualized to the patient and the particulars of the operation (e.g., if the operation was unusually bloody). Having stated that, there is evidence that the following regimens are efficacious in improving outcomes.

Minor Surgery

In patients younger than 40 years undergoing minor surgery with no risk factors, early ambulation decreases risk of deep venous thrombosis, and use of subcutaneous heparin is controversial. In patients between 40 and 60 years or with risk factors, heparin 5000 U administered subcutaneously 2 times per day or enoxaparin 40 mg administered subcutaneously every day is beneficial. In patients older than 60 years or with additional risk factors, heparin can be increased to 3 times per day, or enoxaparin 30 mg administered subcutaneously 2 times per day is beneficial.

Major Surgery

Patients younger than 40 years with no risk factors should receive heparin 5000 U subcutaneously 2 times per day or enoxaparin 40 mg subcutaneously every day. Patients older than 40 years or with risk factors should receive heparin 5000 U subcutaneously 3 times per day or enoxaparin 30 mg subcutaneously 2 times per day.

Orthopedic Surgery

Because of the increased risk of these procedures, aggressive anticoagulation is indicated. Patients undergoing hip fracture repair, total hip replacement, or total knee replacement should receive enoxaparin 30 mg subcutaneously 2 times per day, coumadin to keep international normalized ratio between 2 and 3, or fondaparinux 2.5 mg.

Graded compression stockings and intermittent pneumatic compression boots are often used in combination with pharmacologic therapy, but their benefit is less well established.

TEMPERATURE

Maintenance of normal intraoperative temperature is critical for adequate hemostasis and optimal cardiovascular function. Use of warmed fluids and warming blankets may be necessary for long operations or those in which large body cavities are opened.

POSTOPERATIVE MANAGEMENT

Principles of postoperative management include early mobilization, pulmonary therapy, early nutrition, adequate fluid and electrolyte administration, management of cardiac risk factors, control of blood sugars, and recognition of complications.

Early mobilization is important to prevent muscle wasting and weakness, reduce the risk of venous thromboembolism, reduce the rate of pneumonia, and perhaps speed the return of bowel function. If permitted by the type of surgery, the patient should get out of bed on the day of surgery and be walking on the first postoperative day.

One of the most common postoperative complications is pneumonia. Deep-breathing exercises and the use of an incentive spirometer can decrease this risk.

Early nutrition (within 24 hours of surgery) has been demonstrated in randomized controlled trials to improve outcomes. In most patients, this will amount to having them eat, but many patients may require a nasoenteric tube for this purpose. In patients undergoing surgery on the gastrointestinal tract, the timing of feeds should be individualized to the patient and the type of operation. In general, enteral nutrition is preferable to parenteral nutrition if the gut is functional.

Fluid administration is one of the most important aspects of postoperative care. Adequate resuscitation prevents renal failure and optimizes cardiac function. Excessive fluid can cause congestive heart failure and edema, which in turn inhibits wound healing. Fluid administration must be individualized to the patient and the type of operation; general guidelines are to administer fluid to keep the urine output >30 mL/hr.

Decreasing cardiac risk in patients with preexisting disease requires adequate beta blockade throughout the perioperative period. The heart rate should be kept <70 and lower if hemodynamically tolerated.

Tight control of blood sugars is clearly beneficial in reducing wound infections. This is accomplished initially by aggressive use of sliding-scale insulin and resumption of the patient's home insulin regimen when the patient is eating adequately.

Early recognition of surgical complications is critical to effectively managing them. Common to all but the most minor operations are wound infections, pneumonia, urinary tract infection, catheter infections, deep venous thrombosis, and myocardial infarction. In addition, each operation has its specific complications. Recognition of a complication depends on detailed daily history and physical examination. Wounds should be examined for erythema and discharge. Particularly worrisome is murky brown discharge that may represent a dehiscence or necrotizing fasciitis. Lungs should be examined daily for decreased breath sounds and egophony, and sputum should be examined. Thick green or brown sputum should prompt investigation for pneumonia, including CXR and sputum gram stain and culture. Sites of catheter placement should be examined for erythema and discharge. Urinary symptoms should prompt a urinalysis and culture. Chest pain in the perioperative period should be taken seriously and evaluated with an ECG and cardiac enzymes in the appropriate clinical setting.

Fever is an exceedingly common occurrence in the perioperative period, and early diagnosis is critical. The classic "5 Ws" of wind (pneumonia), wound, walking (deep venous thrombosis), water (urinary tract infection), and wonder drugs (drug reaction) should be considered in all patients. Fevers on the first day after surgery are generally attributed to the inflammatory stress of the surgery or atelectasis. If the fever is not high and history and physical examination are unremarkable, no further workup is indicated. If, on the other hand, the fever is high, the wound should be examined to rule out a rapidly progressive infection, typically caused by Gram-positive cocci. Other diagnostic modalities should be used based on the type of surgery and symptoms. An increasingly common source of fever is *Clostridium difficile* colitis. This should be suspected in any patient with diarrhea after surgery. Three stool samples and a white blood cell count should be sent. Initiation of treatment before laboratory confirmation may be indicated if the suspicion is high.

Examples of complications related to the surgery include fascial dehiscence, breakdown or stricture of enteric anastomoses, thrombosis of vascular grafts, deep space infections, and hernia recurrence. These problems can usually be recognized with careful patient examination.

FLUIDS AND ELECTROLYTES

Understanding fluid and electrolyte replacement begins with knowing the composition of the various body compartments. In a typical 70-kg person, 60% of total body weight is water. Two thirds of this water is contained in the intracellular compartment, and one third is in the extracellular compartment. One quarter of this extracellular water is plasma—approximately 3.5 L in a typical man. Red blood cell volume is approximately 1.5 L. Combined with plasma, this results in a blood volume of approximately 5 L. Electrolyte concentrations in the extracellular and intracellular space are as shown in Table 2-3.

■ TABLE 2-3 Electrolyte Concentrations in the Extracellular and Intracellular Space

Electrolyte	Extracellular (mEq/L)	Intracellular (mEq/L)
Sodium	140	10
Potassium	4.0	150
Calcium	2.5	4.0
Magnesium	1.1	34
Chloride	104	4.0
Carbonate	24	12
Phosphate	2.0	40

Daily maintenance requirements for healthy adults include urinary fluid loss of 1 L, gastrointestinal loss of 200 mL, and insensible losses of 10 mL/kg. Each of these numbers can be adjusted upward in various disease states. Fever, burns, and diarrhea are examples of processes that can dramatically increase fluid losses.

Normal replacement in surgical patients is 1 mEq/kg of sodium and 0.5 mEq/kg of potassium per day. Gastrointestinal losses in patients can be approximated with the information provided in Table 2-4. The composition of various replacement fluids is as shown in Table 2-5.

Common electrolyte abnormalities in the perioperative period include hyponatremia, hypernatremia, hyperkalemia, and hypokalemia. Causes of hyponatremia should be divided into two types, depending on whether there is reduced plasma osmolality. If plasma osmolality is normal or high, the differential diagnosis is hyperlipidemia, hyperproteinemia, hyperglycemia, and mannitol administration. In this case, the treatment focuses on correcting the abnormality in the osmotically active agent.

■ TABLE 2-4 Normal Replacement of Fluids in Surgical Patients (mEq/L)

Type of Fluid	Sodium	Potassium	H+	Bicarbonate
Gastric	20–120	12	30–100	0
Duodenal	110	15	0	10
Ileum (ileostomy)	100	10	0	40
Colon (diarrhea)	120	25	0	45
Bile	140	5	0	25
Pancreas	140	5	0	115

■ **TABLE 2-5** Composition of Various Replacement Fluids (mEq/L)					
Replacement Fluid	**Sodium**	**Potassium**	**Chloride**	**Calcium**	**Lactate**
Normal saline	154	154	0	0	0
Half normal saline	77	77	0	0	0
Lactated Ringer's solution	130	4	109	3	28

More often, the plasma osmolality is reduced. In this case, the question becomes whether the circulating plasma volume is high, as in congestive heart failure, cirrhosis, nephrotic syndrome, and malnutrition; normal, as in syndrome of inappropriate secretion of antidiuretic hormone, paraneoplastic syndromes, endocrine disorders, and various drugs (morphine, aminophylline, indomethacin); or low, with excessive losses or inadequate replacement.

In general, patients with decreased plasma volume should be treated with hypertonic saline if the level is low enough to warrant treatment (<120 mEq/L). In this case, it is critically important to not correct the sodium >0.5 mEq/L per hour. If the patient's are symptomatic, however, it may be advisable to increase the level more quickly. This should only be done in consultation with a neurologist, as faster rates can result in central pontine myelinolysis from the osmotic shift. Patients in whom the effective plasma volume is high should be treated with fluid restriction.

Causes of hypernatremia are divided into water loss and sodium administration. Water loss can result from insensible losses from infection, burns, or fever; renal loss from diabetes insipidus; gastrointestinal losses; or hypothalamic disorders. Sodium administration can be performed via ingestion or intravenously. Treatment consists of addressing the underlying abnormality and administering fluid. Correction of hypernatremia should not progress at a rate >0.5 mEq/L per hour, unless neurologic symptoms are present. Rapid correction of hyponatremia can result in seizures, cerebral edema, and death.

Hypokalemia is usually due to potassium loss. Hypokalemia can result in cardiac arrhythmias, especially in patients taking digoxin. Treatment is with exogenous replacement.

Hyperkalemia is usually due to exogenous administration or from intracellular stores. It can result in weakness and cardiac arrhythmias. If the level is above 6 mEq/L or the patient has ECG changes, treatment with calcium gluconate, sodium bicarbonate, insulin, and glucose can transiently decrease plasma potassium, which may rebound, because these treatments do not alter the total body potassium. Kayexalate decreases total body potassium but takes longer to be effective. Dialysis is extremely effective in decreasing potassium.

KEY POINTS

- Preoperative evaluation is critical to identify modifiable risk factors and provide risk assessment.
- Cardiac history is essential to the evaluation. Goldman criteria can help assess cardiac risk.
- Operation within 3 months of a myocardial infarction is associated with a 30% complication risk.
- Tight glucose control in the perioperative period improves outcomes.
- Anticoagulation in the perioperative period reduces the risk of deep venous thrombosis.
- Enteral nutrition is preferable to parenteral nutrition if the gut is functional.
- Fever in the perioperative period is most commonly caused by the 5 Ws: wind (pneumonia), wound, walking (deep venous thrombosis), water (urinary tract infection), and wonder drugs (drug reaction).

Part II

Gastrointestinal and Abdominal

Stomach and Duodenum

The stomach and duodenum are anatomically contiguous structures, share an interrelated physiology, and have similar disease processes. Peptic ulceration is the most common inflammatory disorder of the gastrointestinal tract and is responsible for significant disability. The stomach and duodenum are principally affected by peptic ulceration.

ANATOMY

The stomach is divided into the fundus, body, and antrum (Fig. 3-1). The fundus is the superior dome of the stomach; the body extends from the fundus to the angle of the stomach (incisura angularis), located on the lesser curvature; and the antrum extends from the body to the pylorus. Hydrochloric acid—secreting parietal cells are found in the fundus, pepsinogen-secreting chief cells are found in the proximal stomach, and gastrin-secreting G cells are found in the antrum.

Six arterial sources supply blood to the stomach: the left and right gastric arteries to the lesser curvature; the left and right gastroepiploic arteries to the greater curvature; the short gastric arteries, branching from the splenic artery to supply the fundus; and the gastroduodenal artery, branching to the pylorus (Fig. 3-2). The vagus nerve supplies parasympathetic innervation via the anterior left and posterior right trunks. These nerves stimulate gastric motility and the secretion of pepsinogen and hydrochloric acid.

The duodenum is divided into four portions (Fig. 3-3). The first portion begins at the pylorus and includes the duodenal bulb. The ampulla of Vater, through which the common bile duct and pancreatic duct drain, is located in the medial wall of the descending second portion of the duodenum. The transverse third portion is traversed anteriorly by the superior mesenteric vessels. The ascending fourth portion terminates at the ligament of Treitz, which defines the duodenal–jejunal junction. The arterial supply to the duodenum is via the superior pancreaticoduodenal artery, which arises from the gastroduodenal artery, and via the inferior pancreaticoduodenal artery, which arises from the superior mesenteric artery.

GASTRIC AND DUODENAL ULCERATION

PATHOGENESIS

The etiology of benign peptic gastric and duodenal ulceration involves a compromised mucosal surface undergoing acid-peptic digestion. Substances that alter mucosal defenses include nonsteroidal anti-inflammatory drugs, alcohol, and tobacco. Alcohol directly attacks the mucosa, nonsteroidal anti-inflammatory drugs alter prostaglandin synthesis, and tobacco restricts mucosal vascular perfusion. However, the most important and remarkable advancement in understanding the pathogenesis of peptic ulceration was the radical idea that infestation with the organism *Helicobacter pylori* was the causative factor in gastric and duodenal ulceration. This discovery destroyed prevailing dogma and profoundly altered the medical and surgical treatment for this disease process. So profound was this discovery that the 2005 Nobel Prize in Medicine was awarded to Drs. Marshall and Warren, two iconoclastic Australian researchers, "for their discovery of the bacterium *Helicobacter pylori* and its role in gastritis and peptic ulcer disease."

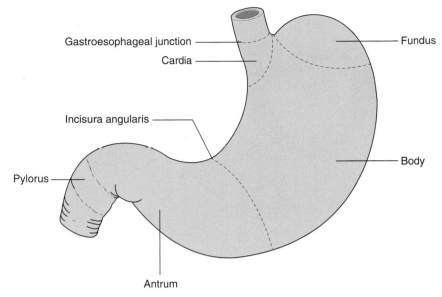

Figure 3-1 • Anatomy of the stomach.

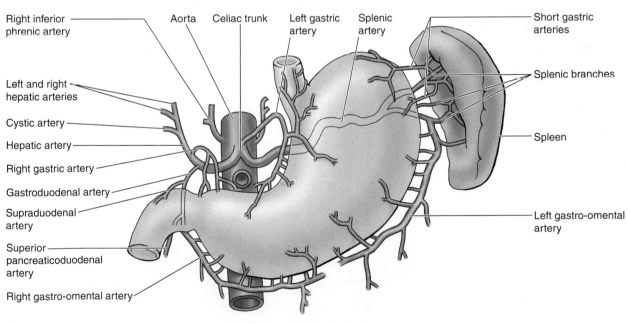

A

Figure 3-2 • Arteries and veins of the stomach and spleen. **A.** Arterial supply. Observe that the stomach receives its main blood supply from branches of the celiac trunk. The fundus of the stomach is supplied by short gastric arteries arising from the splenic artery. The spleen is supplied by the splenic artery, the largest branch of the celiac trunk, which runs a tortuous course to the hilum of the spleen and breaks up into its terminal (splenic) branches.

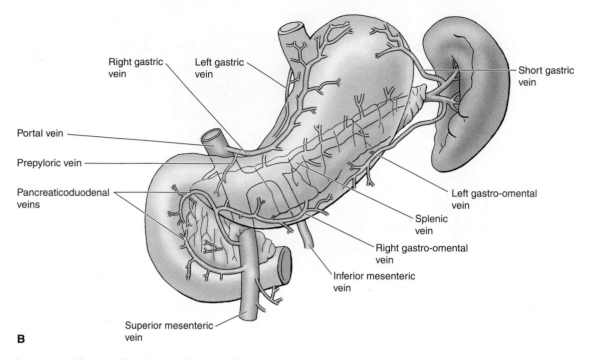

B

Figure 3-2 • *(Continued)* **B.** Venous drainage. The drainage of the stomach is directly or indirectly into the portal vein. The splenic vein usually receives the inferior mesenteric vein and then unites with the superior mesenteric vein to form the portal vein as shown here. From Moore KL, Dalley AF II. *Clinically Oriented Anatomy.* 4th ed. Baltimore: Lippincott Williams & Wilkins, 1999.

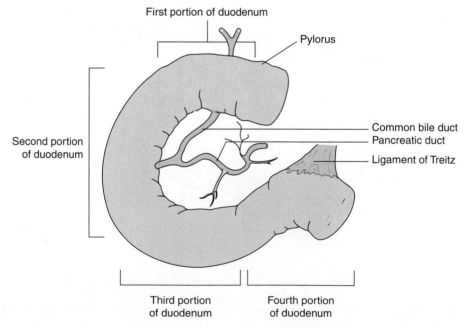

Figure 3-3 • Anatomy of the duodenum.

HISTORY

Patients typically present with epigastric pain relieved by antacids. Sensations of fullness and mild nausea are common, but vomiting is rare unless pyloric obstruction is present secondary to scarring. Physical examination is often benign except for occasional epigastric tenderness.

DIAGNOSTIC EVALUATION

The radiographic evaluation of peptic ulcers entails barium studies that reveal evidence of crater deformities at areas of ulceration. Serum testing determines whether there are antibodies to *H. pylori*, and breath testing confirms infection.

Definitive diagnosis is made by direct visualization of the ulcer using endoscopy (see Color Plate 1). For nonhealing gastric ulcers refractory to medical therapy, it is extremely important that biopsy of the ulcer be performed to rule out gastric carcinoma. Duodenal ulcers are rarely malignant.

TREATMENT

Medical treatment is similar for gastric and duodenal ulceration. The goals of medical therapy are to decrease production of or neutralize stomach acid and to enhance mucosal protection against acid attack. Medications include antacids ($CaCO_3$), H_2-blockers (cimetidine, ranitidine), mucosal coating agents (sucralfate), and proton-pump inhibitors (omeprazole). If *H. pylori* is present, treatment with oral antibiotics is associated with a 90% eradication rate. Treatment regimens may consist of tetracycline/metronidazole/bismuth subsalicylate, amoxicillin/metronidazole/ranitidine, or other combinations.

As a result of the advent of proton pump inhibitors (PPIs) and the increased understanding of the role *H. pylori* plays in peptic ulceration, operations for ulcer disease have become infrequent. Indications for surgical treatment in the acute setting are either perforation or massive bleeding. Indications for elective operation are a chronic nonhealing ulcer after medical therapy or gastric outlet obstruction. The operation chosen must address the indication for which the procedure is performed. Historically, before the era of PPIs and *H. pylori*, the goal of surgery was to permanently reduce acid secretion by removing the entire antrum. In most instances, vagotomy and distal gastrectomy (antrectomy), with Billroth I or II anastomosis, fulfilled these criteria (Figs. 3-4 and 3-5). Because denervation of the

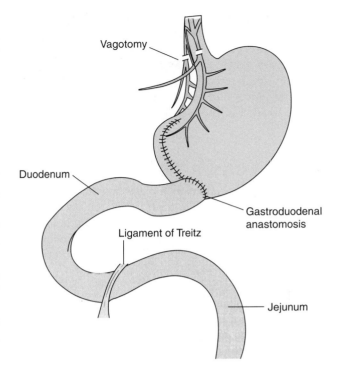

Figure 3-4 • Vagotomy and antrectomy with Billroth I anastomosis.

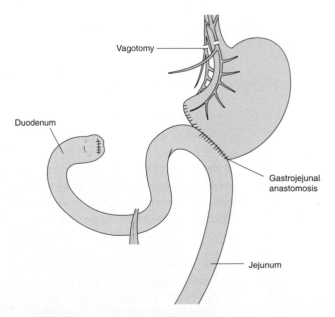

Figure 3-5 • Vagotomy and antrectomy with Billroth II anastomosis.

stomach by truncal vagotomy alters normal patterns of gastric motility and causes gastric atony, surgical drainage procedures are required afterward to ensure satisfactory gastric emptying. Today, most cases of perforation are treated with closure of the defect with omental patch, and cases of bleeding are treated with suture ligation of the bleeding vessel.

STRESS GASTRITIS AND ULCERATION

PATHOGENESIS

Critically ill patients subjected to severe physiologic stress, often in the intensive care unit setting, are at risk for developing gastroduodenal mucosal erosion that can progress to ulceration. The commonly accepted etiology of stress gastritis and ulceration is mucosal ischemia induced by an episode of hypotension from hemorrhage, sepsis, hypovolemia, or cardiac dysfunction. Ischemia disrupts cellular mechanisms of mucosal protection, resulting in mucosal acidification and superficial erosion. Areas of erosion may coalesce and form superficial ulcers. Stress ulcers may be seen throughout the stomach and proximal duodenum.

HISTORY

Patients are usually critically ill and have a recent history of hypotension. Massive upper gastrointestinal bleeding is the usual finding.

DIAGNOSTIC EVALUATION

Sites of hemorrhage can be identified by endoscopy.

TREATMENT

Endoscopy can often control bleeding by either electrocoagulation or photocoagulation. Persistent or recurrent bleeding unresponsive to endoscopic techniques requires surgical intervention. Depending on the circumstances, operations for control of bleeding stress gastritis or ulcer require oversewing of the bleeding vessel. Usually, vagotomy is also performed to reduce acid secretion. In many cases, because bleeding is often diffuse and cannot be controlled by simple suture ligation, partial or total gastrectomy is performed.

PREVENTION

Prevention of stress ulceration involves maintaining blood pressure, tissue perfusion, and acid–base stability, as well as decreasing acid production while bolstering mucosal protection. The incidence of life-threatening hemorrhagic gastritis has decreased as intravenous H_2-blocker therapy and oral cytoprotectants have been introduced to the intensive care setting.

CUSHING'S ULCER

Distinct from stress gastritis, Cushing's ulcers are seen in patients with intracranial pathology (e.g., tumors, head injury). Ulcers are single and deep and may involve the esophagus, stomach, and duodenum. Because of the depth of ulceration, perforation is a common complication. Neuronally mediated acid hypersecretion is thought to be the main cause of Cushing's ulcer.

ZOLLINGER-ELLISON SYNDROME AND GASTRINOMAS

PATHOGENESIS

Zollinger-Ellison syndrome occurs in patients with severe peptic ulceration and evidence of a gastrinoma (non–B-cell pancreatic tumor). Peptic ulceration results from the production of large volumes of highly acidic gastric secretions owing to elevated serum gastrin levels. Ninety percent of gastrinomas are found in the "gastrinoma triangle," defined by the junction of the cystic duct and the common bile duct, the junction of the second and third portions of the duodenum, and the junction of the neck and body of the pancreas.

HISTORY

Gastrin-secreting tumors produce a clinical picture of epigastric pain, weight loss, vomiting, and severe diarrhea.

DIAGNOSTIC EVALUATION

Diagnosis is confirmed by the secretin-stimulation test, in which the injection of intravenous secretin elevates serum gastrin levels to at least 200 pg/mL. Once diagnosed, tumor localization is performed by magnetic resonance imaging, abdominal ultrasound, computed tomography, selective abdominal angiography, or selective venous sampling.

TREATMENT

Acid hypersecretion can be controlled medically with H_2 blockade and PPI. Somatostatin analogs (octreotide) have been found to be effective in decreasing tumor secretion of gastrin and in controlling the growth of tumor metastases.

Gastrinoma is a curable disease, despite the malignant nature of most tumors. Complete resection of tumors results in a near 100% 10-year survival rate. Incomplete resection or unresectability carries <50% 10-year survival rate. When simple excision or enucleation for cure is not feasible, an attempt is made to prolong survival by debulking and performing lymph node dissection to reduce tumor burden and acid hypersecretion.

STOMACH CANCER

Despite the decreasing incidence of gastric carcinoma in Western populations during the past decades, patient survival has not improved. In the United States, fewer than 10% of patients with stomach cancer survive 5 years. Illustrative of geographic variation, stomach cancer is endemic in Japan. Because of the high incidence of disease, mass screening programs are able to detect early-stage lesions, which accounts for a 50% overall survival rate at 5 years.

RISK FACTORS

Environmental and dietary factors are thought to influence the development of gastric cancer. Smoked fish and meats contain benzopyrene, a probable carcinogen to gastric mucosa. Nitrosamines are known carcinogens that are formed by the conversion of dietary nitrogen to nitrosamines in the gastrointestinal tract by bacterial metabolism. Atrophic gastritis, as seen in patients with hypogammaglobulinemia and pernicious anemia, is considered to be a premalignant condition for developing gastric cancer, because high gastric pH encourages bacterial growth. Chronic atrophic gastritis results in achlorhydria, and 75% of patients with gastric cancer are achlorhydric.

PATHOLOGY

Most tumors are adenocarcinomas, and spread is via lymphatics, venous drainage, and direct extension. Most tumors are located in the antral prepyloric region.

Gastric tumors can be typed according to gross appearance. Polypoid fungating nodular tumors are usually well differentiated and carry a relatively good prognosis after surgery. Ulcerating or penetrating tumors are the most common and are often mistaken for benign peptic ulcers because of their sessile nature. Superficial spreading lesions diffusely infiltrate through mucosa and submucosa and have a poor prognosis because most are metastatic at the time of diagnosis.

The pathologic staging of gastric cancer is based on depth of tumor invasion and lymph node status. Survival is closely correlated with the pathologic stage of a specific tumor (Fig. 3-6).

HISTORY

Patients with gastric cancer usually give a history of vague and nonspecific symptoms. Upper abdominal discomfort, dyspepsia, early satiety, belching, weight loss, anorexia, nausea, vomiting, hematemesis, or melena is common. Definite symptoms do not occur until tumor growth causes luminal obstruction, tumor infiltration results in gastric dysmotility, or erosion causes bleeding. By the time of diagnosis, tumors are usually unresectable. Later symptoms indicative of metastatic disease are abdominal distention owing to ascites, resulting from hepatic or peritoneal metastases, and dyspnea and pleural effusions, resulting from pulmonary metastases.

PHYSICAL EXAMINATION

Few findings are noted on physical examination, except in advanced disease. A firm, nontender, mobile epigastric mass can be palpated, and hepatomegaly with ascites may be present. Other distant signs of metastatic disease include Virchow supraclavicular sentinel node, Sister Joseph umbilical node, and Blumer shelf on rectal examination.

DIAGNOSTIC EVALUATION

Anemia is often found on routine blood studies. The anemia is usually hypochromic and microcytic secondary to iron deficiency. Stool is often positive for occult blood.

In recent years, upper endoscopy has replaced the barium-contrast upper gastrointestinal study as the imaging modality of choice. Endoscopy allows direct visualization and biopsy of the tumor.

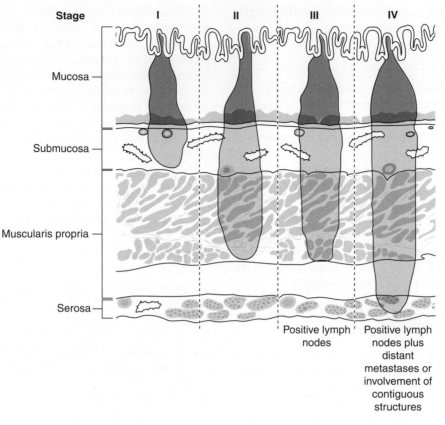

Figure 3-6 • Staging system for gastric carcinoma.

At least four biopsies should be made of the lesion. With 10 biopsies, the diagnostic accuracy approaches 100%. In Japan, the double-contrast air/barium study is used extensively for screening. Once diagnosis is made, computed tomography is performed to evaluate local extension and to look for evidence of ascites or metastatic disease.

STAGING

Staging for stomach cancer is according to TNM classification (Table 3-1).

TREATMENT

The theory behind curative resection involves en bloc primary tumor resection with wide disease-free margins and disease-free lymph nodes. Tumors are located either in the proximal, middle, or distal stomach. The type of operation performed for cure depends on tumor location. Distal lesions located in the antral or prepyloric area are treated with subtotal gastrectomy and Billroth II or Roux-en-Y anastomosis (Fig. 3-7).

Midgastric and proximal lesions are treated with total gastrectomy, with extensive lymph node dissection. The lesser and greater omentum are removed, along with the spleen. If the body or tail of the pancreas is involved, distal pancreatectomy can be performed. Reconstruction is achieved via Roux-en-Y anastomosis (Fig. 3-8).

Proximal lesions carry a poor prognosis, and surgical intervention is usually palliative. If there is extension into the distal esophagus, it is resected, along with the cardia and lesser curvature. The remaining stomach tube is closed, and the proximal aspect is anastomosed to the midesophagus through a right thoracotomy. If extensive esophageal involvement is discovered, radical near-total gastrectomy and a near-complete esophagectomy are performed, with continuity restored using a distal transverse colon and proximal left colon interposition (Fig. 3-9).

TABLE 3-1 American Joint Committee on Cancer (AJCC) TNM Classification of Carcinoma of the Stomach

Primary Tumor (T)

Tis	Carcinoma in situ: intraepithelial tumor without invasion of the lamina propria
T1	Tumor invades lamina propria or submucosa
T2	Tumor invades muscularis propria or subserosa[a]
T2a	Tumor invades muscularis propria
T2b	Tumor invades subserosa
T3	Tumor penetrates serosa (visceral peritoneum) without invasion of adjacent structures[b]
T4	Tumor invades adjacent structures[b]

Regional Lymph Nodes (N)

N0	No regional lymph node metastasis[c]
N1	Metastasis in 1 to 6 regional lymph nodes
N2	Metastasis in 7 to 15 regional lymph nodes
N3	Metastasis in more than 15 regional lymph nodes

Distant Metastasis (M)

M0	No distant metastasis
M1	Distant metastasis

Stage Grouping

Stage 0	Tis	N0	M0
Stage IA	T1	N0	M0
Stage IB	T1	N1	M0
	T2a/b	N0	M0
Stage II	T1	N2	M0
	T2a/b	N1	M0
	T3	N0	M0
Stage IIIA	T2a/b	N2	M0
	T3	N1	M0
	T4	N0	M0
Stage IIIB	T3	N2	M0
Stage IV	T4	N1–3	M0
	T1–3	N1–3	M0
	Any T	Any N	M1

[a]A tumor may penetrate the muscularis propria with extension into the gastrocolic or gastrohepatic ligaments, or into the greater or lesser omentum, without perforation of the visceral peritoneum covering these structures. In this case, the tumor is classified as T2. If there is perforation of the visceral peritoneum covering the gastric ligaments or the omentum, the tumor should be classified as T3.
[b]The adjacent structures of the stomach include the spleen, transverse colon, liver, diaphragm, pancreas, abdominal wall, adrenal gland, kidney, small intestine, and retroperitoneum. Intramural extension to the duodenum or esophagus is classified by the depth of the greatest invasion in any of these sites, including the stomach.
[c]A designation of pN0 should be used if all examined lymph nodes are negative, regardless of the total number removed and examined.
Reprinted with permission from the American Joint Committee on Cancer (AJCC), Chicago, Illinois. Original source: AJCC Cancer Staging Manual. 6th ed. New York, NY: Springer-Verlag; 2002.

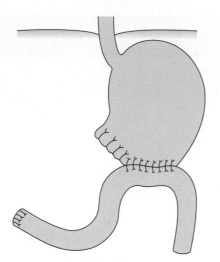

Figure 3-7 • Billroth II reconstruction after antral gastric cancer resection.

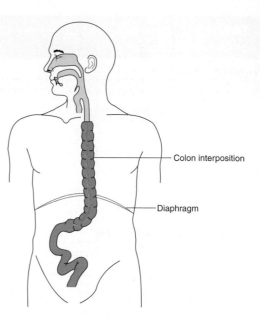

Figure 3-9 • Colonic interposition after near-total esophagectomy and near-total gastrectomy.

PROGNOSIS

The overall 5-year survival rate for gastric cancer in the United States is approximately 10%. Based on pathologic staging of tumors, the survival rate for stage I is 70%; stage II, 30%; stage III, 10%; and stage IV, 0%.

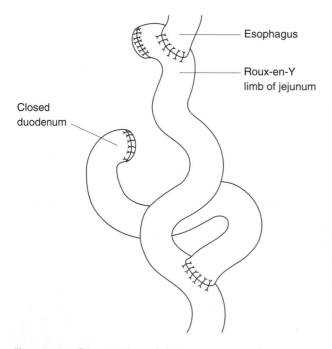

Figure 3-8 • Roux-en-Y esophagojejunostomy reconstruction after total gastrectomy.

KEY POINTS

- Peptic ulceration involves a compromised mucosal surface undergoing acid-peptic digestion. Causes include *Helicobacter pylori* infection (90% of cases), nonsteroidal anti-inflammatory drugs, alcohol, and tobacco. Treatment consists of decreasing stomach acidity and enhancing mucosal protection. *H. pylori* is eradicated with oral antibiotic therapy. Surgery is reserved for perforation, massive bleeding, gastric outlet obstruction, and nonhealing ulcers.

- Stress gastritis and ulceration are secondary to mucosal ischemia caused by hypotension and hypoperfusion.

- Cushing's ulcers occur in patients with intracranial pathology, most probably secondary to neuronally mediated acid hypersecretion.

- Gastrinomas cause Zollinger-Ellison syndrome, which is seen in patients with severe peptic ulceration, elevated serum gastrin levels, or evidence of a tumor within the "gastrinoma triangle." Diagnosis is confirmed by the secretin-stimulation test. Medical treatment includes H_2 blockade, proton pump inhibition, and somatostatin analogs. Complete surgical resection can be curative.

- Pathologic staging of gastric cancer is based on the depth of invasion and lymph node status. Most tumors are located in the antral region. En bloc resection with Billroth II or Roux-en-Y anastomosis is usually performed. Esophageal involvement requires esophagogastrectomy.

Small Intestine

ANATOMY AND PHYSIOLOGY

The small intestine comprises the duodenum, jejunum, and ileum and extends from the pylorus proximally to the cecum distally. Its main function is to digest and absorb nutrients. Absorption is achieved by the large surface area of the small intestine, secondary to its long length and extensive mucosal projections of villi and microvilli. A broad-based mesentery suspends the small intestine from the posterior abdominal wall once the retroperitoneal duodenum emerges at the ligament of Treitz and becomes the jejunum. Arterial blood is supplied from branches of the superior mesenteric artery, and venous drainage is via the superior mesenteric vein (Fig. 4-1). The mucosa has sequential circular folds, called plicae circulares. The plicae circulares are more numerous in the proximal bowel than in the distal bowel. The mucosal villi and microvilli create the surface through which carbohydrates, fats, proteins, and electrolytes are absorbed (Figs. 4-2 and 4-3).

SMALL BOWEL OBSTRUCTION

Although the potential causes of small bowel obstruction (SBO) are varied, the presentation of this disorder is usually quite consistent because of a common mechanism. Obstruction of the small bowel lumen causes progressive proximal accumulation of intraluminal fluids and gas. Peristalsis continues to transport swallowed air and secreted intestinal fluid through the bowel proximal to the obstruction, resulting in small bowel dilation and eventual abdominal distention. Depending on the location of the obstruction, vomiting occurs early in proximal obstruction and later in more distal blockage (Fig. 4-4). Crampy abdominal pain initially occurs as active proximal peristalsis exacerbates bowel dilation. With progressive bowel wall edema and luminal dilation, however, peristaltic activity decreases and abdominal pain lessens. At presentation, patients exhibit abdominal distention and complain of mild diffuse abdominal pain.

ETIOLOGY

The first and second most common causes of SBO are adhesions and hernias, respectively (Table 4-1). Most adhesions are caused by postoperative internal scar formation. Discovering the actual mechanism of obstruction is important for therapeutic planning, because the mechanism of obstruction relates to the possibility of vascular compromise and bowel ischemia. For example, a closed-loop obstruction caused by volvulus with torsion is at higher risk for vascular compromise than an SBO from a simple adhesive band (Fig. 4-5).

A second mechanism causing bowel ischemia is incarceration in a fixed space. Incarceration and subsequent strangulation impedes venous return, causing edema and eventual bowel infarction. Other mechanisms of obstruction that rarely compromise vascular flow are intraluminal obstruction by a gallstone or bezoar and intussusception caused by an intramural or mucosal lesion at the leading edge.

HISTORY

Patients usually present with complaints of intermittent crampy abdominal pain, abdominal distention, obstipation, nausea, and vomiting. Vomiting of feculent material usually occurs later in the course of obstruction. Constant localized pain or pain out of proportion to

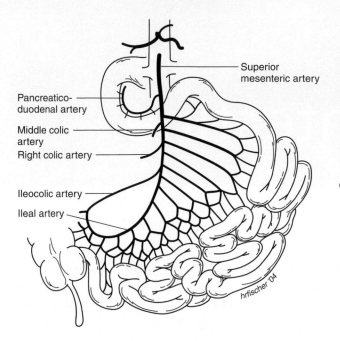

Figure 4-1 • Anatomy of the small intestine demonstrating vascular anatomy of the varying segments. Note longer vasa recta in jejunum versus ileum.

From Lawrence PF, Bell RM, Dayton MT, et al. *Essentials of General Surgery.* 4th ed. Philadelphia: Lippincott Williams & Wilkins, 2005.

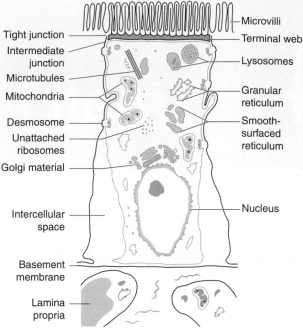

Figure 4-3 • Diagram of a columnar epithelial intestinal absorptive cell with luminal microvilli.

physical findings may indicate ischemic bowel and is a clear indication for urgent surgical exploration.

PHYSICAL EXAMINATION

A distended abdomen with diffuse midabdominal tenderness to palpation is usually found on physical examination. Typically, there are no signs of peritonitis. If constant localized tenderness is apparent, indicating localized peritonitis, then ischemia and gangrene must be suspected. An essential aspect of

the physical examination is to check for abdominal wall hernias, especially in postsurgical patients. Elevation in temperature should not be present in uncomplicated cases. Tachycardia may be present from hypovolemia secondary to persistent vomiting or from toxemia caused by intestinal gangrene.

DIAGNOSTIC EVALUATION

Upright radiographs classically demonstrate distended loops of small bowel with multiple air–fluid interfaces. Occasionally, the radiograph shows the etiology of the obstruction, the site of obstruction, and whether the obstruction is partial or complete. Dilated small bowel in the presence of a dilated colon suggests the diagnosis of paralytic ileus, not SBO. A small bowel contrast study may be necessary to demonstrate transit of contrast into the colon, thereby ruling out SBO. Free air indicates perforation of the intra-abdominal gastrointestinal tract, whereas biliary gas and an opacity near the ileocecal valve indicate gallstone ileus.

Abdominal computed tomography (CT) scans can often demonstrate the transition point, where the dilated bowel proximal to the point of obstruction transitions to the decompressed bowel more distally. Also, in cases where the bowel has twisted on its mesentery, a "swirl sign" can be seen as the mesenteric

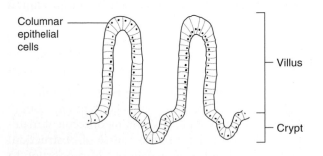

Figure 4-2 • Structure of small intestinal villi.

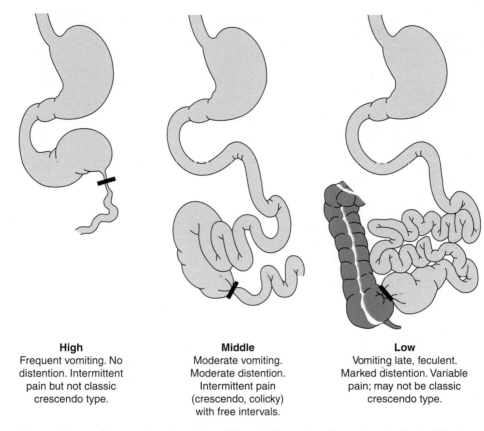

High	Middle	Low
Frequent vomiting. No distention. Intermittent pain but not classic crescendo type.	Moderate vomiting. Moderate distention. Intermittent pain (crescendo, colicky) with free intervals.	Vomiting late, feculent. Marked distention. Variable pain; may not be classic crescendo type.

Figure 4-4 • Variable manifestations of small bowel obstruction depend on the level of blockage.

vasculature twists on itself, creating a distinctive swirling radiographic pattern.

Laboratory examination often reveals a hypokalemic alkalosis owing to dehydration from repeated emesis. White blood cell count and amylase may be mildly elevated. Lactic acidosis is cause for concern and may indicate intestinal necrosis.

TREATMENT

In decades past, most patients presenting with an SBO were taken directly to the operating room for exploration to rule out intestinal necrosis. However, over the past few decades it became apparent that most patients can be safely managed medically in the absence of peritonitis or other worrisome clinical findings. Supportive therapy allows for spontaneous resolution of the obstruction and return of normal bowel function. For patients who are candidates for a trial of nonsurgical therapy, initial treatment consists of nasogastric decompression to relieve proximal gastrointestinal distention and associated nausea and vomiting. Fluid resuscitation and supportive hydration is necessary because patients are typically intravascularly depleted from diminished oral fluid intake and vomiting.

■ TABLE 4-1 Causes of Small Bowel Obstruction
Adhesions
Hernias—abdominal wall, internal
Neoplasms—primary, metastatic
Obturation/strictures—ischemia, radiation,
Crohn's disease, gallstone, bezoar
Intussusception
Meckel's diverticulum
Volvulus
Superior mesenteric artery syndrome
Intramural hematoma

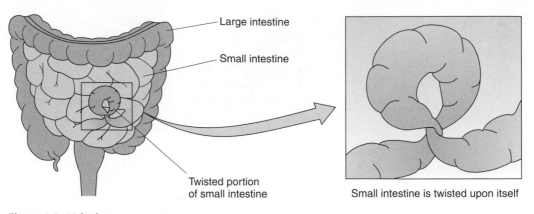

Figure 4-5 • Volvulus.
From Willis MC. *Medical Terminology: A Programmed Learning Approach to the Language of Health Care.* Baltimore: Lippincott Williams & Wilkins, 2002.

The decision to operate is based on the nature of the obstruction and the patient's clinical condition. On initial presentation, if ischemia or perforation is suspected, immediate operation is necessary. Otherwise, patients can be observed with serial physical examinations, serum tests, and abdominal radiographs for evidence of resolution. If the patient's condition worsens or fails to improve with supportive therapy, operative intervention is indicated.

CROHN'S DISEASE

Crohn's disease is a transmural inflammatory disease that may affect any part of the gastrointestinal tract, from the mouth to the anus. Ileal involvement is most common. The disease is characterized by skip lesions that involve discontinuous segments of abnormal mucosa. Granulomata are usually seen microscopically, but not always. Areas of inflammation are often associated with fibrotic strictures, enterocutaneous fistulae, and intra-abdominal abscesses, all of which usually require surgical intervention.

EPIDEMIOLOGY

Crohn's disease occurs throughout the world, although the actual incidence exhibits a geographic and ethnic variability. The incidence in the United States is approximately 10 times that of Japan. Ashkenazi Jews have a far higher incidence of disease than do African Americans.

ETIOLOGY

The cause of Crohn's disease remains unknown. Because of the presence of granulomata, mycobacterial infection has been postulated as the causative agent. Recent investigations with *Mycobacterium paratuberculosis* have proved inconclusive. An immunologic basis for the disease has also been advanced; however, although humoral and cellular immune responses are involved in disease pathogenesis, no specific immunologic disturbance has been identified.

PATHOLOGY

The small intestine is affected in at least 70% of all patients with Crohn's disease. The ileum is typically diseased, with frequent right colon involvement. On gross inspection, the serosal surface of the bowel is hypervascular, and the mesentery characteristically shows signs of "creeping fat." The bowel walls are edematous and fibrotic. The mucosa has a cobblestone appearance, with varying degrees of associated mucosal ulceration (see Color Plates 2 and 3).

Histologically, a chronic lymphocytic infiltrate in an inflamed mucosa and submucosa is seen. Fissure ulcers penetrate deep into the mucosa and are often associated with granulomata and multinucleated giant cells. Granulomata are seen more frequently in distal tissues, which explains why granulomata are seen more often in colonic disease than in ileal disease.

HISTORY

Patients with Crohn's disease of the small bowel present complaining of diarrhea, abdominal pain, anorexia, nausea, and weight loss. The diarrhea is usually loose and watery, without frank blood. Dull abdominal pain is usually in the right iliac fossa or periumbilical region.

Children often present with symptoms of malaise and have noticeable growth failure. Strictures may cause partial SBO, resulting in bacterial overgrowth and subsequent steatorrhea, flatus, and bloating.

PHYSICAL EXAMINATION

Patients may appear to be either generally healthy or may have significant cachexia. Abdominal examination may reveal right iliac fossa tenderness. In acutely ill patients, a palpable abdominal mass may be present, indicating abscess formation. Enterocutaneous fistulae may be present. Oral examination may reveal evidence of mucosal ulceration, whereas perianal inspection may show skin tags, fissures, or fistulae. Extraintestinal manifestations include erythema nodosum, pyoderma gangrenosum, ankylosing spondylitis, and uveitis.

DIAGNOSTIC EVALUATION

Blood studies often show a mild iron-deficiency anemia and a depressed albumin level. If hypoalbuminemia is severe, peripheral edema may be present.

Small intestine Crohn's disease is diagnosed by bariumcontrast enteroclysis. This small intestine enema technique provides better mucosal definition than standard small bowel follow-through studies. This technique illustrates aphthoid ulcers, strictures, fissures, bowel wall thickening, and fistulae. Fistulograms are helpful to define existing fistula tracks, and CT can localize abscesses. Once radiographic evidence of disease is found, colonoscopy should be performed to evaluate the colonic mucosa and to obtain biopsies of the terminal ileum.

DIFFERENTIAL DIAGNOSIS

In addition to the diagnosis of Crohn's disease, one should consider the possibility of acute appendicitis, *Yersinia* infection, lymphoma, intestinal tuberculosis, and Behçet disease.

COMPLICATIONS

Crohn's disease carries a high morbidity and low mortality. Small bowel strictures secondary to inflammation and fibrosis are common complications that present as obstructions. Fistulae from small bowel to adjacent loops of small bowel, large bowel, bladder, vagina, or skin also occur. Ileal Crohn's disease can result in gallstone formation because of the interruption of the enterohepatic circulation of bile salts. Kidney stones may also form because of hyperoxaluria. Normally, calcium and oxalate bind in the intestine and are excreted in the feces. With ileal Crohn's disease, steatorrhea causes ingested fat to bind intraluminal calcium, thus allowing free oxalate to be absorbed. Finally, adenocarcinoma is a rare complication that usually arises in the ileum.

TREATMENT

Mild disease can be controlled with a 4- to 6-week course of sulfasalazine or mesalazine. Alternatively, oral corticosteroids can be used with equivalent results. Metronidazole may also be useful. Patients with bile salt–induced diarrhea after ileal resection may benefit from cholestyramine.

Severe disease is treated with hospitalization, bowel rest, hydration, intravenous nutrition, corticosteroids, and metronidazole. Patients with chronic active disease may benefit from a course of mercaptopurine.

Surgery for Crohn's disease should only be performed for complications of the disease (Table 4-2). Operation should be conservative and should address only the presenting indication, using gentle surgical technique. Resections should be avoided, as overly aggressive intervention can produce surgically induced short bowel syndrome and malnutrition. Some common surgical problems encountered in Crohn's disease and its treatments include ileocolic disease, which is managed by conservative ileocecal resection to grossly normal margins (Fig. 4-6); stricture, managed by stricturoplasty, which entails incising the antimesenteric border of the stricture along the intestinal long axis and then closing the enterotomy transversely (Fig. 4-7); and abscess/fistula, which is managed by open or percutaneous drainage of the abscess and resection of the small bowel segment responsible for initiating the fistula with primary anastomosis (Fig. 4-8).

■ TABLE 4-2 Indications for Surgery in Crohn's Disease
Stricture with Obstructive Symptoms
Fistula
Abscess
Perforation
Bleeding

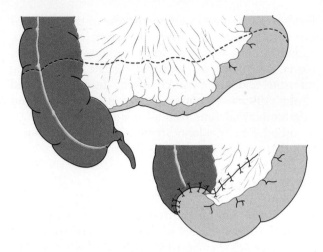

Figure 4-6 • Ileocecal resection for Crohn's disease.

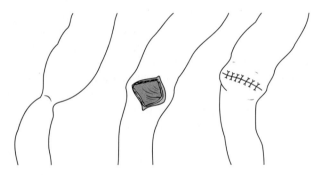

Figure 4-7 • Stricturoplasty of a localized stricture with transverse closure.

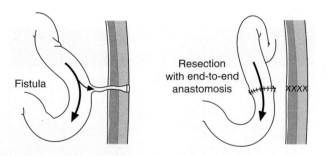

Figure 4-8 • Fistula resection with end-to-end anastomosis.

MECKEL'S DIVERTICULUM

This most common congenital anomaly of the small intestine is an antimesenteric remnant arising from a failure of vitelline duct obliteration during embryonic development. Meckel's diverticula are true diverticula affecting all three intestinal muscle layers. Diverticula are usually <12 cm in length and are found within 100 cm of the ileocecal valve.

Associated abnormalities of the vitelline duct depend on the degree of duct obliteration that occurs during development. Complete ductal obliteration leaves a thin fibrous band connecting ileum to umbilicus, whereas complete duct persistence results in a patent ileoumbilical fistula. Partial obstruction results in cyst or blind sinus formation (Fig. 4-9). Heterotopic tissue (gastric, pancreatic) is found in 30% to 50% of diverticula.

In the United States, Meckel's diverticulum is associated with the "Rule of 2s": it occurs in 2% of the population, is located within 2 ft of the ileocecal valve, is usually 2 in long, contains two types of heterotopic tissue (gastric, pancreatic, duodenal, or intestinal), and is the most common cause of rectal bleeding in infants younger than 2 years.

COMPLICATIONS

Bleeding within the diverticulum may occur from peptic ulceration arising from heterotopic gastric mucosa. In infants, Meckel's diverticulum is the most common cause of major lower gastrointestinal bleeding.

Bowel obstruction may result from one of two mechanisms. Intussusception can occur when an inverted diverticulum functions as a lead point, or small bowel volvulus can occur around a fixed obliterated vitelline duct extending from the ileum to the umbilicus.

DIAGNOSTIC EVALUATION

For Meckel's diverticula containing heterotopic gastric mucosa, the technetium 99 (^{99}Tc) scan is helpful for diagnosis: pertechnetate anions are taken up by ectopic gastric parietal cells and indicate diverticulum location. Diverticula that do not contain heterotopic gastric tissue can occasionally be visualized using standard barium-contrast studies.

TREATMENT

Definitive treatment for Meckel's diverticulum complications is surgical resection. In adult patients incidentally

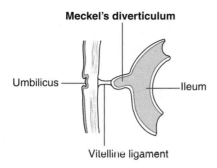
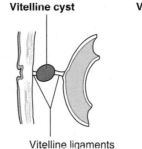
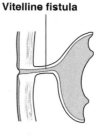

Figure 4-9 • Vitelline duct remnants.

found to have an asymptomatic Meckel's diverticulum during laparotomy, the diverticulum should be left in situ, as the chance of producing surgical morbidity and mortality are respectively 23 and five times higher for resection than when only symptomatic diverticula are removed.

SMALL BOWEL TUMORS

Tumors of the small bowel are rare, accounting for 1% to 5% of all gastrointestinal tumors. Most tumors are benign. Common benign neoplasms of the small bowel include tubular and villous adenomas, lipomas, leiomyomas, and hemangiomas. Telangiectasias of Rendu-Osler-Weber syndrome, neurofibromas of neurofibromatosis, hamartomatous polyps of Peutz-Jeghers syndrome, and heterotopic tissue as in Meckel's diverticulum are also found. Possible explanations for this lack of malignancy include short exposure to ingested carcinogens secondary to rapid transit time, low bacterial counts resulting in fewer endogenously produced carcinogens, and the intraluminal secretion of IgA by small bowel mucosa.

Benign lesions are usually asymptomatic and are incidental findings. Of symptomatic lesions, obstruction is the most common presentation, followed by hemorrhage. In the workup of gastrointestinal bleeding, however, unless other evidence exists, small bowel lesions should be low on the list of differential diagnoses, because >90% of bleeding lesions occur between the esophagus and distal duodenum and between the ileocecal valve and anus. Small bowel lesions should be suspected if careful skin examination reveals café-au-lait spots (neurofibromatosis), telangiectasia (Rendu-Osler-Weber syndrome), or mucocutaneous pigmentation (Peutz-Jeghers syndrome).

Malignant tumors of the small bowel typically present with obstruction or bleeding. The four major malignant tumors are adenocarcinoma, gastrointestinal stromal tumors, carcinoid, and lymphoma.

DIAGNOSTIC EVALUATION

Visual endoscopic identification of small bowel tumors is usually possible for lesions of the proximal duodenum and terminal ileum. The remainder of the small bowel requires examination by barium-contrast studies. For larger lesions, CT may be helpful.

In situations involving active hemorrhage, ^{99}Tc sulfur colloid or ^{99}Tc-labeled red blood cell studies may show the bleeding site. However, a bleeding rate of 1 mL/min is required for accurate localization.

When available diagnostic modalities are insufficient, exploratory laparotomy may be necessary. In addition to external inspection at laparotomy, operative endoscopy can be used for intraluminal evaluation.

CARCINOID TUMORS

Carcinoid tumors are the most common endocrine tumors of the gastrointestinal tract, constituting more than half of all such lesions. They account for up to 30% of all small bowel tumors. Carcinoid tumors arise from neuroendocrine enterochromaffin cells. Hence tumors can secrete serotonin and other humoral substances, such as histamine, dopamine, tachykinins, peptides, and prostaglandins. The metabolite of serotonin, 5-hydroxyindoleacetic acid, is excreted in the urine and is easily detected.

All carcinoids are considered malignant because of their potential for invasion and metastasis. Patients with metastatic disease manifest the carcinoid syndrome, which consists of the systemic effects (flushing, diarrhea, sweating, and wheezing) of secreted vasoactive substances. Presence of the carcinoid syndrome indicates hepatic metastasis, because systemic effects occur when venous drainage from a tumor escapes hepatic metabolism of vasoactive substances.

Approximately 85% of carcinoid tumors are found in the intestine; of these, approximately 50% are found in the appendix, making it the most common site of occurrence, followed by the ileum, jejunum, rectum, and duodenum (see Color Plate 4). Other sites of disease include the lungs and occasionally the pancreas and biliary tract. Appendiceal carcinoids rarely metastasize, whereas lesions of the ileum have the highest association with carcinoid syndrome. Jejunoileal carcinoids are frequently multicentric.

HISTORY

The clinical presentation of patients with carcinoid tumors differs depending on tumor location. Primary tumors may present as SBO, because tumors can incite an intense local fibrosis of the bowel that causes angulation and kinking of the involved segment. As noted, metastatic disease with hepatic spread manifests as the carcinoid syndrome. Occult primary lesions do not cause systemic effects because 5-hydroxytryptamine (serotonin) is metabolized by the liver. Other presenting symptoms can include abdominal pain, upper intestinal or rectal bleeding, intussusception, weight loss, or a palpable abdominal mass.

DIAGNOSTIC EVALUATION

Laboratory studies should include plasma and urine analysis to evaluate for elevated levels of plasma serotonin and urinary 5-hydroxyindoleacetic acid. Barium-contrast studies are also useful for diagnosing carcinoid tumors. Barium enemas can demonstrate lesions of the rectum and large bowel, whereas small bowel enteroclysis may show a discrete lesion or a stricture secondary to fibrosis. Because primary tumors are usually small, CT is usually helpful only for detecting hepatic metastases. Colonoscopy can show tumors from the terminal ileum to the rectum.

Because neuroendocrine tumors often express functional receptors, radiolabeled octreotide imaging can be useful in detecting occult disease. Octreotide scanning is based on physiologic function, rather than on detectable anatomic alterations, and may have better diagnostic sensitivity than conventional imaging modalities.

TREATMENT

Surgical resection of the primary tumor is always undertaken, even in cases of metastatic disease. If the tumor is left in situ, bowel obstruction and intussusception ultimately result. At laparotomy, adequate bowel and mesenteric margins must be obtained, as with any cancer-related operation. Depending on tumor size and the degree of spread, lesions can be treated with simple local excision for small primaries to wide en bloc resection for metastatic disease.

Patients who have carcinoid syndrome can achieve symptomatic relief with subcutaneous injections of somatostatin analogs (e.g., octreotide). Induction with general anesthesia may provoke a life-threatening carcinoid crisis characterized by hypotension, flushing, tachycardia, and arrhythmias. Intravenous somatostatin or octreotide rapidly reverses the crisis.

PROGNOSIS

Carcinoid tumors are relatively indolent, slow-growing neoplasms. Prognosis for patients with carcinoid tumors is directly related to the size of the primary tumor and to the presence of metastasis.

For noninvasive lesions of the appendix and rectum <2 cm in size, the 5-year survival rate nears 100%. As the tumor size increases, the survival rate decreases. The presence of muscle wall invasion and positive lymph nodes are poor prognostic signs.

Patients with hepatic metastases have an average survival of approximately 3 years. Liver lesions are usually multiple. Because incapacitating symptoms of the carcinoid syndrome are proportional to tumor bulk, cytoreductive surgery can ameliorate symptoms, as well as prolong survival. Nonsurgical palliation is achieved with somatostatin analog therapy or chemoembolization of the tumor.

KEY POINTS

- Small bowel obstruction is commonly caused by adhesions and hernias. Bowel infarction occurs with closed-loop obstruction and strangulation. Patients with peritonitis require immediate surgery. Many patients are successfully managed with supportive therapy alone. Surgery is indicated if the obstruction fails to resolve spontaneously.

- Crohn's disease is a transmural inflammatory process that affects any part of the gastrointestinal tract, from mouth to anus. The ileum is most commonly involved. Surgical treatment is reserved mainly for complications.

- Meckel's diverticulum is the most common congenital abnormality of the small intestine and arises from a failure of vitelline duct obliteration. It is a true diverticulum and may contain heterotopic gastric and pancreatic tissue. Peptic ulceration with hemorrhage may develop. It is the most common cause of major lower gastrointestinal bleeding in infants.

- Small bowel tumors are rare and usually benign, often presenting as small bowel obstructions. Benign tumors include adenomas, lipomas, leiomyomas, and hemangiomas. Malignant tumors include adenocarcinoma, gastrointestinal stromal tumors, carcinoid, and lymphoma.

- Carcinoid tumors are the most common endocrine tumors of the gastrointestinal tract and most frequently occur in the appendix. All carcinoid tumors are considered malignant because of their potential for invasion and metastasis.

- Carcinoid tumors secrete serotonin, which is broken down in the liver to the metabolite 5-hydroxyindoleacetic acid, which is, in turn, excreted in the urine. Carcinoid syndrome, manifested by flushing, diarrhea, sweating, and wheezing, invariably indicates hepatic metastases, because vasoactive substances have escaped hepatic metabolism.

- Carcinoid syndrome is treated with somatostatin analogs and chemoembolization to provide symptomatic relief

5 Colon

ANATOMY AND PHYSIOLOGY

The colon begins at the ileocecal valve and extends distally to the anal canal. Its primary function is the reabsorption of water and sodium, secretion of potassium and bicarbonate, and storage of fecal material. The ascending and descending colon are fixed in a retroperitoneal location, whereas the transverse and sigmoid colon are intraperitoneal.

Arterial supply to the cecum, ascending colon, and transverse colon is from the superior mesenteric artery by way of the ileocolic, right colic, and middle colic arteries. The remainder of the colon is supplied by the inferior mesenteric artery by way of the left colic, sigmoid, and superior hemorrhoidal arteries and the middle and inferior hemorrhoidal arteries that arise from the internal iliac artery. The inconstant anastomotic artery between the middle colic of the superior mesenteric artery and left colic of the inferior mesenteric artery is called the anastomosis (or arc) of Riolan. The interconnecting arcades in closer proximity to the mesenteric border of the colon are referred to as the marginal artery of Drummond (Fig. 5-1). This amalgamation of anastomotic branches runs around the medial margin of the entire colon, from the ileocolic artery to the sigmoid arteries. Venous drainage from the colon includes the superior and inferior mesenteric veins. The inferior mesenteric vein joins the splenic vein, which joins the superior mesenteric vein to form the portal vein. In this way, mesenteric blood flow enters the liver, where it is detoxified before entering the central circulation. Lymphatic drainage follows the arteries and veins.

ULCERATIVE COLITIS

Ulcerative colitis is an inflammatory disease of the colon with unknown cause. An autoimmune basis is suspected. Inflammation almost always involves the rectum and extends proximally toward the cecum to varying degrees. The small bowel is uninvolved except in cases of "backwash ileitis" that may occur in proximal colonic disease. Extracolonic manifestations include inflammatory eye and skin disorders, arthritis, blood disorders, and sclerosing cholangitis.

PATHOLOGY

Inflammation is confined to the mucosa and submucosa. Superficial ulcers, thickened mucosa, crypt abscesses, and pseudopolyps may also be present.

EPIDEMIOLOGY

The incidence is six per 100,000. It is more common in developed countries, especially among Caucasians and the Jewish population. There is no predilection for sex. Approximately 20% of patients have first-degree relatives who are affected, suggesting a genetic basis. Linkage analysis has identified an association with HLA-DR2.

HISTORY

Most patients usually present in the second through fourth decade of life. Patients commonly complain

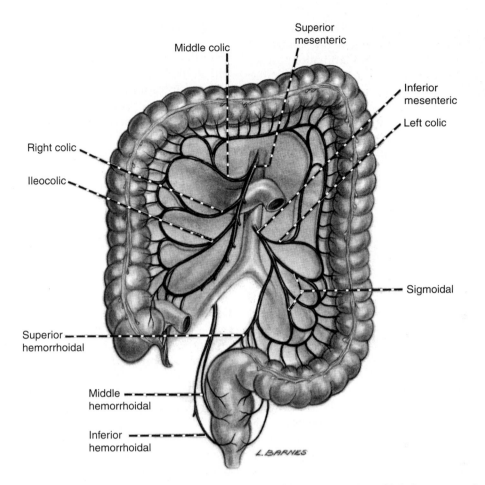

Figure 5-1 • The blood supply to the colon originates from the superior and inferior mesenteric arteries.
From Corman RL. *Colon and Rectal Surgery*. 5th ed. Philadelphia: Lippincott Williams & Wilkins, 2004.

of bloody diarrhea, mucus/pus per rectum, fever, abdominal pain, and weight loss. A history of repeated attacks is common. Numerous diseases are associated with ulcerative colitis, including sclerosing cholangitis in 1% of patients, as well as arthritis, iritis, cholangitis, aphthous ulcers, pyoderma gangrenosum, erythema nodosum, hemolytic anemia, and ankylosing spondylosis. These diseases may be part of the initial presentation.

PHYSICAL EXAMINATION

Abdominal pain is common. Rectal tenderness may occur with rectal fissures. The disease may present with abdominal distention as evidence of massive colonic distention, a situation known as toxic megacolon. This may progress to frank perforation with signs of peritonitis.

DIAGNOSTIC EVALUATION

Plain films may show massive colonic dilation, indicating toxic megacolon. Perforation will result in air under the diaphragm. Barium enema may reveal a "stovepipe colon" owing to loss of haustral folds, as well as mucosal ulcerations.

Endoscopy demonstrates thickened friable mucosa. Fissures and pseudopolyps, if present, almost always involve the rectum and varying portions of the colon. Biopsy shows ulceration limited to the mucosa and submucosa. Crypt abscesses arising from the crypts of Lieberkuhn coalesce to form ulcerations.

COMPLICATIONS

Perforation and hemorrhage may occur during a severe attack. Obstruction may develop from stricture as a result of chronic inflammation. Toxic megacolon is uncommon but is life-threatening if not controlled with medical therapy. Severe inflammation causes destruction of the myenteric plexus and muscular layer, leading to massive distention and perforation. Patients are invariably septic and mortality high unless emergent subtotal colectomy is performed. Colon cancer occurs frequently, with a risk of approximately 10% within 20 years. Once the diagnosis of ulcerative colitis is made, routine colonoscopic surveillance is mandatory.

TREATMENT

Initial therapy is medical, with fluid administration, electrolyte correction, and parenteral nutrition if necessary. Corticosteroids, other immunosuppressives, and sulfasalazine are all effective. Topical mesalamine, in the form of enemas, is effective for mild and moderate disease. Newer immunosuppressive agents—including infliximab, a monoclonal antibody against tumor necrosis factor—may be useful. High-fiber diet and bulking agents are often useful.

Indications for surgery include colonic obstruction, massive blood loss, failure of medical therapy, toxic megacolon, and cancer. The recommendation of prophylactic colectomy for these patients is being reconsidered on the basis of recent data that suggest the incidence of cancer is not as high as once thought. When elective surgery is performed, sphincter-sparing operations allow the ileum to be anastomosed to the rectal stump or anus, preserving continence and bowel movement. The ileum is fashioned into a J-pouch, which serves the fecal reservoir role of the removed rectum.

DIVERTICULOSIS

Diverticulosis refers to the presence of diverticula, outpouchings of the colon that occur at points where the arterial supply penetrates the bowel wall (singular, *diverticulum*; plural, *diverticula*) (Fig. 5-2). These are acquired or false diverticula because not all layers of the bowel wall are included. Most diverticula occur in the sigmoid colon (Figs. 5-3 and 5-4). Diverticulosis is the most common cause of lower gastrointestinal hemorrhage, usually from the right colon. Of people with diverticulosis, 15% will have a significant episode of bleeding.

EPIDEMIOLOGY

Diverticular disease is common in developed nations and is likely related to low-fiber diets. Because of reduced intraluminal stool volume, the normal segmental colonic peristaltic contractions are extra forceful, which increases intraluminal pressure and causes herniation of the mucosa through the circular muscles of the bowel wall where the marginal artery branches penetrate. Men and women are equally affected, and the prevalence increases dramatically with age. Approximately one third of the population has diverticular disease, but this number increases to more than half of those older than 80 years of age.

HISTORY

Patients usually present with bleeding from the rectum without other complaints. They may have had previous episodes of bleeding or crampy abdominal pain, commonly in the left lower quadrant.

DIAGNOSTIC EVALUATION

For patients who stop bleeding spontaneously, elective colonoscopy should be performed to determine the cause of the bleeding. If bleeding continues, diagnostic

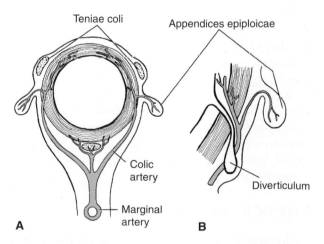

Figure 5-2 • Blood supply to the colon (**A**) and formation of the diverticulum (**B**). Note the passage of the mucosal diverticulum through the muscle coat along the course of the artery.
From Snell RS. *Clinical Anatomy*. 7th ed. Philadelphia: Lippincott Williams & Wilkins, 2003.

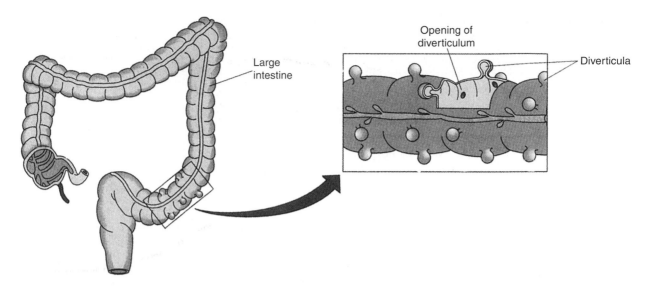

Figure 5-3 • Diverticulosis, diverticulitis.
Reprinted with permission from Willis MC. *Medical Terminology: The Language of Health Care.* 1st ed. Baltimore: Williams & Wilkins; 1996:374.

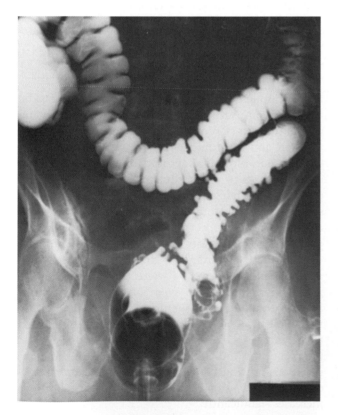

Figure 5-4 • Extensive sigmoid diverticular disease with slight spasm but no stigmata of acute inflammation. In the absence of classic symptoms and signs of diverticulitis, surgery is not advised solely on the basis of this radiographic appearance.
From Corman RL. *Colon and Rectal Surgery.* 5th ed. Philadelphia: Lippincott Williams & Wilkins, 2004.

and therapeutic modalities include radioisotope bleeding scans, which have variable success rates, and mesenteric angiography, which has an excellent success rate in the presence of active bleeding.

TREATMENT

Asymptomatic individuals require no treatment. In the event of a bleed, 80% will stop spontaneously. Elective segmental or subtotal colectomy is not usually recommended at first episode. However, depending on the ability to accurately determine the site of bleeding, the severity of the initial bleeding episode, and the general status of the patient, it may be indicated. Patients with recurrent bleeding are usually offered surgical resection. Active bleeding is treated colonoscopically if the colon can be cleaned and the bleeding site identified. Embolization of the bleeding vessel may be possible using selective angiography. In the face of massive bleeding, if the above methods fail and no bleeding site is identified, emergent subtotal colectomy is performed. Before embarking on such an irreversible procedure, which involves removing most of the colon, it is of utmost importance to ensure that the bleeding source is not from hemorrhoids or a rectal source. If a colonic bleeding site is identified, segmental colectomy can be performed, usually based on the arterial branch feeding the bleeding site.

DIVERTICULITIS

The narrow neck of a diverticulum predisposes it to infection, which occurs either from increased intraluminal pressure or inspissated food particles. Infection leads to localized or free perforation into the abdomen. Diverticulitis most commonly occurs in the sigmoid and is rare in the right colon. Approximately 20% of patients with diverticula experience an episode of diverticulitis. Each attack makes a subsequent attack more likely and increases the risk of complications.

HISTORY

Patients usually present with left lower quadrant pain; right-sided diverticulitis causes right-sided pain but is less common. The pain is usually progressive over a few days and may be associated with diarrhea or constipation.

PHYSICAL EXAMINATION

Abdominal tenderness, usually in the left lower quadrant, is the most common finding. Local peritoneal signs of rebound and guarding may be present. Significant colonic inflammation may present as a palpable mass. Diffuse rebound tenderness and guarding as evidence of generalized peritonitis suggests free intra-abdominal perforation.

DIAGNOSTIC EVALUATION

Elevation of the white blood cell count is usual. Radiographs of the abdomen are typically normal, except for cases of perforation or obstruction. In cases of perforation, free air is seen under the diaphragms on chest x-ray. Computed tomography (CT) may demonstrate pericolic fat stranding, bowel wall thickening, or abscess. Colonoscopy and barium enema should not be performed during an acute episode because of the risk of causing or exacerbating an existing perforation.

COMPLICATIONS

Stricture, perforation, or fistulization with the bladder, skin, vagina, or other portions of the bowel may develop.

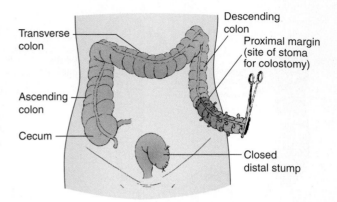

Figure 5-5 • The Hartmann procedure for diverticulitis: primary resection for diverticulitis of the colon. The affected segment (clamp attached) has been divided at its distal end. In a primary anastomosis, the proximal margin (dotted line) is transected and the bowel attached end-to-end. In a two-stage procedure, a colostomy is constructed at the proximal margin with the distal stump oversewn (Hartmann procedure, as shown) or brought to the outer surface as a mucous fistula. The second stage consists of colostomy takedown and anastomosis.
From Smeltzer SC, Bare BG. Brunner & Suddarth's *Textbook of Medical-Surgical Nursing*. 9th ed. Philadelphia: Lippincott Williams & Wilkins, 2000.

TREATMENT

Most episodes of diverticulitis are mild and can be treated on an outpatient basis with broad-spectrum oral antibiotics. Combination treatment with ciprofloxacin and metronidazole (Flagyl) is appropriate to cover aerobic and anaerobic organisms. For severe cases or cases in older adult patients or debilitated patients, hospitalization with bowel rest and broad-spectrum intravenous antibiotics (e.g., ampicillin, ciprofloxacin, and metronidazole) are required. For patients who do not improve in 24 to 48 hours, repeat CT scan with percutaneous drainage of any identifiable abscess cavity may obviate the need for emergency operation. In the event of free perforation or failure of medical management, surgical exploration with resection and colostomy is usually required (Hartmann procedure; Fig. 5-5). In addition, surgical intervention is indicated in the presence of the complications previously described. With repeated attacks of diverticulitis, the risk of developing complications increases significantly.

COLONIC NEOPLASMS

Recent evidence suggests that colon cancer follows an orderly progression in which adenomatous polyps undergo malignant transformation over a variable time period (Fig. 5-6). For this reason, these polyps are considered premalignant lesions. Fifty percent of carcinomas have a *ras* gene mutation, whereas 75% have a *p53* gene mutation.

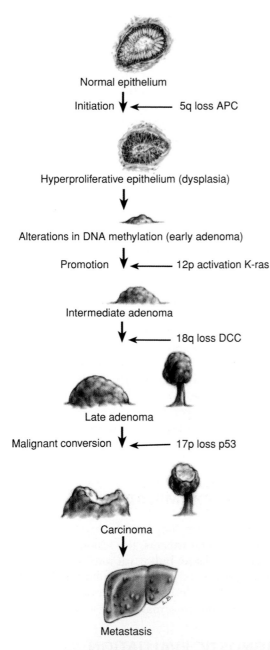

Figure 5-6 • Model of colorectal carcinogenesis. (Redrawn from Fearon ER, Vogelstein B. A genetic model of colorectal cancer tumorigenesis. *Cell* 1990;61:759.)
From Corman RL. *Colon and Rectal Surgery*. 5th ed. Philadelphia: Lippincott Williams & Wilkins, 2004.

EPIDEMIOLOGY

Colon cancer is the second most common cause of cancer-related death in the United States. Risk factors include high-fat and low-fiber diets, age, and family history. Ulcerative colitis, Crohn's disease, and Gardner syndrome all predispose to cancer, and cancer develops in all patients with familial polyposis coli if they are not treated.

PATHOLOGY

Adenomatous polyps are either tubular or villous, with some lesions exhibiting features of both. The higher the villous component, the higher the risk of malignancy. As the lesion grows in size, the likelihood of its having undergone malignant transformation increases significantly. Although tubular adenomas <1 cm contain malignancy in only 1% of cases, lesions >2 cm contain malignancy 25% of the time. For villous adenomas, the numbers are 10% and 50%, respectively. Ninety percent of colon cancers are adenocarcinomas, and 20% of these are mucinous, carrying the worst prognosis. Other types include squamous, adenosquamous, lymphoma, sarcoma, and carcinoid. Three percent of tumors are synchronous (occurring simultaneously), and metachronous tumors (multiple primary cancers developing at intervals) also occur in 3% of cases.

SCREENING

Screening is aimed at detecting polyps and early malignant lesions. In theory, colon cancer is a preventable disease, because if all patients underwent thorough screening and timely polyp removal, the mortality rate from colon cancer would be drastically reduced. The current screening recommendations from the American Gastroenterological Association divide people into two groups: average risk and increased risk. Average-risk persons lack any identifiable risk factors. Increased-risk persons have either a personal history of adenomatous polyps or colorectal cancer, first-degree relatives with colorectal cancer or adenomatous polyps, a family history of multiple cancers, or a history of inflammatory bowel disease. Screening should begin at age 50 years for average-risk patients and age 40 years for increased-risk patients. American Cancer Society guidelines for the early detection of colorectal cancer include the following:

- yearly fecal occult blood test or fecal immuno-chemical test

- flexible sigmoidoscopy every 5 years
- yearly fecal occult blood test or fecal immunochemical test, plus flexible sigmoidoscopy every 5 years
- double-contrast barium enema every 5 years
- colonoscopy every 10 years

Patients with positive test results should be followed up with colonoscopy.

STAGING

Generations of medical students have been confused by the various staging systems used for classifying colon cancer. Although the Dukes classification system devised in 1932 was simple and uncomplicated, it was eventually found to be inferior with respect to prognostication than the subsequently developed Astler-Coller system. Since 1991, the American Society of Colon and Rectal Surgeons have endorsed the TNM staging system, which has become the standard for modern cancer staging (Fig. 5-7).

The TNM (tumor, nodes, metastases) classification system is as follows:

Tis: Carcinoma in-situ
T1: Tumor invades submucosa.
T2: Tumor invades muscularis propria.
T3: Tumor invades through the muscularis propria into the subserosa or into the pericolic or perirectal tissue.
T4: Tumor directly invades other organs or structures and/or perforates the visceral peritoneum.
N0: No regional lymph node metastasis.
N1: Metastasis in one to three regional lymph nodes.
N2: Metastasis in four or more regional lymph nodes.
M0: No distant metastasis or residual tumor.
M1: Distant metastasis present.

Staging is based on a combined evaluation of characteristics involving the tumor, lymph nodes, and presence of metastasis.

HISTORY

The clinical presentation of colon cancer is often dependent on the location of the lesion. Small proximal ascending colonic neoplasms are often asymptomatic. Occult blood in the stool and weight loss from metastatic disease may be the only signs. As the size of a lesion increases, right colon cancers usually cause bleeding that is more significant, whereas lesions in the left colon typically present with obstructive symptoms, including a change in stool caliber, tenesmus, or constipation. In general, this is due to fecal matter entering the right colon in liquid form and easily transiting a large cecal lesion, whereas desiccated stool in the left colon tends to obstruct when confronted with malignant luminal narrowing.

Rectal bleeding from a low rectal cancer should never be mistakenly explained away as symptomatic hemorrhoids. Simple digital rectal examination will demonstrate the tumor and prevent delay in diagnosis. Rectal cancer also can present with passage of mucus per rectum, arising from tumor surface secretions.

Complete acute large bowel obstruction may also occur. Any older adult patient who lacks a history of prior abdominal surgery or recent colonoscopy who presents with a large bowel obstruction must be considered to have obstructing colon cancer until proven otherwise. Any sizable lesion may produce abdominal pain. Perforation typically causes frank peritonitis. Constitutional symptoms, including weight loss, anorexia, and fatigue, are common with metastatic disease.

PHYSICAL EXAMINATION

Rectal examination may reveal occult or gross blood, and for low rectal cancers, the lesion can be directly palpated. For large bulky tumors, a mass may be noted on abdominal examination. Stigmata of hereditary disorders, including familial polyposis syndrome or Gardner syndrome, may be present.

DIAGNOSTIC EVALUATION

Laboratory evaluation should include a hematocrit, which often reveals microcytic anemia from chronic occult blood loss. The liver is the most common site

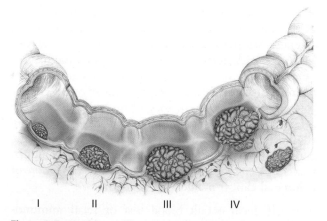

| I | II | III | IV |

Figure 5-7 • Understanding cancer: the stages of cancer (I-IV).

for metastases, and liver function tests may be abnormal. Carcinoembryonic antigen may also be obtained; although it is not a useful screening test, it is valuable as a marker for recurrent cancer.

Colonoscopy has the advantage of examining the entire colon while also performing confirmatory biopsy for tissue diagnosis. Flexible sigmoidoscopy reaches up to 70 cm of the most distal large intestine, whereas colonoscopy can examine the entire colon and even intubate the distal ileum. Approximately 70% of lesions should be detected by flexible sigmoidoscopy. Rigid sigmoidoscopy is only useful for examining the lower 25 cm and is therefore often used to evaluate rectal cancers.

Radiologic evaluation can be performed with double-contrast barium enema, which uses both a radio-opaque contrast medium (barium) to coat the colon wall and air to provide luminal distention. The classic finding on barium enema is a constricting filling defect, known as an apple core lesion (Fig. 5-8). CT is useful for evaluating extent of disease and the presence of metastases, particularly in the liver.

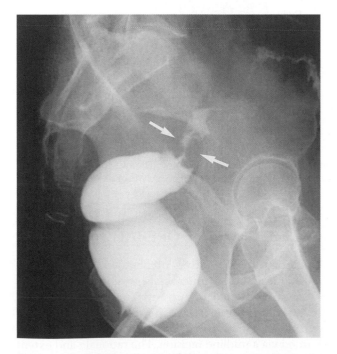

Figure 5-8 • Adenocarcinoma of the colon presenting as an "apple core" lesion. Image from a barium enema study demonstrates a circumferential mass (arrows). This mass has disrupted the normal mucosal pattern and has irregular overhanging edges.
From Kelsen DP, Daly JM, Kern SE, et al. *Gastrointestinal Oncology: Principles and Practice*. Philadelphia: Lippincott Williams & Wilkins, 2002.

Magnetic resonance imaging may be better for evaluating liver metastases but usually does not add more overall information than that which is obtained with CT.

Positron-emission tomography scan is useful for showing metastatic disease or else late recurrence in a patient who previously underwent resection and who has an increasing carcinoembryonic antigen level. For rectal lesions, endorectal ultrasound is the standard of care for assessing the depth of tumor invasion and the presence of lymph node metastases.

TREATMENT

Surgical therapy of colon cancer is based on complete removal of the malignant lesion and associated lymph nodes. The oncologic principles underlying segmental colon resection for malignancy are based on the blood supply of the segment of colon containing the lesion, as well as the distribution of the parallel draining lymph node network. For cancers of the cecum and ascending colon, right hemicolectomy is indicated. Tumors of the transverse colon require transverse colectomy, with removal of the hepatic and splenic flexures. Descending colon tumors require left colectomy, and sigmoid tumors are treated with sigmoidectomy. Most rectal tumors are treated with low anterior resection, whereas the very low rectal cancers near the anus occasionally require abdominoperineal resection, which entails resection of the anus with closure of the perianal skin and creation of a permanent end colostomy, because anastomosis may not be technically feasible. Examples of the extent of resection for different types of colectomy are shown in Figure 5-9.

Historically, open surgery has been the standard approach for colon resection; however, the laparoscopic technique has gained rapid acceptance, given the reduced morbidity compared with open surgery, in addition to studies showing the less invasive approach to be equally effective as open surgery in terms of survival. The widely quoted randomized trial results by the Clinical Outcomes of Surgical Therapy (COST) Study Group, published in 2004, showed no difference in either recurrence or 3-year survival between laparoscopic or open groups. These findings were subsequently supported by other randomized trials, such as the Conventional Versus Laparoscopic-Assisted Surgery in Colorectal Cancer (CLASSIC) trial from the United Kingdom, published in 2007. In summary, despite the development of new surgical techniques, the basic oncologic

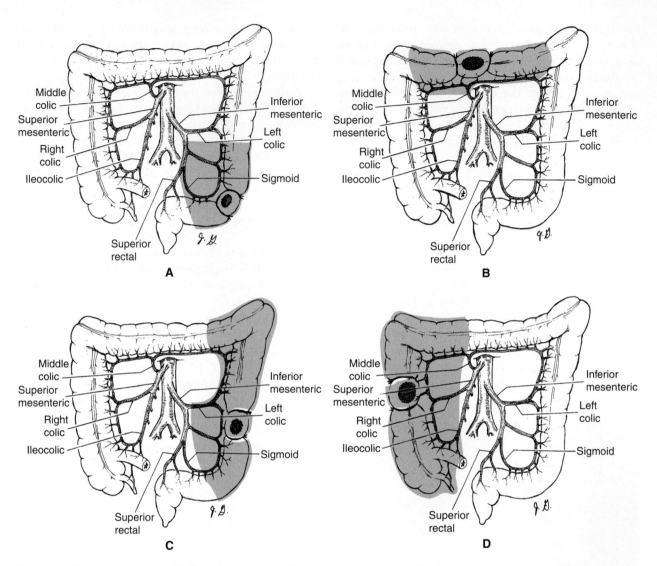

Figure 5-9 • Types of colectomy. **(A)** Sigmoid colectomy; **(B)** transverse colectomy; **(C)** left colectomy; **(D)** right colectomy.
Adapted from Kelsen DP, Daly JM, Kern SE, et al. *Gastrointestinal Oncology: Principles and Practice*. Philadelphia: Lippincott Williams & Wilkins, 2002.

goals and extent of resection should be identical, regardless of the approach.

With respect to the extent of resection, guidelines from the American Joint Committee on Cancer, the American College of Pathology, and the National Comprehensive Cancer Network recommend 12 or more lymph nodes to be sampled during surgery. Thorough sampling and examination of the draining lymph nodes is thought to improve staging accuracy, which allows more appropriate adjuvant chemotherapy administration. By upstaging patients, some investigators believe patients will therefore be offered more aggressive treatment that will likely result in improved overall survival.

COLECTOMY: THE OPERATION

Traditional preoperative preparation has included mechanical and antimicrobial bowel cleansing; however, this practice is currently undergoing critical review (see Preoperative Issues in Chapter 1 for expanded discussion). Most open resections are performed via a midline incision. The rationale and extent of excision for various tumors is described above and in Figure 5-9.

Mobilization of the right or left colon involves incising the white line of Toldt on the respective side. Care is taken to avoid the ureter, which can be injured as the colon is mobilized. Consideration of a ureteral stent should be made if the tumor is bulky and there is concern about identifying the ureter intraoperatively. The transverse colon is intraperitoneal and does not require mobilization. Once adequate length of colon has been mobilized, the peritoneum overlying the mesentery is incised to its root, and all the mesenteric vessels in the specimen are ligated. In the open technique, noncrushing clamps are usually placed alongside the resection margin to reduce spillage, and the ends of the bowel are usually stapled and the specimen removed. Reconstruction of bowel continuity is performed with either hand-sewn or stapled anastomosis. For low colon or rectal anastomosis, use of an end-to-end anastomosis stapler placed through the anus is a preferred technique.

ANGIODYSPLASIA

Angiodysplasia is being recognized with increasing frequency as a significant source of lower gastrointestinal hemorrhage. These anomalous vascular lesions are histologically similar to telangiectasia and arise most commonly in the cecum and right colon.

EPIDEMIOLOGY

Angiodysplasia is one of the most common causes of lower gastrointestinal bleeding. The prevalence increases with age, to an incidence of approximately one fourth of the older adult population. Age and resulting bowel wall strain are thought to cause vascular tissue proliferation, leading to angiodysplastic lesions.

HISTORY

Patients usually present with multiple episodes of low-grade bleeding. In 10% of cases, patients present with massive bleeding.

DIAGNOSTIC EVALUATION

Diagnosis can be made with arteriography, nuclear scans, or endoscopy.

TREATMENT

Endoscopic treatment includes electrocautery and argon plasma coagulation. Angiography with highly selective embolization or vasopressin infusion is often effective. Because many angiodysplastic lesions rebleed, definitive treatment may occasionally require segmental colectomy.

VOLVULUS

Volvulus occurs when a portion of the colon rotates on the axis of its mesentery, compromising blood flow and creating a closed-loop obstruction (Fig. 5-10). The sigmoid colon (75%) and cecum (25%) are most commonly involved. The relative redundancy of the sigmoid loop causes torsion around the mesenteric axis, whereas poor fixation of the cecum in the right iliac fossa leads to either axial torsion (cecal volvulus) or anteromedial folding (cecal bascule).

EPIDEMIOLOGY

The incidence of volvulus is approximately two in 100,000. Risk factors include age, chronic constipation, previous abdominal surgery, and neuropsychiatric disorders.

HISTORY

The patient usually relates the acute onset of crampy abdominal pain and distention.

PHYSICAL EXAMINATION

The abdomen is tender and distended, and peritoneal signs of rebound and involuntary guarding may be present. Frank peritonitis and shock may follow.

DIAGNOSTIC EVALUATION

Abdominal radiographs may reveal a massively distended colon with a "corkscrew" or "bird's beak" at

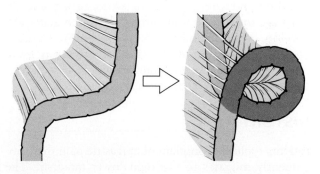

Figure 5-10 • Volvulus.

the point of torsion. The distended colonic loop has the appearance of a bent tire or large coffee bean.

TREATMENT

Sigmoid volvulus may be reduced by enemas or endoscopy. Rectal tubes are sometimes used to prevent acute recurrence and aid decompression. Because of the high rate of recurrence, operative repair after resolution of the initial episode is recommended. In the acute setting and depending on the operative findings, fixation of the untwisted loop to the respective fossa may suffice for cases of viable bowel; otherwise, resection is performed with either primary anastomosis or end colostomy (Hartmann procedure) in cases of sepsis and gangrene. Treatment of cecal volvulus is usually operative at the outset, because nonoperative intervention is rarely successful, and the incidence of gangrenous ischemic changes is high.

APPENDICITIS

Appendicitis is the most common reason for urgent abdominal operation. The causes of appendiceal inflammation and infection are related to processes that obstruct the appendiceal lumen, thereby causing distal swelling, decreased venous outflow, and ischemia. The most common extraluminal cause of obstruction is the swelling of submucosal lymphoid tissue in the wall of the appendix in response to a viral infection. This is illustrated by the incidence of viral syndromes often seen in pediatric patients shortly before developing appendicitis. The most common intraluminal cause of obstruction is from a fecalith (small, firm ball of stool). Cases of obstruction with fecaliths have a higher incidence of perforation.

EPIDEMIOLOGY

Children and young adults between ages 5 and 35 years are most commonly affected. Appendicitis will develop in approximately 5% of people over their lifetime. Perforation at the time of surgery is more often seen in very young children and in older adults as a result of delayed diagnosis.

HISTORY

Patients typically complain of epigastric pain that subsequently migrates to the right lower quadrant. The initial discomfort is thought to be due to obstruction

and swelling of the appendix and the latter due to peritoneal irritation. Retrocecal appendicitis may cause pain higher in the right abdomen, whereas appendicitis located in the pelvis may cause vague pelvic discomfort. Anorexia is an almost universal complaint. Nausea and emesis may occur after the onset of pain. Up to 20% of patients report experiencing diarrhea, which often leads the examiner to make an incorrect diagnosis of gastroenteritis. Generalized abdominal pain may signify rupture and diffuse peritonitis.

PHYSICAL EXAMINATION

Low-grade fever is typical. Nearly all patients have right lower quadrant tenderness, classically located at McBurney's point, two thirds the distance from the umbilicus to anterior superior iliac spine. Rebound and guarding develop as the disease progresses and the peritoneum becomes inflamed. Signs of peritoneal irritation include the obturator sign (pain on external rotation of the flexed thigh) and the psoas sign (pain on right thigh extension). Rovsing's sign is eliciting pain in the right lower quadrant on palpation of the left lower quadrant. In cases of contained perforation, the omentum walls off the infectious process, occasionally resulting in a palpable mass in thin patients. If the perforation is free and not contained, then diffuse peritonitis and septic shock may develop. Rectal examination may reveal tenderness if the appendix hangs low in the pelvis.

DIAGNOSTIC EVALUATION

The white blood cell count is usually mildly to moderately elevated. Urinalysis should be performed to rule out a urinary tract infection.

Depending on a patient's age, presenting history and physical examination, and available resources, radiologic studies may include ultrasound or CT scanning. Plain abdominal x-rays (supine and upright) usually provide no useful information in confirming the diagnosis of appendicitis. Ultrasonographic evidence of appendicitis includes appendiceal wall thickening, luminal distention, and lack of compressibility. Ultrasound is also useful in female patients for demonstrating ovarian or other gynecologic pathology. CT scanning may show appendiceal enlargement, periappendiceal inflammatory changes, free fluid, or right lower quadrant abscess (Fig. 5-11).

CT scanning is also useful for ruling in or out alternative diagnoses, thereby reducing the negative appendectomy rate in many hospitals.

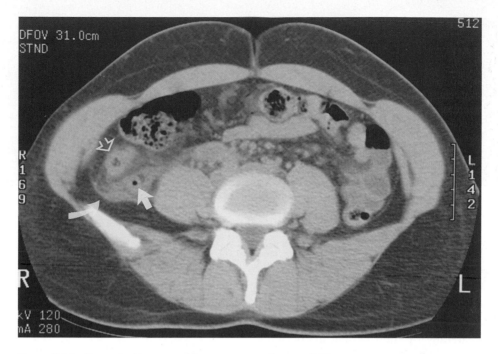

Figure 5-11 • Computed tomographic appearance of appendicitis.
From Harwood-Nuss A, Wolfson AB, Linden CH, et al. *The Clinical Practice of Emergency Medicine.* 3rd ed. Philadelphia: Lippincott Williams & Wilkins, 2001.

TREATMENT

Uncomplicated appendicitis requires appendectomy. Both open and laparoscopic techniques are appropriate. Laparoscopic appendectomy is associated with less postoperative pain, a shorter hospital course, better cosmesis, and faster return to work. Selected advanced cases with appendiceal abscess may initially be managed nonoperatively with antibiotics and percutaneous CT-guided abscess drainage. Once the infection has abated and the inflammatory process resolved, interval appendectomy may be performed at a later date.

KEY POINTS

- Surgery for ulcerative colitis is indicated for intractable bleeding, obstruction, failure of medical therapy, toxic megacolon, and risk of cancer.
- Diverticulosis is the most common cause of lower gastrointestinal bleeding. Prevalence of diverticula increases with age. Cause is related to low-fiber dietary intake.
- Elective surgical therapy for diverticulitis is indicated for repeated attacks because of the high recurrence and complication rate. Emergent surgical therapy is indicated for free perforation and usually requires segmental colon resection and end colostomy (Hartmann procedure).
- Colon cancer follows a progression from adenoma to carcinoma. Adenomatous polyps are considered premalignant and must be removed entirely. Screening for colon cancer should begin at age 50 for normal-risk patients.
- Surgical therapy for colon cancer is predicated on removal of the malignant lesion and the draining lymph nodes. Both open and laparoscopic techniques are accepted surgical therapies for resection.
- Angiodysplasia is common in older adult patients and is one of the most common causes of lower gastrointestinal bleeding.
- Volvulus is a life-threatening condition that presents with abdominal pain and distention.
- Appendicitis is the most common reason for urgent abdominal operation. Right lower quadrant abdominal pain, fever, and leukocytosis are hallmarks of the disease. Appendectomy can be performed with either open or laparoscopic techniques.

6 Liver

ANATOMY AND PHYSIOLOGY

The liver is located in the right upper quadrant of the abdomen and is bounded superiorly and posteriorly by the diaphragm, laterally by the ribs, and inferiorly by the gallbladder, stomach, duodenum, colon, kidney, and right adrenal. It is covered by Glisson capsule and peritoneum. The right and left lobes of the liver are defined by the plane formed by the gallbladder fossa and the inferior vena cava. The falciform ligament between the liver and diaphragm is a landmark between the lateral and medial segments of the left lobe. The coronary ligaments continue laterally from the falciform and end at the right and left triangular ligaments. These ligaments define the bare area of the liver, an area devoid of peritoneum. The liver parenchyma is divided into eight segments on the basis of arterial and venous anatomy (see Color Plate 5). Segment 1 is also known as the caudate lobe. It is not visible from the ventral surface of the liver, being tucked behind segment 4. The caudate is juxtaposed to the inferior vena cava and has venous branches that drain directly into the cava. These branches are quite fragile and must be carefully controlled if resection of the caudate is required. Segments 2, 3, and 4 form the left lobe of the liver, whereas segments 5, 6, 7, and 8 comprise the right lobe. Segment 4 may be divided into cranial segment 4a and caudal segment 4b.

The hepatic circulation is based on a portal circulation that provides the liver with first access to all intestinal venous flow. Seventy-five percent of total hepatic blood flow is derived from the portal vein, which is formed from the confluence of the splenic and superior mesenteric veins. The remaining blood supply comes from the hepatic artery via the celiac axis. The right hepatic artery arises from the superior mesenteric artery in 15% of patients. When this occurs, the artery will run posterior to the bile duct on the right side of the hilum, and it is termed a replaced right hepatic artery. The left hepatic artery arises from the left gastric in 15% of patients, called a replaced left hepatic artery. In this instance, the artery will run in the cranial portion of the gastrohepatic ligament. Other arterial variants include a completely replaced hepatic artery, which arises from the superior mesenteric artery, and a middle hepatic artery, which occurs when the segment 4 branch arises in the hilum. Blood leaving the liver enters the inferior vena cava via the right, middle, and left hepatic veins. Often there is an accessory right hepatic vein that leaves the liver caudad to the principle right hepatic vein. This vein must be controlled separately during right hepatic lobectomy.

The hepatic hilum can be palpated by placing a finger through the foramen of Winslow (epiploic foramen) into the lesser sac (Fig. 6-1). This is an important maneuver because it provides control of the hepatic hilum (hepatoduodenal ligament), within which runs the hepatic artery, portal vein, and bile duct. A Pringle maneuver, which involves placing a clamp on the hilum, disrupts most blood flow to the liver and can greatly reduce bleeding during liver resection (Fig. 6-2). This maneuver also makes the liver ischemic and can cause arterial thrombosis. As a result, it should be used for a limited amount of time and only when necessary.

The liver is the site of many critical events in energy metabolism and protein synthesis. Glucose is taken up and stored as glycogen, and glycogen is broken down, as necessary, to maintain a relatively constant level of serum glucose. The liver is able to initiate gluconeogenesis during stress, and the liver can oxidize fatty acids to

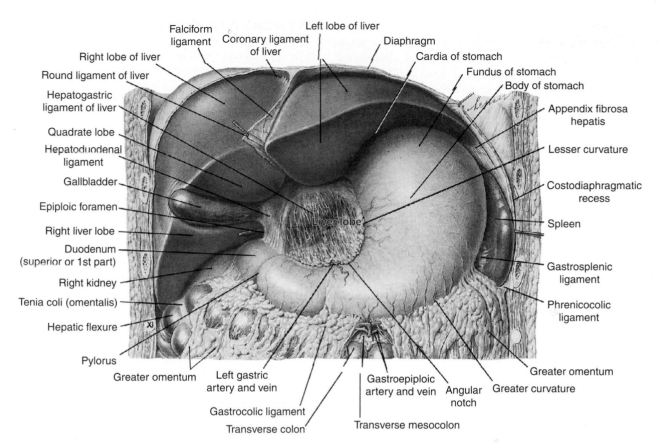

Figure 6-1 • The lesser sac. The lesser sac is behind the hepatoduodenal and hepatogastric ligaments. Entry is through the epiploic foramen (foramen of Winslow).
From Sadler T. *Langman's Medical Embryology, Ninth Edition Image Bank.* Baltimore: Lippincott Williams & Wilkins, 2003.

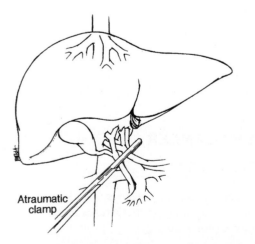

Figure 6-2 • Pringle maneuver. Occlusion of the porta hepatis decreases blood flow to the liver to slow bleeding during liver surgery.
From Blackbourne LH. *Advanced Surgical Recall.* 2nd ed. Baltimore: Lippincott Williams & Wilkins, 2004.

ketones, which the brain can use as an energy source. Proteins synthesized in the liver include the coagulation factors fibrinogen, prothrombin, prekallikrein, high-molecular-weight kininogen, and factors V, VII, VIII, IX, X, XI, and XII. Of these, prothrombin and factors VII, IX, and X are dependent on vitamin K. The anticoagulant warfarin (Coumadin) affects these vitamin K–dependent pathways, resulting in an increased prothrombin time. Albumin and alpha globulin are produced solely in the liver.

The digestive functions of the liver include bile synthesis and cholesterol metabolism. Heme is used to form bilirubin, which is excreted in the bile after conjugation with glycine or taurine. Bile emulsifies fats to aid their digestion and plays a role in vitamin uptake. Bile salts excreted into the intestine are reabsorbed into the portal circulation. This cycle of bile excretion and absorption is termed the enterohepatic circulation. Total body bile circulates approximately

10 times per day in this loop. More than 95% of excreted bile is reabsorbed, and the remainder must be resynthesized. The rate-limiting step of cholesterol synthesis involving the enzyme 3-hydroxy-3-methyl-glutaryl–coenzyme A reductase occurs in the liver, as does cholesterol metabolism to bile salts.

Detoxification occurs in the liver through two pathways. Phase I reactions involve cytochrome P450 and include oxidation, reduction, and hydrolysis. Phase II reactions consist of conjugation. These reactions are critical to destruction or renal clearance of toxins. The dosing of all oral drugs is determined only after considering the first-pass effect of the drug through the liver. The initial hydroxylation of vitamin D occurs in the liver. Immunologic functions are mediated by Kupffer cells, the resident liver macrophages.

BENIGN LIVER TUMORS

PATHOLOGY

Benign liver tumors include hepatocellular adenoma (see Color Plate 6), focal nodular hyperplasia, hemangioma, and lipoma. Hemangiomas are categorized into capillary and cavernous types, the former being of no clinical consequence and the latter capable of attaining large size and rupturing.

EPIDEMIOLOGY

Only 5% of liver tumors are benign, with hemangioma being the most common. Approximately 7% of people have a cavernous hemangioma at autopsy. The incidence of adenoma is one per million in women without a history of oral contraceptive use. These medicines increase the risk by a factor of 40. This lesion most commonly occurs in women between 30 and 50 years of age. Adenoma and focal nodular hyperplasia are five times more common in female patients.

HISTORY

Patients with adenomas and hemangiomas can be asymptomatic or present with dull pain; rupture can produce sudden onset of severe abdominal pain. These lesions can also become large enough to cause jaundice or symptoms of gastric outlet obstruction, including nausea and vomiting. Focal nodular hyperplasia is rarely symptomatic.

PHYSICAL EXAMINATION

Large lesions can be palpated. Jaundice may occur in patients if the tumor causes bile duct obstruction.

DIAGNOSTIC EVALUATION

These lesions are most often found incidentally at laparotomy or on imaging studies requested for other reasons. Laboratory evaluation is often unremarkable, although hemorrhage in an adenoma can lead to hepatocellular necrosis and a subsequent increase in transaminase levels. Hemangioma can cause a consumptive coagulopathy. Ultrasound differentiates cystic from solid lesions. Triple-phase computed tomography (CT) is the best study for distinguishing between various types of benign and malignant lesions, but in certain cases, this determination is not possible. Adenomas are typically low-density lesions; focal nodular hyperplasias may appear with a filling defect or central scar, whereas hemangiomas have early peripheral enhancement after contrast administration. Hemangiomas should not be biopsied because of the risk of bleeding.

TREATMENT

Patients with adenoma who are using oral contraceptives should stop. If the lesion does not regress, resection should be considered in otherwise healthy individuals because of the risk of malignant degeneration or hemorrhage. Relative contraindications to resection include a tumor that is technically difficult to resect or tumors of large size in which a large portion of the liver would need to be removed. Symptomatic hemangiomas should be resected, if possible. Because focal nodular hyperplasia is not malignant and rarely causes symptoms, it should not be resected unless it is found incidentally at laparotomy and is small and peripheral enough to be wedged out easily.

LIVER CANCER

PATHOLOGY

Liver cancers are hepatomas, also known as hepatocellular carcinoma, or metastases from other primaries (see Color Plate 7).

EPIDEMIOLOGY

Ninety-five percent of liver tumors are malignant. Hepatoma is one of the most common malignancies in the world, but rates in the United States are relatively low (approximately two per 100,000). It is more common in male than in female patients.

ETIOLOGY

Cirrhosis is a predisposing factor to hepatoma; as such, hepatitis B, the leading cause of cirrhosis, and alcoholism are associated with hepatoma development. Fungal-derived aflatoxins have been implicated as causes of hepatoma, as have hemochromatosis, smoking, vinyl chloride, and oral contraceptives.

HISTORY

Patients with hepatoma may complain of weight loss, right upper quadrant or shoulder pain, and weakness. Hepatic metastases are often indistinguishable from primary hepatocellular carcinoma.

PHYSICAL EXAMINATION

Hepatomegaly may be appreciable, and signs of portal hypertension, including splenomegaly and ascites, may be present. Jaundice occurs in approximately half of patients.

DIAGNOSTIC EVALUATION

Laboratory examination may reveal abnormal liver function tests. α-Fetoprotein is a specific marker for hepatoma but can also be elevated in embryonic tumors. Radiographic studies are used to differentiate benign and malignant lesions. Ultrasonography can distinguish cystic from solid lesions, whereas CT or magnetic resonance imaging can reveal multiple lesions and clarify anatomic relationships (Fig. 6-3). They can also demonstrate nodularity of the liver, hypersplenism, and portal hypertension, indicative of underlying liver disease. Hepatic arteriography can diagnose a hemangioma. Because most cancers occur in the setting of liver disease and cirrhosis, it is important to perform viral studies for hepatitis.

TREATMENT

Before consideration of resection, the underlying health of the liver should be assessed using the Child-Turcotte-Pugh scoring system (Table 6-1). Patients with Child class C disease will generally not tolerate a resection; patients with Child class B disease may tolerate a limited resection.

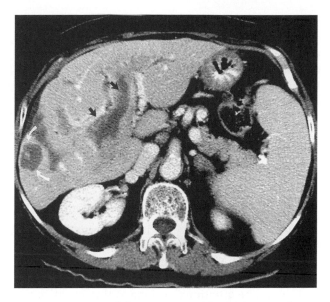

Figure 6-3 • Hepatocellular carcinoma with portal venous thrombosis. Computed tomography image demonstrates portal vein thrombus (black arrows on thrombosed right and left portal veins). A mass (curved white arrows) is present in the right lobe of the liver.
From Kelsen DP, Daly JM, Kern SE, et al. *Gastrointestinal Oncology: Principles and Practice.* Philadelphia, PA: Lippincott Williams & Wilkins; 2002:10–16.

If the patient is a surgical candidate, treatment involves resection of the tumor. Survival without treatment averages 3 months; resection can extend survival to 3 years, with a 5-year survival rate of 11% to 46%.

■ **TABLE 6-1** Child-Turcotte-Pugh Scoring System for Cirrhosis

Clinical Variable	1 Point	2 Points	3 Points
Encephalopathy	None	Stage 1–2	Stage 3–4
Ascites	Absent	Slight	Moderate
Bilirubin (mg/dL)	<2	2–3	>3
Bilirubin in PBC or PSC (mg/dL)	<4	4–10	10
Albumin (g/dL)	>3.5	2.8–3.5	<2.8
Prothrombin time (seconds prolonged or INR)	<4 sec or INR <1.7	4–6 sec or INR 1.7–2.3	>6 sec or INR >2.3

Child class A = 5–6 points; Child class B = 7–9 points; Child class C = 10–15 points.
PBC, primary biliary cirrhosis; PSC, primary sclerosing cholangitis; INR, international normalized ratio.

The decision to resect the tumor depends on comorbid disease and the location and size of the tumor. When possible, wedge resection should be performed, because formal hepatic lobectomy does not provide any additional survival benefit. Patients with small tumors who are not candidates for resection because of tumor location or concomitant cirrhosis should be considered for liver transplantation. Liver transplantation is becoming an increasingly attractive option for these patients, providing good long-term survival. Patients who meet the Milan criteria (tumor <5 cm or no more than three tumors, the largest of which is <3 cm) will receive extra points on the liver transplant list.

Metastatic disease occurs in decreasing frequency from lung, colon, pancreas, breast, and stomach. When colon cancer metastasizes to the liver, resection of up to three lesions has been shown to improve survival and should be attempted as long as the operative risk is not prohibitive. In general, liver metastases from other tumors should not be resected.

LIVER ABSCESSES

ETIOLOGY

Liver abscesses are most frequently due to bacteria, amebas, or the tapeworm *Echinococcus*. Bacterial abscesses usually arise from an intra-abdominal infection in the appendix, gallbladder, or intestine but may be due to trauma or a complication of a surgical procedure. Causative organisms are principally gut flora, including *Escherichia coli*, *Klebsiella*, enterococci, and anaerobes (including *Bacteroides*). Amebic abscesses owing to *Entamoeba histolytica* are an infrequent complication of gastrointestinal amebiasis.

EPIDEMIOLOGY

Pyogenic abscesses are responsible for fewer than one in 500 adult hospital admissions. Amebic abscesses occur in 3% to 25% of patients with gastrointestinal amebiasis (Fig. 6-4). Risk factors include HIV, alcohol abuse, and foreign travel. *Echinococcus* is most commonly seen in Eastern Europe, Greece, South Africa, South America, and Australia; although rare in the United States, it is the most common cause of liver abscesses worldwide (Fig. 6-5).

HISTORY

Patients with pyogenic or amebic abscesses usually have nonspecific complaints of vague abdominal pain,

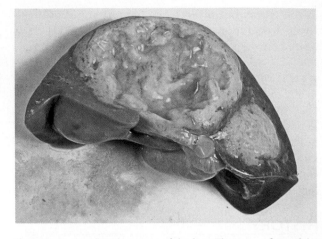

Figure 6-4 • Amebic abscesses of the liver. The cut surface of the liver shows multiple abscesses containing "anchovy paste" material.
From Rubin E, Farber JL. *Pathology*. 3rd ed. Philadelphia, PA: Lippincott Williams & Wilkins; 1999:9–75.

weight loss, malaise, anorexia, and fever. Travel to an endemic region may suggest *Echinococcus*.

PHYSICAL EXAMINATION

The liver may be tender or enlarged, and jaundice may occur. Rupture of an abscess can lead to peritonitis, sepsis, and circulatory collapse.

DIAGNOSTIC EVALUATION

The white blood cell count and transaminase levels are elevated. Antibodies to ameba are found in 98% of patients with amebic abscesses but in fewer than 5% of those with pyogenic abscesses. Echinococcal infection

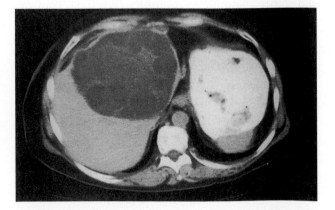

Figure 6-5 • A computed tomography scan shows a multilocular cyst in the liver of a patient with hydatid disease.
From Sun, Tsieh MD. *Parasitic Disorders: Pathology, Diagnosis, and Management*. 2nd ed. Baltimore: Lippincott Williams & Wilkins, 1999.

produces eosinophilia and a positive heme agglutination test. Ultrasonography is approximately 90% sensitive for demonstrating a lesion; CT is slightly better. The presence of multiple cysts, or "sand," on CT is suggestive of *Echinococcus*. Sampling of the cyst contents with CT or ultrasound guidance reveals the causative organism in the case of pyogenic abscesses but does not usually lead to a diagnosis in amebic abscesses. Aspiration of echinococcal cysts is contraindicated because of the risk of contaminating the peritoneal cavity.

TREATMENT

Pyogenic abscesses require antibiotics alone or in combination with percutaneous or open drainage. Amebic abscesses are treated with metronidazole (Flagyl), with or without chloroquine, and surgical drainage is reserved for complications, including rupture. Echinococcal abscesses require an open procedure. Scolecoidal agents (e.g., ethanol or 20% sodium chloride) are instilled directly into the cyst, followed by drainage, with care not to spill the organisms into the peritoneum.

PORTAL HYPERTENSION

ETIOLOGY

Portal hypertension is caused by processes that impede hepatic blood flow, either at the presinusoidal, sinusoidal, or postsinusoidal levels. Presinusoidal causes include schistosomiasis and portal vein thrombosis. The principal sinusoidal cause in the United States is cirrhosis, usually caused by alcohol but also by hepatitis B and C. Cirrhosis develops in approximately 15% of alcoholics. Postsinusoidal causes of portal hypertension include Budd-Chiari syndrome (hepatic vein occlusion), pericarditis, and right-sided heart failure.

COMPLICATIONS

Bleeding varices are a life-threatening complication of portal hypertension. When portal pressures increase, flow through the hemorrhoidal, umbilical, or coronary veins becomes the low-resistance route for blood flow. The coronary vein empties into the plexus of veins draining the stomach and esophagus (Fig. 6-6). Engorgement of these veins places the patient at risk of bleeding into the esophagus or stomach.

HISTORY

Alcoholism, hepatitis, or previous variceal hemorrhage are common.

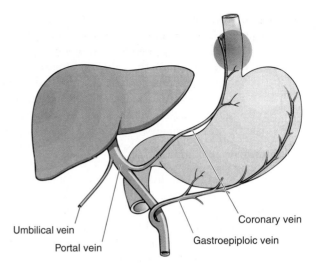

Figure 6-6 • Selected collateral circulation in portal hypertension.

PHYSICAL EXAMINATION

A variety of physical findings, including ascites, jaundice, "cherubic face," spider angioma, testicular atrophy, gynecomastia, and palmar erythema, may suggest the diagnosis.

DIAGNOSTIC EVALUATION

Laboratory examination may reveal increased liver enzymes, which may return to normal with advanced cirrhosis as the amount of functioning hepatic parenchyma decreases. Tests of liver synthetic function, including clotting times and serum albumin, may be abnormal.

TREATMENT

Patients with portal hypertension are placed on beta-blockers to decrease the risk of bleeding. Endoscopic surveillance and banding are useful in preventing bleeding episodes.

For patients with upper gastrointestinal bleeds, large-bore intravenous lines and volume resuscitation should be started immediately. A nasogastric tube should be placed to confirm the diagnosis. If the patient cannot be lavaged clear, suggesting active bleeding, emergency endoscopy is both diagnostic and therapeutic. Endoscopy is >90% effective in controlling acute bleeding from esophageal varices. Should this fail, balloon tamponade with a Sengstaken-Blakemore tube and vasopressin infusion should be considered. Use of the Sengstaken-Blakemore tube involves passing the gastric balloon into the stomach, exerting gentle traction on the tube, and then inflating the esophageal balloon to tamponade bleeding. Although effective in stopping life-threatening hemorrhage, the tube can produce gastric and esophageal ischemia and must be used with extreme caution. Transjugular intrahepatic portosystemic shunting has a high rate of success in controlling acute bleeding and is usually preferred to an emergent surgical shunt, although this is also an option (Fig. 6-7).

Approximately 40% of patients with varices will develop a bleeding complication. Seventy percent of patients with a first episode will rebleed. For this reason, a definitive procedure should be considered after the initial episode is controlled.

Patients with bleeding varices and cirrhosis will ordinarily be considered for liver transplantation. If there is no cirrhosis, or if the patient has good residual liver function,

surgical shunts have better long-term patency than transjugular intrahepatic portosystemic shunting. Surgical shunts are divided into nonselective and selective shunts. Nonselective shunts divert the entire portal blood flow into the systemic circulation. An example is an end-to-side portacaval shunt, in which the portal vein is divided and drained directly into the inferior vena cava. Selective shunts divert only a portion of the portal blood away from the liver. The most common is the distal splenorenal shunt, in which portal blood is shunted through the renal vein and into the cava. Because there is still blood going to the liver to be detoxified, patients with selective shunts have less encephalopathy and equivalent success in preventing rebleeding.

As a last resort in patients with bleeding esophageal varices, a Sugiura procedure can be performed. During this procedure, the varices are disconnected from the portal circulation by complete esophageal transection and reanastomosis. This procedure also includes splenectomy, proximal gastric devascularization, vagotomy, and pyloroplasty.

In patients with Budd-Chiari syndrome, side-to-side portacaval shunt can be life-saving.

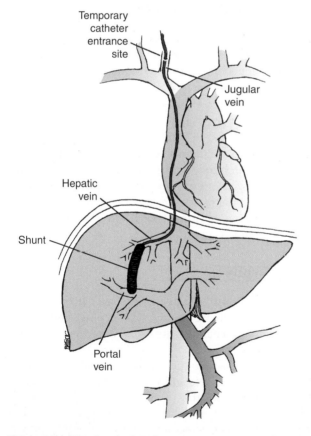

Figure 6-7 • Transjugular intrahepatic portosystemic shunting. A metallic shunt is placed from the hepatic vein to the right portal vein via a catheter introduced through the internal jugular vein. The shunt will typically continue into the main portal vein.
From Blackbourne LH. *Advanced Surgical Recall.* 2nd ed. Baltimore, MD: Lippincott Williams & Wilkins; 2004.

KEY POINTS

- The liver performs an array of functions involving energy metabolism, protein synthesis, digestion, and detoxification.

- Only 5% of liver tumors are benign.

- Hepatocellular carcinoma is extremely common worldwide but is relatively rare in the United States.

- Causes of hepatocellular carcinoma include cirrhosis, aflatoxin, smoking, and vinyl chloride.

- The prognosis for hepatocellular carcinoma is poor.

- Liver abscesses are most commonly caused by bacteria, amebas, or *Echinococcus*.

- Portal hypertension has presinusoidal, sinusoidal, and postsinusoidal causes.

- Variceal hemorrhage is life-threatening, but endoscopy is usually successful in controlling bleeding.

- Because of the high recurrence rate, a definitive procedure should be considered after the first episode of variceal bleeding.

- Surgical shunts may have better long-term patency than transjugular intrahepatic portosystemic shunting and should be considered in patients with preserved liver function.

Gallbladder

ANATOMY AND PHYSIOLOGY

The gallbladder is located in the right upper quadrant of the abdomen beneath the liver. The cystic duct exits at the neck of the gallbladder and joins the common hepatic duct to form the common bile duct, which empties into the duodenum at the ampulla of Vater. This is surrounded by the sphincter of Oddi, which regulates bile flow into the duodenum (Fig. 7-1).

Bile produced in the liver is stored in the gallbladder. Bile is important for the absorption of fat-soluble vitamins (A, D, E, and K). Cholecystokinin stimulates gallbladder contraction and release of bile into the duodenum. The spiral valves of Heister in the cystic duct prevent bile reflux into the gallbladder. Arterial supply is from the cystic artery, which most commonly arises from the right hepatic artery and courses through the triangle of Calot, which is bounded by the cystic duct laterally, the common hepatic duct medially, and the edge of the liver superiorly (Fig. 7-2).

GALLSTONE DISEASE

Cholelithiasis is the presence of gallstones within the gallbladder. Choledocholithiasis refers to stones in the common bile duct (Fig. 7-3). Biliary colic is pain produced when the gallbladder contracts against a transiently obstructing stone in the neck of the gallbladder. There is no inflammatory or infectious process in biliary colic. Acute cholecystitis produces a constant pain and refers to inflammation and infection of the gallbladder; total or partial occlusion of the cystic duct is thought to be required. The most common organisms cultured during acute cholecystitis are *Escherichia coli*, *Klebsiella*, enterococci, *Bacteroides fragilis*, and *Pseudomonas*.

Gallstones within the common bile duct are a major cause of pancreatitis, known as gallstone pancreatitis.

PATHOGENESIS

Gallstones are composed of cholesterol, calcium bilirubinate (pigment), or a mixture of both. Cholesterol stones make up approximately 75% of gallstones in Western countries. Stone formation occurs when bile becomes supersaturated with cholesterol. Cholesterol crystals then precipitate out of solution and agglomerate to form stones.

A high-cholesterol diet causes increased concentrations of cholesterol and may have a role in the pathogenesis of cholesterol stones. Pigment stones are composed of calcium bilirubinate and are either black or brown. Black pigment stones are usually found in the gallbladder and are associated with cirrhosis and hemolytic processes, such as sickle cell anemia, thalassemia, and spherocytosis. Brown stones are associated with chronic biliary tract infection and are often found in the bile ducts. Patients with indwelling biliary stents or with intraluminal nonabsorbable sutures in the ducts from prior surgery are prone to developing brown stones.

EPIDEMIOLOGY

Approximately 10% of the U.S. population has gallstones. The vast majority of people with stones are asymptomatic. Nevertheless, more than 600,000 cholecystectomies are performed in the United States annually.

Gallstones are found more commonly in women. Risk factors include obesity, multiparity, chronic total

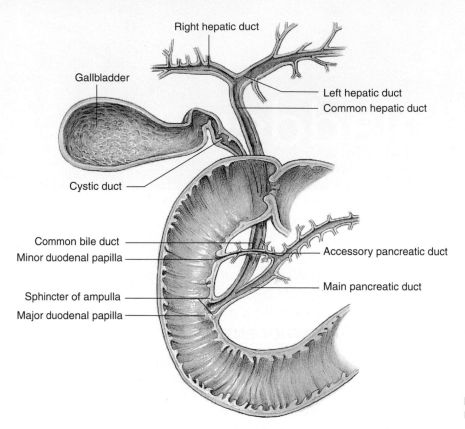

Figure 7-1 • Duct system.
From Anatomical Chart Company.

parenteral nutrition use, high-dose estrogen oral contraceptives, rapid weight loss, diabetes, and increasing age. Some ethnic groups such as American Indians have very high prevalence rates. Spinal cord injury predisposes to cholesterol stones.

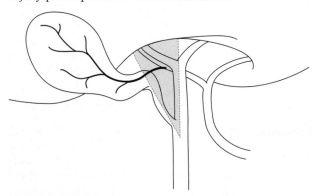

Figure 7-2 • The hepatocystic triangle (of Calot) is defined by three structures: cystic duct, common hepatic duct and lower liver edge.
From Blackbourne LH. *Advanced Surgical Recall*. 2nd ed. Baltimore: Lippincott Williams & Wilkins, 2004.

HISTORY

As stated, most patients with gallstones are asymptomatic. Patients with biliary colic usually complain of right upper quadrant or epigastric pain, often radiating around the right flank to the back. The pain is usually postprandial (occurring after eating). Pain episodes may be precipitated by fatty food intake and last several hours before resolving spontaneously. Associated nausea and vomiting are common.

Cholecystitis implies infection and inflammation of the gallbladder. The pain of cholecystitis is usually constant, with progressive worsening. Patients may have fever, chills, or sweats.

Choledocholithiasis can result in transient or complete blockage of the common bile duct. Patients may relate episodes of passing dark urine or light-colored stools caused by the inability of bile pigments to reach the gastrointestinal tract and from subsequent renal clearance. Choledocholithiasis can also lead to ascending cholangitis, demonstrated by right upper quadrant abdominal pain, fever, and chills.

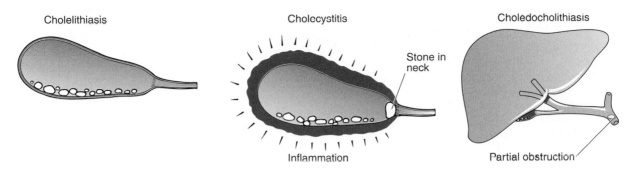

Figure 7-3 • Biliary pathology.

Pancreatitis owing to choledocholithiasis (gallstone pancreatitis) typically manifests with epigastric pain radiating to the back.

PHYSICAL EXAMINATION

Physical examination in simple biliary colic reveals right upper quadrant tenderness but no fever. Cholecystitis may be associated with fever and signs of peritoneal irritation, including right upper quadrant rebound and guarding. The classic finding in acute cholecystitis is the arrest of inspiration on deep right upper quadrant palpation as pressure from the examiner's hand contacts the inflamed gallbladder and peritoneum (Murphy sign). Choledocholithiasis may be associated with jaundice, in addition to signs of biliary colic. Cholangitis is classically marked by fever, right upper quadrant pain, and jaundice (Charcot triad). Progression of cholangitis to sepsis defines Reynolds pentad by adding hypotension and mental status changes to the triad. Patients with gallstone pancreatitis have epigastric tenderness. A palpable, nontender, distended gallbladder in the clinical setting of jaundice indicates malignant biliary obstruction (Courvoisier law).

DIAGNOSTIC EVALUATION

Laboratory examination in biliary colic is usually unremarkable. Cholecystitis usually manifests with increased white blood cell count and minor liver function test abnormalities. Choledocholithiasis is classically associated with increased serum bilirubin and alkaline phosphatase. Cholangitis usually causes elevated serum bilirubin and transaminase levels, as well as leukocytosis. Gallstone pancreatitis is accompanied by elevations in serum amylase and lipase.

Ultrasound is the best modality for imaging the gallbladder and bile ducts, having a sensitivity and specificity of 98% for the detection of gallstones. On ultrasound, the gallstones appear as opacities, with echoless shadows posteriorly (Fig. 7-4). Moving the patient during ultrasound examination often demonstrates migration of the stones to the dependent portion of the gallbladder. Ultrasound is also used for diagnosing acute cholecystitis. Fluid around the gallbladder (pericholecystic fluid), a thickened gallbladder wall, and an ultrasonographic Murphy sign all support the diagnosis of acute cholecystitis.

When ultrasound findings are equivocal or acalculous cholecystitis is suspected, cholescintigraphy (e.g., hepatobiliary iminodiacetic acid scan) is almost 100% sensitive and 95% specific for acute cholecystitis.

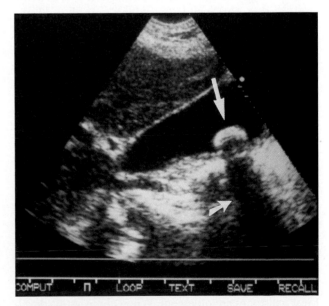

Figure 7-4 • Gallstone. There is a hyperechoic stone (large arrow) in the dependent portion of the gallbladder, with a posterior shadow (small arrow). There is no thickening of the gallbladder wall or fluid around the gallbladder.
From Harwood-Nuss A, Wolfson AB, Linden CH, et al. *The Clinical Practice of Emergency Medicine*. 3rd ed. Philadelphia: Lippincott Williams & Wilkins, 2001.

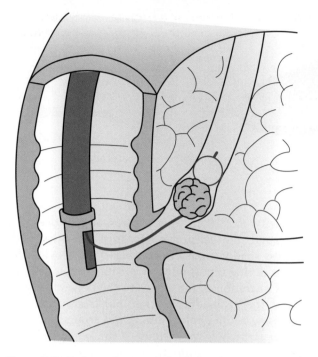

Figure 7-5 • Endoscopic retrograde cholangiopancreatography removal of common bile duct stone using balloon-tip catheter.

In this test, a radionucleotide that is injected intravenously is taken up in the liver and excreted into the biliary tree. If the cystic duct is obstructed, as in acute cholecystitis, the gallbladder does not fill, and the radionucleotide passes directly into the duodenum.

Choledocholithiasis can be diagnosed by intraoperative cholangiography at the time of surgery or preoperatively or postoperatively by endoscopic retrograde cholangiopancreatography (ERCP). ERCP is performed by using a specialized side-viewing endoscope to visualize the ampulla, where the pancreatic and biliary ducts enter the duodenum. Using a catheter passed through the endoscope, contrast media is injected retrograde and outlines the biliary tree and pancreatic duct (Fig. 7-5). Magnetic resonance cholangiopancreatography can noninvasively detect common bile duct stones; however, it lacks the therapeutic advantage of ERCP for stone extraction.

COMPLICATIONS

Most gallstones are quiescent. When cholecystitis develops, however, delayed diagnosis may result in gangrenous necrosis of the gallbladder wall with perforation, leading to localized abscess or frank biliary peritonitis. Emphysematous cholecystitis owing to *Clostridium perfringens* can be seen in diabetic patients.

Gallstone pancreatitis may occur as a result of a common duct stone causing blockage of the ampulla, theoretically resulting in bile reflux into the pancreatic duct or increased intraductal pressure. (See Chapter 9, Pancreas.)

Chronic perforation may result in a bilioenteric fistula. This occurs in older adult patients when a large gallstone erodes through the gallbladder wall and causes a fistula to form between the gallbladder and bowel (usually duodenum, rarely colon). The large stone can then pass out of the gallbladder, through the fistula and into the bowel, resulting in distal bowel obstruction (gallstone ileus). Stone obstruction of the small bowel typically occurs at the terminal ileum, whereas the large bowel obstruction typically occurs at the sigmoid colon. Pneumobilia and a smooth obstructing mass on imaging studies are classic findings.

TREATMENT

For patients with asymptomatic stones found on workup for other problems, the incidence of symptoms or complications is approximately 2% per year. Cholecystectomy is usually not advised for these patients. For individuals with biliary colic, laparoscopic cholecystectomy is a safe and effective procedure. This is performed electively in most cases. If the preoperative workup suggests that common duct stones may be present, either ERCP or intraoperative cholangiography should be performed. (See Appendix for a description of a typical laparoscopic cholecystectomy.)

Patients with acute cholecystitis should be adequately fluid resuscitated before surgery, as vomiting and diminished oral intake often results in dehydration. Intravenous antibiotics should be administered.

Laparoscopic cholecystectomy is the procedure of choice for removal of the gallbladder (Fig. 7-6). In the acute setting with gallbladder inflammation and infection, the procedure tends to be technically more difficult and has a higher rate of conversion to the open technique when compared with elective operations for biliary colic. Rarely, when patients are too ill to tolerate surgery, a cholecystostomy tube may be considered. This involves placing a percutaneous drain into the gallbladder lumen for decompression and drainage of pus. Cholecystectomy can then be performed when the patient is stable.

Patients with gallstone pancreatitis require aggressive fluid resuscitation and close observation. Fortunately, mild episodes account for 80% of cases; however, severe fulminant cases can be lethal. Intravenous antibiotics are

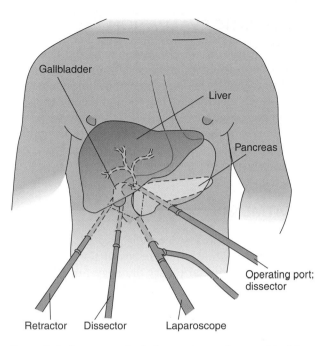

Figure 7-6 • Laparoscopic cholecystectomy: four small incisions allow insertion of laparoscope and instruments for retraction & dissection.
From Smeltzer SC, Bare BG. *Textbook of Medical-Surgical Nursing.* 9th ed. Philadelphia: Lippincott Williams & Wilkins, 2000.

only indicated in severe cases with pancreatic necrosis, infected necrosis, or infectious complications. Early ERCP is indicated in patients with signs of common bile duct obstruction (cholangitis, jaundice, dilated common duct on imaging studies) and in patients with severe disease. Once pancreatic inflammation subsides, cholecystectomy with intraoperative cholangiography should be performed during the same hospitalization to reduce the risk of recurrent pancreatitis and to rule out residual common duct stones. If stones are present, intraoperative common duct exploration or postoperative ERCP is performed. The risk of recurrent pancreatitis is approximately 40% within 6 weeks (see Chapter 9, Pancreas).

Cholangitis, usually caused by choledocholithiasis, requires rapid diagnosis and treatment. Gram-negative organisms are the most common cause. Prompt treatment with intravenous antibiotics, fluid resuscitation, and urgent biliary decompression and drainage are indicated. ERCP with sphincterotomy is the primary intervention. If the obstructing stone is unable to be extracted, an indwelling biliary stent can be passed proximal to the stone to allow decompression and drainage of infected bile into the duodenum. Other methods of decompression include percutaneous transhepatic drainage or open surgical drainage with common bile duct exploration and T-tube placement. Overall mortality is approximately 15%.

GALLBLADDER CANCER

EPIDEMIOLOGY

Carcinoma of the gallbladder is the most common malignancy of the biliary tract. Cancer of the gallbladder is three times more common in females. The incidence is 2.5 in 100,000. Risk factors include gallstones, porcelain gallbladder, and adenoma. One percent of all patients who undergo cholecystectomy for gallstones will be found to have gallbladder carcinoma.

PATHOLOGY

Adenocarcinoma is the most common histologic type. Approximately 80% are adenocarcinomas, 10% are anaplastic, and 5% are squamous cell.

HISTORY

Unfortunately, most patients usually present with late-stage disease complaining of vague right upper quadrant pain. Weight loss, anorexia, and nausea may also be present.

PHYSICAL EXAMINATION

A right upper quadrant mass may be present. Obstructive jaundice represents invasion or compression of the common bile duct. Ascites is seen in advanced cases.

STAGING

Staging of gallbladder carcinoma is as follows:

Stage I: confined to mucosa/submucosa
Stage II: involvement of muscle layer of gallbladder wall
Stage III: lymph node involvement or extension into the liver (<2 cm liver invasion)
Stage IV: liver invasion >2 cm or distant metastasis.

TREATMENT

The mainstay of treatment for gallbladder cancer is surgical, because early detection and complete resection provide the only chance for cure. The extent of resection is controversial but is based on the stage of disease. Options include simple cholecystectomy, radical resection of the gallbladder including partial hepatic resection, or palliative operation as symptoms arise.

Most cases of early-stage disease are found incidentally after elective laparoscopic cholecystectomy. If the cancer is stage I and confined to the mucosa/submucosa, then no additional surgery is indicated. For stage II and III lesions, where the muscle layer is involved, the en-bloc resection of the gallbladder with hepatic segments 4 and 5 as well as radical lymph node dissection is indicated. Overall, stage IV cancers show no benefit from attempts at radical resection (except perhaps in patients with T4N0 disease).

PROGNOSIS

Unless cancer is found incidentally at cholecystectomy for symptomatic gallstones, the chance of long-term survival is low. For all patients diagnosed with gallbladder cancer, only 4% will be alive after 5 years. Patients found to have incidentally noted in situ disease on cholecystectomy have survival rates of 88%. Overall survival rates of patients with American Joint Committee on Cancer stage I disease is 60%; stage II, 24%; stage III, 9%; and stage IV, 1%.

BILE DUCT CANCER

EPIDEMIOLOGY

Bile duct cancer (cholangiocarcinoma) is rare. Risk factors include ulcerative colitis, sclerosing cholangitis, and infection with *Clonorchis sinensis*. Patients with sclerosing cholangitis should be observed closely for evidence of cancer.

HISTORY

Patients with advanced disease typically complain of right upper quadrant pain. Biliary obstruction may lead to jaundice and pruritus.

PHYSICAL EXAMINATION

The patient may be jaundiced, with a palpable nontender distended gallbladder. If so, Courvoisier law states that the site of obstruction is in the common bile duct, distal to the confluence of the hepatic and cystic ducts.

DIAGNOSTIC EVALUATION

Laboratory studies are consistent with the chemical findings of obstructive jaundice. Ultrasound and computed tomography show evidence of biliary obstruction with dilated ducts, but percutaneous transhepatic cholangiography or ERCP is usually necessary to demonstrate the lesion. With access to the biliary tree, brushings or biopsies can be performed for cytologic diagnosis.

TREATMENT

Unresectable tumors are usually treated with either endoluminal stenting to relieve obstruction or else with percutaneous catheter biliary drainage. Surgical treatment mostly depends on the location of the tumor within the extrahepatic bile duct. Tumors of the proximal and middle thirds of the duct are best treated with resection and reconstruction with Roux-en-Y hepaticojejunostomy (Fig. 7-7). Tumors of the distal lower third are best treated with pancreaticoduodenectomy (Whipple procedure; Fig. 7-8).

PROGNOSIS

Overall mortality is 90% at 5 years. The 5-year survival rate after proximal duct resection is approximately 5%, after middle duct resection is 10%, and after Whipple procedure for distal duct lesions is 30%.

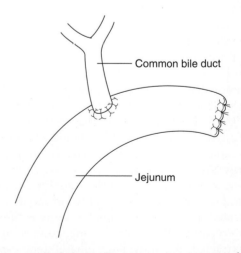

Figure 7-7 • Choledochojejunostomy. Anastomosis of common bile duct to jejunum.
From Blackbourne LH. *Advanced Surgical Recall.* 2nd ed. Baltimore: Lippincott Williams & Wilkins, 2004.

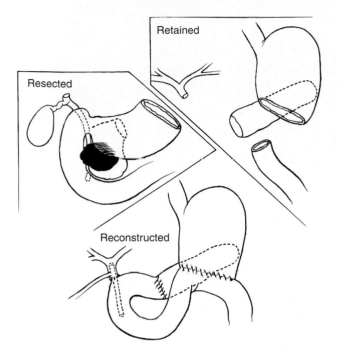

Figure 7-8 • Classic pancreaticoduodenectomy. Top left: The structures resected include the distal stomach; pylorus; entire duodenum; head, neck, and uncinate process of the pancreas with tumor (black); gallbladder; and distal extrahepatic biliary tree. Top right: The structures retained include the proximal stomach, body and tail of the pancreas, proximal biliary tree, and jejunum distal to ligament of Treitz. Bottom: The reconstruction is shown as a proximal end-to-end pancreaticojejunostomy, end-to-side hepaticojejunostomy, and a distal gastrojejunostomy. From Yeo C, Cameron JL. The pancreas. In: Hardy J, ed. *Hardy's Textbook of Surgery.* 2nd ed. Philadelphia: JB Lippincott Co, 1988:717-718.

KEY POINTS

- Cholelithiasis is asymptomatic gallstones within the gallbladder.
- Biliary colic is symptomatic gallstones causing transient right upper quadrant pain without inflammation or infection.
- Cholecystitis is inflammation and often infection of the gallbladder; symptoms include persistent right upper quadrant pain and signs of infection.
- Choledocholithiasis is stones in the common bile duct; serum studies often show elevated liver function tests.
- Cholangitis is infection in the bile ducts extending into the liver; patients have right upper quadrant pain, fever, and jaundice.
- Gallstone pancreatitis is a complication of gallstone disease (choledocholithiasis).
- Gallbladder and bile duct cancers are rare and usually fatal.
- A jaundiced patient with a distended palpable nontender gallbladder indicates distal common bile duct obstruction (Courvoisier law).
- Surgical therapy for cholangiocarcinoma (bile duct cancer) depends on tumor location: resection with Roux-en-Y reconstruction (proximal tumors) or Whipple operation (distal tumors).

8 Spleen

The spleen is a lymphatic organ located in the left upper abdominal quadrant. It contains the largest accumulation of lymphoid cells in the body. In addition to filtering the blood, it plays an important role in host defense. Splenic lymphocytes are involved in antigen recognition and plasma cell production, whereas splenic endothelial macrophages extract bacteria and damaged red blood cells from circulation by phagocytosis. White pulp of the spleen contains high concentrations of antigen-presenting cells and receives arterial blood supply first. Blood then travels through an open-type circulation known as the red pulp, where foreign particles are filtered and antibody-coated cells are removed. Removal of red blood cell imperfections is another function of the spleen. These include Howell-Jolly bodies (Fig 8-1), which are nuclear remnants, Pappenheimer bodies, which are iron inclusions, and Heinz bodies, which are denatured hemoglobin. Splenectomy or hyposplenism is associated with the presence of these abnormalities in the peripheral blood.

Surgical issues regarding the spleen are multiple and varied. Life-threatening hemorrhage from a lacerated spleen resulting from trauma is a common problem, requiring swift surgical intervention. Certain disease states, such as immune thrombocytopenic purpura (ITP) and the hemolytic anemias, are often treated with splenectomy when medical management fails. Splenectomy may be necessary as part of another operation, such as distal pancreatectomy. In addition, the traditional staging workup for Hodgkin disease has involved removal of the spleen to determine extent of disease, although this is now rarely performed.

ANATOMY

The spleen is embryologically derived from condensations of mesoderm in the dorsal mesogastrium of the developing gastrointestinal tract. In the mature abdomen, the spleen is found attached to the stomach by the gastrosplenic ligament and to the left kidney by the splenorenal ligament. Other supporting attachments include the splenocolic and splenophrenic ligaments (Fig. 8-2).

Accessory spleens are present in approximately 25% of patients. They are most often found in the splenic hilum and in the supporting splenic ligaments and greater omentum.

Arterial blood is mostly supplied via the splenic artery, which is one of three branches of the celiac axis (splenic, left gastric, common hepatic). At the hilum, the splenic artery divides into smaller branches that supply the several splenic segments. Additional arterial blood is supplied via the short gastric and left gastroepiploic vessels (Fig. 8-3).

Venous drainage is from segmental veins that join at the splenic hilum to form the splenic vein. Running behind the upper edge of the pancreas, the splenic vein joins with the superior mesenteric vein to form the portal vein.

SPLENIC HEMORRHAGE

The most common cause of splenic hemorrhage is blunt abdominal trauma. Nonpenetrating injury may cause disruption of the splenic capsule or frank laceration of the splenic parenchyma. Displaced rib fractures

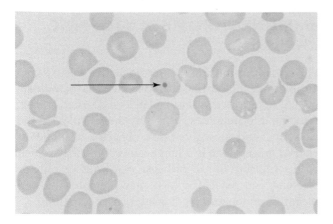

Figure 8-1 • Howell-Jolly bodies. These are round nuclear fragments that are chromosomes separated from the mitotic spindle during abnormal mitosis.
From Anderson SC. *Anderson's Atlas of Hematology.* Philadelphia: Lippincott Williams & Wilkins, 2003.

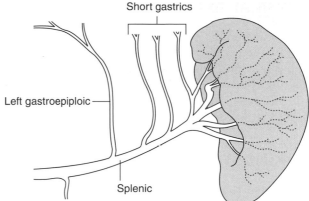

Figure 8-3 • Arterial supply of the spleen.

of the left lower chest often cause splenic laceration. Splenic injuries are graded from I to V based on the extent of laceration and hematoma (Table 8-1).

Splenic hemorrhage may also be iatrogenic. Intraoperative damage to the spleen may occur during unrelated abdominal surgery that results in bleeding controlled only by splenectomy. Estimates are

that 20% of splenectomies result from iatrogenic causes. Infectious diseases (e.g., mononucleosis, malaria) may damage the spleen to the point that unnoticed blunt trauma can cause "spontaneous" splenic rupture and hemorrhage.

HISTORY

Patients typically present with a recent history of trauma, usually to the left upper abdomen or left flank.

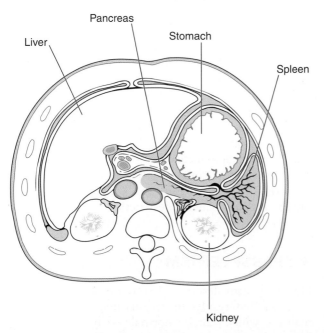

Figure 8-2 • Normal anatomic relations of the spleen. The spleen lies behind the stomach and above the left kidney. It is an intra-abdominal organ, although its blood supply courses through the retroperitoneum.

Grade	Description
I	Hematoma: Subcapsular <10% surface area Laceration: <1 cm deep
II	Hematoma: Subcapsular 10%–50% surface area Parenchymal <5 cm diameter Laceration: 1–3 cm deep, not involving trabecular vessels
III	Hematoma: Subcapsular >50% surface area Parenchymal >5 cm diameter Any expanding or ruptured Laceration: >3 cm deep or involving trabecular vessels
IV	Laceration: Segmental vessels involved with devascularization <50%
V	Completely shattered spleen or hilar vascular injury with devascularization.

TABLE 8-1 Grades of Splenic Injury

From PF Lawrence. *Essentials of General Surgery.* 4th ed. Philadelphia: Lippincott Williams & Wilkins, 2006.

PHYSICAL EXAMINATION

Depending on the degree of splenic injury and hemoperitoneum, a physical examination may reveal left upper quadrant abdominal tenderness, left lower rib fractures, abdominal distention, peritonitis, and hypovolemic shock. Pain on the left shoulder is referred to as Kerr's sign and is referred pain from peritoneal irritation.

DIAGNOSTIC EVALUATION

Computed tomography (CT) scan, abdominal ultrasound, and peritoneal lavage (see Chapter 27, Trauma) can be used to detect intraperitoneal blood. In hemodynamically stable patients, CT can demonstrate the degree of both splenic injury and hemoperitoneum.

TREATMENT

For patients with splenic injury who are hemodynamically stable and without evidence of ongoing hemorrhage, nonoperative management with close hemodynamic monitoring has become the accepted treatment of choice. In children, nonoperative management is widely applied as a result of the incidence of overwhelming postsplenectomy sepsis seen in the pediatric population. Recent advances in interventional radiology have made it possible to embolize the spleen, or a portion, to obviate the need for laparotomy. This can have the advantage of salvaging enough of the spleen to prevent major complications, such as postsplenectomy sepsis, but splenic abscess may occur. For patients with known or suspected splenic injury who are hemodynamically unstable, operative intervention is indicated to control ongoing hemorrhage.

Once in the operating room, the decision to perform splenic repair (splenorrhaphy) versus splenectomy is based on the degree of injury to the parenchyma and blood supply of the organ. Relatively minor injuries, such as a small capsular laceration with minor oozing, may be repaired, whereas a fragmented spleen with involvement of the hilar vessels necessitates surgical removal. If splenic repair is contemplated, the spleen must be mobilized completely to determine the extent of injury and the likelihood of success. If there are other organs injured in addition to the spleen, splenectomy is generally recommended.

IMMUNE THROMBOCYTOPENIC PURPURA

ITP is an autoimmune hematologic disease in which antiplatelet IgG antibodies, produced largely in the spleen, are directed against a platelet-associated antigen, resulting in platelet destruction by the reticuloendothelial system and subsequent thrombocytopenia. The disease is typically seen in young women, who may present with complaints of menorrhagia, easy bruising, mucosal bleeding, and petechiae. Men may present with complaints of prolonged bleeding after shaving trauma.

TREATMENT

Initial therapy is with corticosteroids, which improve platelet counts after 3 to 7 days of therapy. Initial doses are 1 mg/kg orally until the platelet count is normal, followed by a 4- to 6-week taper. High-dose dexamethasone or methylprednisolone is also an option. Intravenous immunoglobulin can be used to support the platelet count, as can anti-Rh(D) if patients have Rh(D) positive platelets. For prolonged active bleeding, platelet transfusions should be administered to achieve hemostasis. If patients are asymptomatic, platelet counts of <30,000 can be tolerated. Once patients become symptomatic or the platelet count decreases to <10,000, therapy should be considered. Patients with chronic refractory ITP may benefit from rituximab or thrombopoiesis-stimulating agents, but these are considered experimental at this time.

Few patients enjoy complete and sustained remission with corticosteroid treatment alone. Patients typically become refractory to medical treatment, and thrombocytopenia recurs. Splenectomy is then indicated. After splenectomy, normal platelet counts develop in approximately 80% of patients because the organ of both significant antiplatelet antibody production and platelet destruction is removed.

HYPERSPLENISM

Hypersplenism describes a state of increased splenic function that results in various hematologic abnormalities, which can be normalized by splenectomy. Elevated splenic function causes a depression of the formed blood elements, leading to a compensatory hyperplasia of the bone marrow.

HISTORY

As in ITP, most patients are women who present with signs of anemia, recurrent infections, or easy bruising.

PHYSICAL EXAMINATION

Abdominal examination reveals splenomegaly.

DIAGNOSTIC EVALUATION

Peripheral-blood smear may reveal leukopenia, anemia, thrombocytopenia, or pancytopenia. Bone marrow biopsy shows pancellular hyperplasia.

TREATMENT

Splenectomy may produce hematologic improvement.

HEMOLYTIC ANEMIAS

Hemolytic anemias are characterized by an elevated rate of red blood cell destruction from either a congenital or acquired etiology. Congenital hemolytic anemias result from basic defects of the cell membrane (hereditary spherocytosis), hemoglobin synthesis (thalassemia), hemoglobin structure (sickle cell anemia), or cellular metabolism (glucose-6-phosphate dehydrogenase deficiency). Acquired autoimmune hemolytic anemias result when antibodies are produced that are directed against the body's own red blood cells.

DIAGNOSTIC EVALUATION

A positive direct Coombs test demonstrates complexed antibodies on the red blood cell membrane. Warm-reactive antibodies are IgG, and cold-reactive antibodies are IgM.

TREATMENT

The role of splenectomy in treating hemolytic anemias depends on the particular disease process. For example, red blood cell survival normalizes after splenectomy for hereditary spherocytosis, whereas operative intervention has no role in the treatment of anemia of glucose-6-phosphate dehydrogenase deficiency that is secondary to a defect of metabolism, not cellular structure. Occasionally, splenectomy may be useful in selected patients with sickle cell anemia and thalassemia. Patients with autoimmune hemolytic anemias undergo initial corticosteroid treatment and progress to splenectomy only after medical treatment failure.

HODGKIN DISEASE STAGING

Because of a greater reliance on CT scans and the favorable success of salvage chemotherapy in the treatment of Hodgkin lymphoma, the need for determining whether disease is present across the diaphragm by means of laparotomy and splenectomy has sharply declined. Treatment with salvage chemotherapy after local radiation failure still carries a highly favorable outcome in most cases. Therefore, splenectomy for staging Hodgkin disease is now rarely performed.

OVERWHELMING POSTSPLENECTOMY SEPSIS

Asplenic individuals are at greater risk for developing fulminant bacteremia because of decreased opsonic activity, decreased levels of IgM, and decreased clearance of bacteria from the blood after splenectomy. As a rule, children are at greater risk for development of sepsis than are adults, and fatal sepsis is more common after splenectomy for hematologic disorders than after trauma. The risk of sepsis is higher in the first postoperative year, and, for adults, each subsequent year carries approximately a 1% chance of developing sepsis. Other data show a mortality of less than one per 1,000 patient-years. The clinical picture of overwhelming postsplenectomy sepsis is the onset of high fever followed by circulatory collapse from septic shock. Disseminated intravascular coagulation often occurs. The offending pathogens are the encapsulated bacteria *Streptococcus pneumoniae*, *Haemophilus influenzae*, and *Neisseria meningitidis*.

SPLENECTOMY CONSIDERATIONS

Any patient scheduled to undergo splenectomy should receive immunization against Steptococcus pneumoniae, Haemophilus influenzae, and Neisseria meningitidis, preferably at least 2 weeks before surgery. Straightforward splenectomy can be performed laparoscopically, whereas complicated splenectomy in patients with massive spleens or severe thrombocytopenia are more likely to require laparotomy. During surgery, the spleen is mobilized from the splenorenal, phrenosplenic, and lienocolic ligaments. The main artery is found on the superior border of the pancreas and should generally be taken early. Care must be taken to control the short gastric arteries entering the greater curve of the stomach. The tail of the pancreas nestles into the splenic hilum and can be damaged, causing a pancreatic leak or fistula. Patients generally have nasogastric decompression to prevent the stomach from distending and hemorrhage along the greater curve. Patients with compromised immune systems, including young children and transplant recipients, should be considered for long-term oral penicillin prophylaxis.

SPLENIC ABSCESS

Splenic abscesses most commonly occur as a consequence of other intra-abdominal infection. They can also occur after arterial embolization of either the liver or spleen. Diabetes seems to be a risk factor. Patients generally present with left upper quadrant pain, fever, and leucocytosis. Antibiotics, catheter-based drainage, and splenectomy are all appropriate management options.

KEY POINTS

- The spleen is a lymphatic organ that plays roles in antigen recognition and blood filtering.
- Accessory spleens occur in 25% of patients and are most commonly found in the splenic hilum.
- Arterial blood is supplied via the splenic artery, the short gastric arteries, and branches of the left gastroepiploic artery.
- Hemorrhage secondary to trauma is the most common indication for splenectomy.
- Nonoperative management or organ-sparing splenorrhaphy can be attempted to avoid the risk of overwhelming postsplenectomy sepsis, especially in children.
- Hemodynamically stable patients with splenic injury can be managed nonoperatively.
- Immune thrombocytopenic purpura, hypersplenism, and specific hemolytic anemias are disease states for which splenectomy may be indicated.
- Splenectomy for staging Hodgkin disease is now rarely performed, because of improved imaging modalities (computed tomography scan) and the success of chemotherapy.
- The risk of overwhelming postsplenectomy sepsis is greater in children than in adults. High fever and septic shock are often accompanied by disseminated intravascular coagulation.
- Vaccination against *Streptococcus pneumoniae*, *Haemophilus influenzae*, and *Neisseria meningitidis* should be administered to all surgically and functionally asplenic patients, because these encapsulated organisms are responsible for causing overwhelming postsplenectomy sepsis.

9 Pancreas

The pancreas is a key regulator of digestion and metabolism through both endocrine and exocrine functions. Disorders of surgical importance include acute pancreatitis, chronic pancreatitis, and pancreatic cancer.

EMBRYOLOGY

Formation of the pancreas begins during the first few weeks of gestation, with the development of the ventral and dorsal pancreatic buds. Clockwise migration of the ventral bud allows fusion with the larger dorsal bud, creating the duct of Wirsung, which is the main pancreatic duct. Failure of this process results in pancreas divisum, wherein the duct of Santorini drains a portion of the exocrine pancreas through a separate minor duodenal papilla (Fig. 9-1). This anatomic variant is associated with pancreatitis. Annular pancreas occurs when the ventral bud fails to rotate, resulting in pancreatic tissue completely or partially encircling the second portion of the duodenum. This situation may result in duodenal obstruction, requiring duodenojejunostomy or gastrojejunostomy in some cases.

ANATOMY AND PHYSIOLOGY

The pancreas is a retroperitoneal structure located posterior to the stomach and anterior to the inferior vena cava and aorta. This yellowish, multilobed gland is divided into four portions: head, which includes the uncinate process; neck; body; and tail (Fig. 9-2). It lies in a transverse orientation, with the pancreatic head in intimate association with the C loop of the duodenum, the body draped over the spine, and the tail nestled in the splenic hilum.

The arterial blood supply to the pancreatic head is derived from the anterior and posterior pancreaticoduodenal arteries (Fig. 9-3). These arteries arise from the superior pancreaticoduodenal artery, which is a continuation of the gastroduodenal artery, and from the inferior pancreaticoduodenal artery, which arises from the superior mesenteric artery. The body and tail are supplied from branches of the splenic and left gastroepiploic arteries. Venous drainage follows arterial anatomy and enters the portal circulation.

Sympathetic innervation is responsible for transmitting pain of pancreatic origin, whereas efferent postganglionic parasympathetic fibers innervate islet, acini, and ductal systems. In patients with intractable pain from chronic pancreatitis who have failed operative drainage or resection, splanchnicectomy (sympathectomy) can be performed to interrupt sympathetic nerve fibers.

The functional units of the endocrine pancreas are the islets of Langerhans, which are multiple small endocrine glands scattered throughout the pancreas that make up only 1% to 2% of the total pancreatic cell mass. The bulk of the pancreatic parenchyma is exocrine tissue. Four islet cell types have been identified: A cells (alpha), B cells (beta), D cells (delta), and F cells (pancreatic polypeptide [PP] cells).

Alpha cells produce glucagon, which is secreted in response to stimulation by amino acids, cholecystokinin, gastrin, catecholamines, and sympathetic and parasympathetic nerves. The role of alpha cells is to ensure an ample supply of circulating nutritional fuel during periods of fasting. It promotes hepatic gluconeogenesis and glycogenolysis and inhibits gastrointestinal motility and gastric acid secretion.

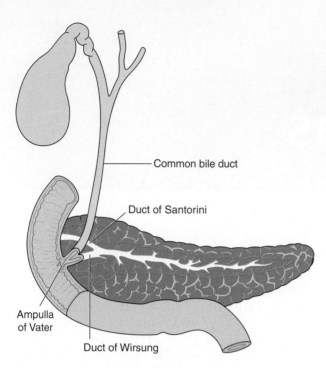

Figure 9-1 • Pancreas divisum. Instead of draining through a common pancreatic duct, the ducts of Wirsung (major duct) and Santorini (minor duct) enter the duodenum separately.

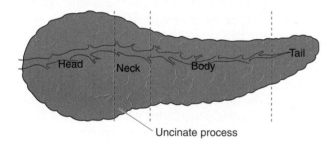

Figure 9-2 • Regional anatomy of the pancreas.

The largest percentage of islet volume is occupied by the insulin-producing beta cells. The main function of insulin is to promote the storage of ingested nutrients. Insulin is released into the portal circulation in response to glucose, amino acids, and vagal stimulation. Insulin has both local and distant anabolic and anticatabolic activity. Local paracrine function is the inhibition of glucagon secretion by alpha cells. In the liver, insulin inhibits gluconeogenesis, promotes the synthesis and storage of glycogen, and prevents glycogen breakdown. In adipose tissue, insulin increases glucose uptake by adipocytes, promotes triglyceride storage, and inhibits lipolysis. In muscle, it promotes the synthesis of glycogen and protein.

Somatostatin is secreted by islet delta cells in response to the same stimuli that promote insulin release. Pancreatic somatostatin slows the movement of nutrients from the intestine into the circulation by decreasing pancreatic exocrine function, reducing splanchnic blood flow, decreasing gastrin and gastric acid production, and reducing gastric emptying time. Somatostatin also has paracrine-inhibitory effects on insulin, glucagon, and PP secretion.

F cells secrete PP after ingestion of a mixed meal. The function of PP is unknown; however, it may be important in priming hepatocytes for gluconeogenesis. Patients with pancreatic endocrine tumors have been noted to have elevated levels of circulating PP.

The basic functional unit of the exocrine pancreas is the acinus. Acinar cells contain zymogen granules in the apical region of the cytoplasm. Acini are drained by a converging ductal system that terminates in the main pancreatic excretory duct. The centroacinar cells of individual acini form the origins of the ducts, with intercalated duct cells lining the remainder.

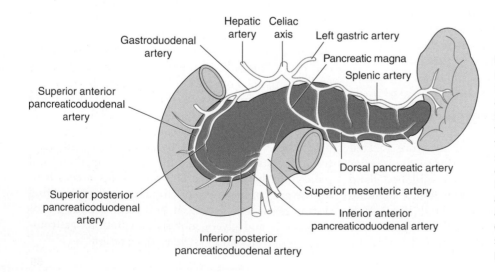

Figure 9-3 • Blood supply of the pancreas. The celiac axis gives rise to the common hepatic artery and splenic artery. The common hepatic artery gives rise to the gastroduodenal artery, which supplies the head of the pancreas, and the splenic artery gives rise the pancreatic magna and many small branches into the body and tail. In addition, the superior mesenteric artery gives rise to the inferior pancreaticoduodenals arteries, which supply the head and the uncinate process.

Exocrine pancreatic secretions are products of both ductal and acinar cells. Ductal cells contribute a clear, basic-pH, isotonic solution of water and electrolytes, rich in bicarbonate ions. Secretion of pancreatic fluid is principally controlled by secretin, a hormone produced in the mucosal S cells of the crypts of Lieberkühn in the proximal small bowel. The presence of intraluminal acid and bile stimulates secretin release, which binds pancreatic ductal cell receptors, causing fluid secretion.

Pancreatic digestive enzymes are synthesized by and excreted from acinar cells after stimulation by secretagogues (cholecystokinin, acetylcholine). Excreted enzymes include endopeptidases (trypsinogen, chymotrypsinogen, and proelastase) and exopeptidases (procarboxypeptidase A and B). Other enzymes produced are amylase, lipase, and colipase. All peptidases are excreted into the ductal system as inactive precursors. Once in the duodenum, trypsinogen is converted to the active form, trypsin, by interaction with duodenal mucosal enterokinase. Trypsin, in turn, serves to activate the other excreted peptidases. In contrast to the peptidases, the enzymes amylase and lipase are excreted into the ductal system in their active forms.

ACUTE PANCREATITIS

PATHOGENESIS

Acute pancreatitis is a disease of glandular enzymatic autodigestion that has varying presentations, ranging from mild parenchymal edema to life-threatening hemorrhagic pancreatitis. Multiple causes have been identified, with alcoholism and gallstone disease accounting for 80% to 90% of cases among Western populations. The remaining cases are attributed to hyperlipidemia, hypercalcemia, trauma, infection, ischemia, trauma from endoscopic retrograde cholangiopancreatography (ERCP), and cardiopulmonary bypass (Table 9-1). The exact pathogenesis of acute pancreatitis remains unclear. One possibility is that obstruction of the ampulla of Vater by gallstones, spasm, or edema causes elevated intraductal pressure and bile reflux into the pancreatic duct. Activation and extravasation of intraparenchymal enzymes results in tissue destruction and ischemic necrosis of the pancreas and retroperitoneal tissues.

HISTORY

Because of the different degrees of pancreatic tissue destruction seen in cases of pancreatitis, the presentation

TABLE 9-1 Causes of Acute Pancreatitis

Alcohol
Biliary tract disease
Hyperlipidemia
Hypercalcemia
Familial
Trauma—external, operative, ERCP
Ischemic—hypotension, cardiopulmonary bypass
Pancreatic duct obstruction—tumor, pancreas divisum, ampullary stenosis, *Ascaris* infestation
Duodenal obstruction
Infection—mycoplasma, mumps, Coxsackie

ERCP, endoscopic retrograde cholangiopancreatography.

of acute disease is varied, and diagnosis may be difficult. Important past medical history includes information regarding prior episodes of pancreatitis, alcoholism, and biliary colic. Patients present with upper abdominal pain (often radiating to the back), nausea, vomiting, and a low-grade fever. A severe attack of pancreatitis is manifested by hypotension, sepsis, and multiorgan failure. Patients with an alcoholic cause usually experience pain 12 to 48 hours after alcohol ingestion.

PHYSICAL EXAMINATION

Patients have upper abdominal tenderness, usually without peritoneal signs. The abdomen may be slightly distended secondary to a paralytic ileus. Low-grade fever and tachycardia are common.

DIFFERENTIAL DIAGNOSIS

Acute pancreatitis is often difficult to differentiate from other causes of upper abdominal pain. The clinical presentation may mimic that of a perforated peptic ulcer or acute biliary tract disease. Other conditions that may have similar presentations are acute intestinal obstruction, acute mesenteric thrombosis, and a leaking abdominal aortic aneurysm.

DIAGNOSTIC EVALUATION

More than 90% of patients who present with acute pancreatitis have an elevated serum amylase. However, amylase levels are relatively nonspecific, because many other intra-abdominal conditions, including intestinal obstruction and perforated peptic ulcer, may cause amylase elevation. If the diagnosis is unclear, a lipase level should also be measured, because it is solely of pancreatic origin.

Leukocytosis >10,000/mL is common, and hemo-concentration with azotemia may also be present because of intravascular depletion secondary to significant third-space fluid sequestration. Hyperglycemia frequently occurs as a result of hypoinsulinemia, and hypocalcemia occurs from calcium deposition in areas of fat necrosis.

Routine chest x-ray may reveal a left pleural effusion, known as a sympathetic effusion, secondary to peripancreatic inflammation. Air under the diaphragm indicates perforation of a hollow viscus, such as a perforated peptic ulcer.

The classic radiographic finding on abdominal x-ray is a sentinel loop of dilated mid- to distal duodenum or proximal jejunum located in the left upper quadrant, adjacent to the inflamed pancreas. In cases of gallstone pancreatitis, radiopaque densities (gallstones) may be seen in the right upper quadrant.

Ultrasonography is the preferred modality for imaging the gallbladder and biliary ductal system, because it is more sensitive as compared with computed tomography (CT) scan. Ultrasound is the study of choice for the detection of cholelithiasis during the workup of gallstone pancreatitis.

CT is the most sensitive radiologic study for confirming the diagnosis of acute pancreatitis. Virtually all patients show evidence of either parenchymal or peripancreatic edema and inflammation. CT is also valuable in defining parenchymal changes associated with pancreatitis, such as pancreatic necrosis and pseudocyst formation. For severe cases, CT scanning with intravenous contrast is important for determining the percentage of pancreatic necrosis, which is a predictor of infectious complications. CT-guided interventional techniques can also be performed to tap peripancreatic fluid collections to rule out infection.

ERCP is useful for imaging the biliary ductal system and can be a diagnostic, as well as a therapeutic, modality. In the case of gallstone pancreatitis, the presence of common bile duct stones (choledocholithiasis) can be confirmed and the stones extracted endoscopically. Magnetic resonance cholangiopancreatography is a newer noninvasive technique that is a diagnostic, but not therapeutic, modality.

DISEASE SEVERITY SCORES

Because the clinical course of pancreatitis can vary from mild inflammation to fatal hemorrhagic disease, prompt identification of patients at risk for development of complications may improve final outcomes. The Ranson criteria are well-known prognostic signs used for predicting the severity of disease on the basis of clinical and laboratory results (Table 9-2). The ability to predict a patient's risk of infectious complications and mortality at the time of admission and during the initial 48 hours allows appropriate therapy to be instituted early in hospitalization. Mortality is correlated with the number of criteria present at admission and during the initial 48 hours after admission: 0 to two criteria, 1% mortality; three to four criteria, 16%; five to six criteria, 40%; and seven to eight criteria, 100%. Since the publication of the Ranson criteria in 1974, newer severity scores have been developed (Acute Physiology and Chronic Health Evaluation II score) to estimate mortality risk in critically ill patients. This calculation uses 12 variables in intensive care unit patients to predict mortality.

TREATMENT

Medical treatment of pancreatitis involves supportive care of the patient and treatment of complications as they arise. No effective agent exists to reverse the inflammatory response initiated by the activated zymogens. With adequate care, however, most cases are self-limited and resolve spontaneously.

■ **TABLE 9-2** Ranson Criteria for Acute Pancreatitis

At Admission	During Initial 48 Hours
Age >55 years	Hematocrit decrease >10%
WBC >16,000/μL	Blood urea nitrogen increase >5 mg/dL
Serum glucose >200 mg/dL	Calcium decrease to <8 mg/dL
Serum LDH >350 U/L	Arterial PO$_2$ <60 mm Hg
AST >250 U/mL	Base deficit <4
	Fluid sequestration <6 L

WBC, white blood cells; LDH, lactate dehydrogenase; AST, aspartate aminotransferase.

Hydration is the most important early intervention in treating acute pancreatitis, because significant third-spacing occurs secondary to parenchymal and retroperitoneal inflammation. Hypovolemia must be avoided because pancreatic ischemia may quickly develop secondary to inadequate splanchnic blood flow.

Traditional treatment calls for putting the pancreas "to rest" by not feeding the patient (NPO). The goal is to decrease pancreatic stimulation, thereby suppressing pancreatic exocrine function. Nasogastric suction can be instituted to treat symptoms of nausea and vomiting.

Antibiotics should be initiated if there is infected pancreatic necrosis, as confirmed by biopsy. In the absence of this, antibiotics are widely used for pancreatitis, but their efficacy is controversial.

If the severity of disease necessitates a prolonged period of remaining NPO, an alternative method of administering nutrition must be instituted. Intravenous nutrition (total parenteral nutrition/hyperalimentation) is commonly initiated. Once pancreatic inflammation resolves, gradual advancement of oral intake proceeds, beginning with low-fat, high-carbohydrate liquids to avoid pancreatic stimulation.

Oxygen therapy may be necessary for treatment of hypoxia, which often occurs secondary to pulmonary changes thought to be due to circulating mediators. Evidence of atelectasis, pleural effusion, pulmonary edema, and adult respiratory distress syndrome may be seen on chest radiograph.

Surgical treatment of acute pancreatitis is directed at complications that develop secondary to the underlying disease process. During the early phase of pancreatitis, areas of necrosis may form because of tissue ischemia from enzyme activation, inflammation, and edema. Necrotic areas eventually liquefy and may become infected if they are unable to reabsorb and heal. CT scanning with intravenous contrast is the key test for defining the extent of pancreatic necrosis. Nonenhancement of 50% or more of the pancreas on CT scan is a strong predictor for the development of infectious complications. Infected collections require surgical debridement and drainage to avoid fatal septic complications.

Initially, collections around the pancreas during episodes of pancreatitis are termed acute pancreatic fluid collections. Peripancreatic collections that persist after the inflammatory phase has subsided may develop a thickened wall, or "rind." Such collections are called pancreatic pseudocysts. To alleviate symptoms or prevent major complications, surgical drainage is usually required for cysts >6 cm in diameter that have persisted for more than 6 weeks. Standard therapy

is internal drainage into the stomach, duodenum, or small intestine.

During the later stage of disease, abscess formation may occur. The pathogenesis is a progression: an ischemic parenchyma progresses to necrosis and is seeded by bacteria, with eventual abscess formation. Most bacteria are of enteric origin, and standard antibiotic therapy is insufficient treatment. If surgical drainage and debridement are not performed, the mortality nears 100%. Percutaneous drainage is usually inadequate, because only the fluid component is removed and the necrotic infected tissue remains. These patients are often remarkably sick. Multiple debridements may be required when the episode is severe. It is not uncommon for anasarca to result from massive volume resuscitation, and it may be difficult to close the abdomen. In this case, a temporary closure should be used. Definitive closure is performed as early as possible after the infection is controlled and the edema has improved. Operations to remove infected pancreatic tissue can be extremely bloody and adequate access and blood should be available.

Hemorrhage secondary to erosion of blood vessels by activated proteases can be a life-threatening complication. Often it is the main hepatic, gastroduodenal, or splenic artery that bleeds. All efforts should be made to control this with angiography, because it can be exceedingly difficult to control this lesion in the operating room.

CHRONIC PANCREATITIS

Of patients with acute pancreatitis, a small number progress to chronic pancreatitis. The chronic form of disease is characterized by persistent inflammation that causes destructive fibrosis of the gland. The clinical picture is of recurring or persistent upper abdominal pain with evidence of malabsorption, steatorrhea, and diabetes.

PATHOGENESIS

Chronic pancreatitis can be categorized into two forms: calcific pancreatitis, usually associated with persistent alcohol abuse, and obstructive pancreatitis, secondary to pancreatic duct obstruction. Alcohol-induced calcific pancreatitis is the most common form of disease in Western populations. Proposed mechanisms of disease include ductal plugging and occlusion by protein and mineral precipitates. The resulting inflammation and patchy fibrosis subsequently lead to parenchymal destruction and eventual atrophy of the gland. Obstructive chronic pancreatitis is due to ductal blockage secondary to scarring from acute pancreatitis or trauma, papillary stenosis, pseudocyst, or tumor. This blockage results in upstream duct dilatation and inflammation.

HISTORY

Abdominal pain is the principal presenting complaint and the most frequent indication for surgery. The pain is upper abdominal, is either intermittent or persistent, and frequently radiates to the back. Patients are often addicted to narcotic pain relievers. Other symptoms result from exocrine insufficiency (malabsorption) and endocrine insufficiency (diabetes mellitus).

DIAGNOSTIC EVALUATION

Given the functional reserve of the pancreas, the diagnosis of chronic pancreatitis is best made using imaging techniques that detect pancreatic morphologic changes rather than tests of glandular function. Exocrine function may be evaluated by the secretin cholecystokinin test, which is now rarely used.

The radiologic signs of chronic pancreatitis include a heterogeneously inflamed or atrophied gland, a dilated and strictured pancreatic duct, and the presence of calculi. Ultrasonography and CT are useful initial imaging procedures; however, ERCP is the most accurate means of diagnosing chronic pancreatitis, because it clearly defines the pathologic changes of the pancreatic ductal system and the biliary tree.

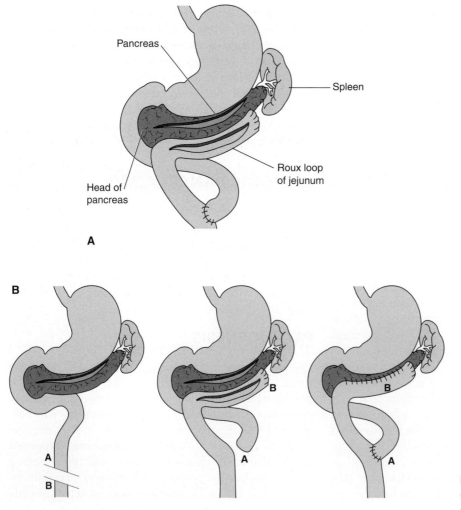

Figure 9-4 • Longitudinal pancreaticojejunostomy used in the treatment of chronic pancreatitis.

TREATMENT

Effective treatment of chronic abdominal pain is often the focus of care for patients with chronic pancreatitis. Opiates are useful for controlling visceral pain; however, many patients become opiate dependent over the long term. Alcohol nerve blocks of the celiac plexus have only moderate success.

Pancreatic exocrine insufficiency is treated with oral pancreatic enzymes, and insulin is used to treat diabetes mellitus. Ethanol intake by the patient must cease.

Surgical intervention is undertaken only if medical therapy has proved unsuccessful in relieving chronic intractable pain. Functional drainage of the pancreatic duct and the resection of diseased tissue are the goals of any procedure. Given ERCP and CT findings, the correct operation can be planned.

For patients with a "chain of lakes"–appearing pancreatic duct, caused by sequential ductal scarring and dilatation, a longitudinal pancreaticojejunostomy (Puestow procedure) is indicated to achieve adequate drainage. A Roux-en-Y segment of proximal jejunum is anastomosed side-to-side with the opened pancreatic duct, facilitating drainage (Fig. 9-4). Distal pancreatic duct obstruction causing localized distal parenchymal disease is best treated by performing a distal pancreatectomy.

ADENOCARCINOMA OF THE PANCREAS

EPIDEMIOLOGY

Pancreatic adenocarcinoma is a leading cause of cancer death, trailing other cancers such as lung and colon. Men are affected more than women by a two-to-one ratio. Risk factors for development of pancreatic cancer are increasing age and cigarette smoking. The peak incidence is in the fifth and sixth decades. Ductal adenocarcinoma accounts for 80% of the cancer types and is usually found in the head of the gland. Local spread to contiguous structures occurs early, and metastases to regional lymph nodes and liver follow.

HISTORY

The signs and symptoms of carcinoma of the head of the pancreas are intrinsically related to the regional anatomy of the gland. Patients classically complain of obstructive jaundice, weight loss, and constant deep abdominal pain owing to peripancreatic tumor infiltration. Patients may present with jaundice and a palpable nontender gallbladder, indicating tumor obstruction of the distal common bile duct (Courvoisier sign). Pruritus often accompanies the development of jaundice.

DIFFERENTIAL DIAGNOSIS

The differential diagnosis of malignant obstructive jaundice includes carcinomas of the ampulla of Vater, pancreatic head, distal common bile duct, or duodenum.

DIAGNOSTIC EVALUATION

The most common laboratory abnormalities are elevated alkaline phosphatase and direct bilirubin levels, indicating obstructive jaundice. The average bilirubin level in neoplastic obstruction is typically higher than that seen in bile duct obstruction from gallstone disease.

CT and ERCP are the modalities of choice for evaluating pancreatic cancer. CT reveals the location of the mass, the extent of tumor invasion or metastasis, and the degree of ductal dilatation (Fig. 9-5). ERCP defines

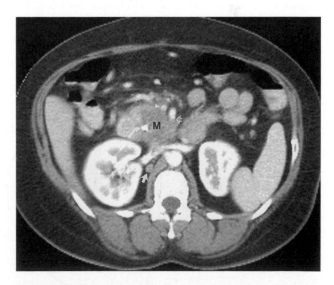

Figure 9-5 • Pancreatic adenocarcinoma. Computed tomography image demonstrates an endoscopically placed biliary stent (curved arrow), passing through a mass (M) in the head of the pancreas. The pancreatic adenocarcinoma has almost obliterated the superior mesenteric vein (arrowhead) and abuts the superior mesenteric artery (open arrow). A retrocaval lymph node is noted (thick arrow).
From Kelsen DP, Daly JM, Kern SE, et al. *Gastrointestinal Oncology: Principles and Practice.* Philadelphia: Lippincott Williams & Wilkins, 2002.

the ductal anatomy and the extent of ductal obstruction and provides biopsy specimens for tissue diagnosis. Drainage stents can be placed into the common bile duct during ERCP for biliary tree decompression. Imaging information suggesting unresectability includes local tumor extension, contiguous organ invasion, superior mesenteric vein or portal vein invasion, ascites, and distant metastases.

TREATMENT

The operation for resectable tumors in the head of the pancreas is pancreaticoduodenectomy (Whipple procedure; Fig. 9-6). This major operation entails the en bloc resection of the antrum, duodenum, proximal jejunum, head of pancreas, gallbladder, and distal common bile duct.

PROGNOSIS

Long-term survival for pancreatic cancer remains dismal, and most patients die within 1 year of diagnosis. The 5-year survival rate for all patients with tumors of the head of the pancreas is approximately 3%. For individuals with tumors amenable to Whipple resection, the 5-year survival rate is only 10% to 20%. Tumors of the body and tail are invariably fatal, because diagnosis is usually made at a more advanced stage as a result of the lack of early obstructive findings.

OTHER PANCREATIC NEOPLASMS

Approximately 20% of all pancreatic cystic lesions will not be pseudocysts. These lesions may be benign or malignant, but even the malignant ones carry better prognosis than adenocarcinoma. Simple cysts are usually congenital. When they appear in children, no treatment is necessary. In patients with polycystic kidney disease, 10% will also have pancreatic cysts. They do not require treatment.

More complicated cystic disease of the pancreas includes serous cystadenoma and mucinous cystic neoplasms. Serous cystadenomas most often occur in women between 30 and 50 years of age. They are generally asymptomatic. Ultrasound reveals a complex low-density mass with fine septae. The fluid is generally clear. Resection is generally curative. Mucinous cystic neoplasms have malignant potential and should be resected with a margin, usually requiring formal partial pancreatectomy. Survival is excellent at 5 years at approximately 70%.

Solid and cystic papillary neoplasms tend to present as large lesions in young women. Resection is often curative.

Intraductal papillary mucinous neoplasms are distinguished from the other cystic lesions of the pancreas in that the pancreatic duct is enlarged because of mucin deposition. ERCP demonstrates mucin in the duct. These lesions have malignant potential and require resection. Long-term prognosis is excellent with resection.

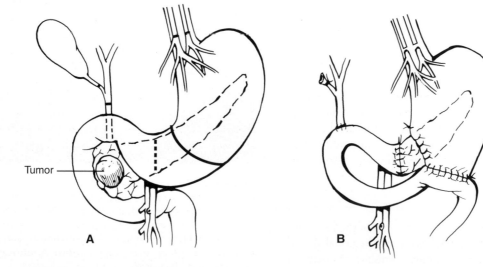

Figure 9-6 • Pancreaticoduodenectomy (Whipple procedure). Preoperative anatomic relationships (A) and postoperative reconstruction (B).

FUNCTIONAL TUMORS OF THE PANCREAS

INSULINOMA

This is the most common tumor of pancreatic islet cells. It is more common in women than men and commonly affects middle-aged patients. Hypersecretion of insulin causes symptoms. Diagnosis is made from the classic Whipple triad of low fasting blood sugars (less than 45 mg/dL); symptoms of hypoglycemia, including palpitations, tachycardia, and shaking; and resolution by administration of exogenous glucose. Patients can lose consciousness or experience seizures. Although most are sporadic, any patient with this syndrome should be suspected of having multiple endocrine neoplasia (MEN) type I, especially if the lesions are multiple. Patients will have an immunoreactive insulin-to-glucose ratio of greater than 0.3 and elevated proinsulin and C-peptide levels. These lesions may be difficult to find because of their small size. Workup includes CT or magnetic resonance imaging to localize the lesion and determine whether metastases are present. Somatostatin receptor scintigraphy may be useful but often fails to localize the lesion. Even if the lesion is not localized, surgical exploration is indicated to try to locate and resect the tumor. Intraoperative ultrasound should be used in this case. Even when metastatic disease is present, resection may be indicated for symptomatic relief.

GASTRINOMA

This tumor is defined by gastrin hypersecretion, causing the severe peptic ulcer disease of Zollinger-Ellison syndrome. The syndrome is slightly more common in men than in women and generally affects patients in middle age. Eighty percent of cases are sporadic, whereas 20% will occur in association with MEN type I. These lesions most commonly occur in the pancreas or duodenum, but can also occur in other areas. Patients present with symptoms of acid hypersecretion, ulcers, and secretory diarrhea. This lesion accounts for less than 1% of all ulcer disease. Patients will have elevated gastrin levels and basal acid output. Secretin stimulation test is used to confirm the diagnosis. CT, magnetic resonance imaging, and ultrasound all have some utility in localizing the tumor, but somatostatin scintigraphy is the test of choice. In sporadic cases not associated with MEN type I, treatment is medical management of gastric hypersecretion and then resection, given the malignant potential

of the lesion. In patients with MEN type I, management must be coordinated with treatment of the other abnormalities.

OTHER TUMORS

Other, rarer types of neuroendocrine tumors that may affect the pancreas may elaborate vasoactive intestinal peptide, pancreatic polypeptide, adrenocorticotropic hormone, and growth hormone–releasing factor.

KEY POINTS

- The pancreas is a retroperitoneal structure consisting of a head, neck, body, and tail.
- The duct of Wirsung drains the mature pancreas. Occasionally, a duct of Santorini drains through a separate minor papilla.
- Congenital variants arise from aberrant pancreatic bud migration.
- The islets of Langerhans of the endocrine pancreas include alpha cells (glucagon), beta cells (insulin), delta cells (somatostatin), and pancreatic polypeptide cells.
- In Western populations, alcohol ingestion and gallstone disease are primarily responsible for acute pancreatitis, and alcohol use is primarily responsible for chronic pancreatitis.
- Ranson criteria are used to predict the severity of the disease and to estimate mortality.
- Pancreatitis is usually self-limiting and resolves with supportive care; however, complications such as chronic pseudocyst, abscess, necrosis, or hemorrhage are treated surgically.
- Surgical treatment includes drainage procedures (longitudinal pancreaticojejunostomy [Puestow procedure]) or pancreatic resection (distal pancreatectomy).
- In pancreatic cancer, obstructive jaundice, weight loss, and abdominal pain are common findings.
- The Courvoisier sign is jaundice and a nontender palpable gallbladder, indicating tumor obstruction of the distal common bile duct.
- Computed tomography and endoscopic retrograde cholangiopancreatography are used to determine tumor resectability.
- Resectable tumors of the head of the pancreas are removed by pancreaticoduodenectomy (Whipple procedure). Prognosis is generally poor.

Bariatric Surgery

Bariatric surgery, or weight loss surgery, limits the amount of food the stomach can hold by reducing the stomach's capacity to a few ounces. In addition to reducing food intake, some weight loss surgeries also alter the digestive process, which curbs the amount of calories and nutrients absorbed.

ANATOMY

The relevant anatomy involves the stomach and proximal small bowel. These are well-vascularized organs, and although they can withstand significant transections and bypass, it remains critical not to compromise the blood supply. See Chapter 3, Stomach and Duodenum, and Chapter 4, Small Intestine.

MORBID OBESITY

EPIDEMIOLOGY

The increased risk for morbidity and mortality is proportional to the degree of a person's excess weight. The most common way to quantify obesity is by the body mass index (BMI), which is calculated as [weight (kilograms)/height (meters)^2]. The BMI associated with lowest mortality is between 20 and 25 kg/m^2. An adult with a BMI >25 kg/m^2 is considered overweight; an adult with BMI >30 kg/m^2 is considered obese. Morbid obesity, approximately equivalent to a person being 100 pounds overweight, can be a life-threatening condition. A person is classified as being morbidly obese if he or she has a BMI ≥40 kg/m^2, or a BMI of ≥35 kg/m^2 with an obesity-related disease, such as type 2 diabetes, heart disease, or sleep apnea.

Approximately 100 million Americans are obese, and 15 million are morbidly obese. Obesity is rapidly becoming an epidemic in the United States, with prevalence rates of 15% in 1980, and increasing to 33% in 2004. Obesity costs the U.S. healthcare system an estimated $117 billion annually, according to the National Institute of Diabetes and Digestive and Kidney Diseases. After tobacco, obesity is the second leading cause of preventable death in the United States.

PATHOPHYSIOLOGY

The ultimate biologic basis of obesity is unknown. A sedentary lifestyle and the availability of high-caloric foods certainly contribute to this disease process. This disorder, nevertheless, is accompanied by a reduction in life expectancy, which is due in large part to the complications associated with diabetes, hypertension, and sleep apnea.

HISTORY

The approach to the morbidly obese patient has to take into account the weight history, dietary habits, lifestyle, exercise tolerance, and medical comorbidities of the individual. Previous attempts at nonsurgical weight loss should be documented. The dietary and weight history should focus on identifying eating disorders, as well as any emotional or psychiatric conditions that may be linked. Counseling a patient to engage in an active exercise regimen is also critical.

The medical history should aim at ruling out any metabolic causes of obesity, such as hypothyroidism and Cushing's syndrome. Obesity is also related to a host of medical comorbidities that should be identified and

■ **TABLE 10-1** Medical Comorbidities of Obesity	
Diabetes mellitus	Hypertension
Obstructive sleep apnea	Hyperlipidemia
Coronary artery disease	Asthma
Pseudotumor cerebri	Infertility (men and women)
Polycystic ovary syndrome	Thromboembolism
Osteoarthritis	Low back pain
Gout	Gastroesophageal reflux
Gallstones	Nonalcoholic steatohepatosis
Urinary incontinence	Skin infections/ulcerations
Depression	Cancer (colorectal, breast, prostate, endometrial)
Pulmonary hypertension	

stabilized preoperatively. These are listed in Table 10-1. As with any other major operation, surgical risk should be individually assessed on the basis of the medical history.

PHYSICAL EXAMINATION

A general physical examination should be performed preoperatively. Specific to the bariatric population, the airway should be evaluated for difficulty of intubation as well as risk for obstructive sleep apnea. The abdomen should be assessed for the degree of central obesity, as well as prior surgical incisions, which may make laparoscopic surgical approaches difficult.

DIAGNOSTIC EVALUATION

Patients are considered suitable candidates for bariatric surgery if they meet criteria set by the 1991 National Institutes of Health consensus conference on bariatric surgery. Patients must:

- Have a BMI >40, or a BMI >35 with significant weight-related comorbidities, such as diabetes, hypertension, or sleep apnea.
- Have no metabolic abnormalities that could cause weight gain.
- Have attempted and failed at nonsurgical weight loss.
- Be psychologically stable with no identifiable eating disorders.

As for any major surgical procedure, the preoperative workup should include an ECG and possibly stress testing to rule out cardiac disease. A chest radiograph may show an enlarged heart or pulmonary congestion. A sleep study may be necessary to evaluate for sleep apnea, which may necessitate the use of a continuous positive airway pressure machine during sleep. Patients with a significant history of heartburn or reflux should undergo an upper gastrointestinal radiograph to rule out a hiatal or paraesophageal hernia, which may alter the surgical plan.

TREATMENT

Nonsurgical Options

Before surgery, all potential candidates should have attempts at lifestyle modifications, including supervised diet and exercise plans. Pharmacologic options include sympathomimetic drugs, such as phentermine or sibutramine (Meridia), or drugs that alter fat digestion, such as orlistat (Xenical). However, most studies have shown that medical management of obesity fails in up to 95% of cases and that most patients regain a substantial portion of their excess weight as soon as medications are discontinued.

Surgical Options

Bariatric surgery has been recognized by the National Institutes of Health as the most effective method to achieve long-term weight loss. A myriad of bariatric surgical procedures have been devised over the years and may be classified as either being restrictive, malabsorptive, or a combination thereof. Restrictive procedures include adjustable gastric banding (AGB), sleeve gastrectomy, and vertical banded gastroplasty. Malabsorptive procedures such as the jejunal-ileal bypass or biliopancreatic diversion have largely fallen out of favor because of issues with malnutrition and organ failure.

The two most commonly performed bariatric surgical procedures in modern practice are AGB and the Roux-en-Y gastric bypass (RYGB). RYGB, the most popular operation in the United States, is both restrictive and malabsorptive. Both AGB and RYGB can be performed either in traditional open fashion or laparoscopically, although the latter approach has significant advantages in decreasing pain, recovery time, and wound complications. Performing these procedures laparoscopically is technically challenging and associated with a significant learning curve.

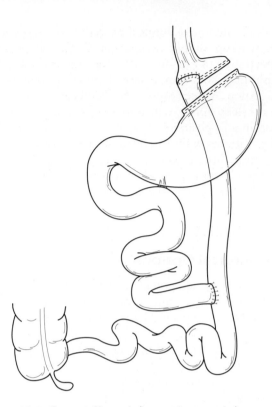

Figure 10-1 • Roux-en-Y gastric bypass. In a gastric bypass, the stomach is transected unevenly, creating a small proximal pouch. A Roux-en-Y gastrojejunostomy is then created. Weight loss occurs as a result of decreased food intake as well as some malabsorption. Gastric bypass is currently the most common bariatric procedure performed in the United States.
From Lawrence PF. *Essentials of General Surgery*. 4th ed. Philadelphia: Lippincott Williams & Wilkins, 2006.

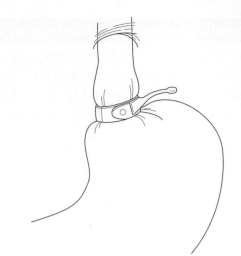

Figure 10-2 • Adjustable gastric band. A band is placed laparoscopically around the stomach with a subcutaneus port to adjust constriction; this results in a smaller gastric reservoir.
From Blackbourne LH. *Advanced Surgical Recall*. 2nd ed. Baltimore: Lippincott Williams & Wilkins, 2004.

RYGB involves the creation of a proximal gastric pouch of approximately 30 mL capacity. Intestinal continuity is restored by attaching a limb of proximal jejunum to this gastric pouch with biliopancreatic continuity established via a jejunojejunostomy (Fig. 10-1).

Patients may experience dumping syndrome postoperatively with RYGB, especially with consumption of highly concentrated sweets. Dumping syndrome is manifested by abdominal cramps, nausea, vomiting, and flushing. In a way, this may be used as an effective form of negative reinforcement to limit the consumption of sweets. Other risks of this procedure include leakage from the intestinal anastomoses, as well as ulcers, strictures, and internal hernias.

Morbidly obese patients are inherently high risk given their propensity for deep venous thrombosis formation and higher incidence of diabetes, hypertension, obstructive sleep apnea, and undiagnosed heart conditions. These all have to be taken into consideration when planning for RYGB. Mortality rate averages 0.5%.

AGB involves placing a silicone band around the upper portion of the stomach (Fig. 10-2). A catheter connects the band to an injection chamber, which is implanted subcutaneously. In the postoperative period, this chamber is used to inflate the band gradually to progressively narrow the gastric inlet and limit caloric intake by controlling portion size. Because no intestines are bypassed, dumping syndrome does not occur. Complications of this procedure include slippage of the stomach around the band, erosion of the band into the lumen of the stomach, and infection, leakage, and migration of the band and injection chamber. Mortality rate averages 0.05%.

RESULTS

Bariatric surgical procedures achieve variable weight loss results. RYGB, whether performed laparoscopically or open, is associated with 75% to 80% excess weight loss (EWL). Excess weight is defined as preoperative weight minus a person's ideal body weight. More importantly, this is associated with resolution of diabetes in approximately 80% to 85% of patients, hypertension in 70% to 80%, and obstructive sleep apnea in 75%. Significant improvements are also seen in lipid profiles and other cardiac risk factors. Long term, there is a 40% decrease in all causes of mortality. Patients need to be monitored long term for any signs of mineral and vitamin deficiency. There are case reports of comatose patients as a result of B-complex vitamin deficiencies, as well as problems with calcium deficiencies and transient hair loss; patients usually recover after the first 6 months postoperatively. In the long term, up to 50% of patients who undergo RYGB may have some weight regain, such that the effective long-term excess weight loss is approximately 65% EWL.

AGB achieves 30% to 40% EWL within a year. However, long-term weight loss is approximately 50% to 55% EWL at 5 to 10 years postoperatively. Diabetes improves in approximately 60% of patients, as do most other comorbidities. Good weight loss results with AGB are particularly dependent on compliance with healthy dietary habits, as patients will not develop any dumping syndrome to dissuade them from consuming inordinate amounts of sweets.

Regardless of the surgical procedure, success in terms of postoperative weight loss is still highly dependent upon patient behavior in terms of pursuing healthy dietary and exercise behavior. Patients who continue to overeat and disregard restrictions on portion size run the risk of dilating the gastric pouch in either a RYGB or AGB. Weight regain in the long term can often be attributed not to any technical surgical failure, but to the fact that patients may revert back to unhealthy lifestyle habits.

KEY POINTS

- Morbid obesity is defined as a body mass index >40 kg/m^2 or a body mass index of 35 to 40 kg/m^2 with comorbidities such as hypertension, diabetes, or sleep apnea.
- Pharmacologic options such as phentermine, sibutramine, or orlistat may result in some weight loss but rarely achieve sustained results in the long term.
- Surgical options are generally categorized into restrictive and malabsorptive options.
- The two most commonly performed bariatric procedures are the Roux-en-Y gastric bypass and the adjustable gastric band.
- Excess weight loss is approximately 65% to 80% with Roux-en-Y gastric bypass and 50% with adjustable gastric band.
- Both procedures are associated with significant improvements in medical comorbidities.

11 Hernias

HERNIAS

A hernia occurs when a defect or weakness in a muscular or fascial layer allows tissue to exit a space in which it is normally contained. Hernias are categorized as reducible, incarcerated, or strangulated. Reducible hernias can be returned to their body cavity of origin. Incarcerated hernias cannot be returned to their body cavity of origin. Strangulated hernias contain tissue with a compromised vascular supply. These are particularly dangerous because they lead to tissue necrosis. If the bowel is involved, this can progress to perforation, sepsis, and death.

EPIDEMIOLOGY

Between 500,000 and 1,000,000 hernia repairs are performed each year. Five percent of people have an inguinal hernia repair during their lifetime. Half of all hernias are indirect inguinal, and one fourth are direct inguinal. In decreasing incidence are incisional and ventral (10%), femoral (6%), and umbilical hernias (3%). Obturator hernias are rare. Indirect inguinal hernias are the most common in both males and females; overall, hernias have a five:one male predominance. Femoral hernias are more common in females than in males.

INGUINAL HERNIAS

ANATOMY

The abdominal contents are kept intraperitoneal by fascial and muscular layers: the innermost layer is the transversalis fascia, with the three more superficial musculofascial layers being the transversus abdominis, the internal oblique, and the external oblique (see Color Plate 8).

During normal development, the testes begin in an intra-abdominal position and descend through the internal ring, taking with them a layer of peritoneum that is stretched into a hollow tube called the processus vaginalis. This invagination of peritoneum, exiting through the deep and superficial inguinal rings and extending into the scrotum to where the testicle has terminated its descent, will result in an indirect inguinal hernia unless the following occurs: the tubular processus vaginalis must collapse upon itself, fusing opposing peritoneal surfaces and obliterating the tube into a cord-like structure. If this obliteration/fusion of the peritoneal layers does not occur completely, an indirect inguinal hernia will result (Fig. 11-1A).

A direct inguinal hernia results from a weakness in the abdominal wall (specifically, the transversalis) in the area just deep to the superficial ring where the spermatic cord exits the inguinal canal before traveling down into the scrotum (Fig. 11-1B). This area is medial to the epigastric vessels and is called Hesselbach triangle (defined as the edge of the rectus sheath medially, the inguinal ligament inferiorly, and the inferior epigastric vessels laterally; Fig. 11-2).

Progressive structural weakening and loss of integrity of the transversalis at this location allows bulging of the weakened abdominal wall through the area of Hesselbach triangle, the most medial aspect and back wall of the inguinal canal itself. Once the defect is large enough, bowel or other abdominal contents can protrude directly through the fascia and out the superficial ring. Direct inguinal hernias are typically seen in older individuals, whereas indirect inguinal hernias predominate in the pediatric population. Also, the

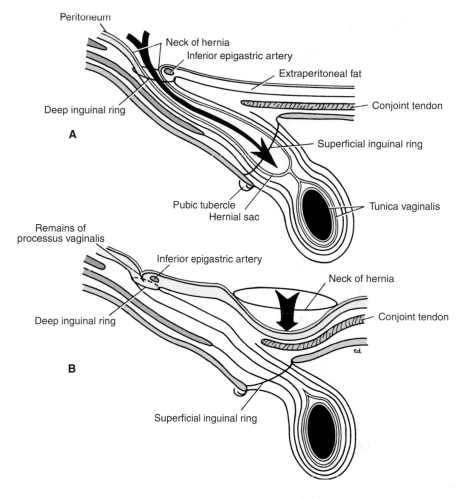

Figure 11-1 • **A.** Indirect inguinal hernia. **B.** Direct inguinal hernia. Note that the neck of the indirect inguinal hernia lies lateral to the inferior epigastric artery, and the neck of the direct inguinal hernia lies medial to the inferior epigastric artery.
From Snell RS. *Clinical Anatomy.* 7th ed. Lippincott Williams & Wilkins, 2003.

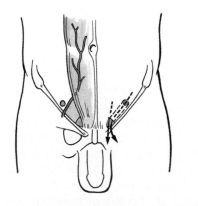

Figure 11-2 • An inguinal hernia is a protrusion of parietal peritoneum and viscera, such as part of the intestine, through a normal or abnormal opening from the abdominal cavity. There are two major categories of inguinal hernia: indirect and direct; approximately 75% are indirect hernias.
From Moore KL, Agur A. *Essential Clinical Anatomy.* 2nd ed. Philadelphia: Lippincott Williams & Wilkins, 2002.

external oblique, which inserts onto the pubic tubercle and bounds the external superficial ring, has no function in the pathogenesis of hernias.

HISTORY

Patients with reducible inguinal hernias describe an intermittent bulge in the groin or scrotum. Persistence of the bulge with nausea or vomiting raises concern for incarceration. Severe pain at the hernia site with nausea or vomiting may occur with strangulation.

PHYSICAL EXAMINATION

With the patient in a standing position, a fingertip is directed upward to find the superficial ring. This is facilitated in male patients by entering the loose scrotum at its base and following the course of the

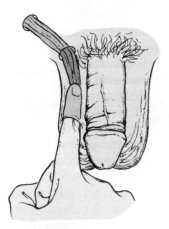

Figure 11-3 • Inguinal canal palpation. Gloved hand palpates inguinal canal by invaginating loose scrotal skin with right index finger at bottom of scrotal sack. Image shows finger following spermatic cord.

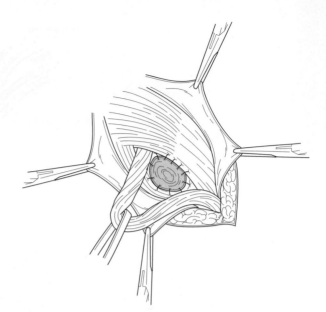

Figure 11-4 • Plug and patch inguinal hernia repair. Plug.
From Blackbourne LH. *Advanced Surgical Recall*. 2nd ed. Baltimore: Lippincott Williams & Wilkins, 2004.

spermatic cord until the superficial ring is encountered. With the fingertip inserted into the ring, a bulge is felt in small hernias as the patient coughs or bears down (Fig. 11-3).

In larger hernias, the herniated sac can be palpated without the aid of Valsalva maneuvers. With the patient in the supine position, reducible hernias can be reduced into the abdomen, whereas incarcerated hernias cannot. Strangulated hernias are tender as a result of peritoneal inflammation. Abdominal distention is often encountered as a result of bowel obstruction.

TREATMENT

Traditionally, the simple presence of an inguinal hernia was indication enough for a surgeon to advise elective repair. Conventional thinking was that the benefit of preventing a hernia accident (i.e., acute incarceration with bowel obstruction or strangulation of abdominal contents) clearly outweighed the potential risks and complications of elective hernia repair. However, the natural history of untreated inguinal hernias and the risks they posed had never been precisely determined until recently. In 2006, a landmark clinical trial involving 720 men with minimally symptomatic inguinal hernias randomly assigned patients to either watchful waiting or surgery with standard open tension-free repair. The key study finding was that the rate of hernia accidents are extremely rare (1.8 per 1,000 patient-years), leading to the study's conclusion that, "A strategy of watchful waiting is a safe and acceptable option for men with asymptomatic or minimally symptomatic inguinal hernias. Acute hernia incarcerations occur rarely, and patients who develop symptoms have no greater risk of operative complications than those undergoing prophylactic hernia repair."

Modern hernioplasty is based on the idea of tension-free repair using an implantable biocompatible prosthesis to reconstruct the fascial hernia defect (Figs. 11-4 and 11-5). The superiority of the concept of mesh tension-free repair versus traditional nonmesh tension-producing repair was validated by a Cochrane Group review published in 2002. The use of mesh was found to significantly reduce the risk of hernia recurrence by an astounding 50% to 75%. Reducible inguinal hernias can be repaired on an elective basis depending on the degree of patient symptoms. Both open and laparoscopic techniques are acceptable, although a recent Veterans Affairs study (2004) showed a higher recurrence rate with laparoscopic repair (10%) when compared with open repair (4%) of primary hernias. The usual indications for laparoscopic repair are bilaterality and recurrence. Interestingly, the Veterans Affairs study showed the rates of recurrence after repair of recurrent hernias as being similar with laparoscopic versus open repairs (10.0% versus 14.1%). Inguinal hernias in adult men should typically be repaired with mesh to avoid recurrence. In women, the round ligament is ligated and the ring closed so mesh use is variable.

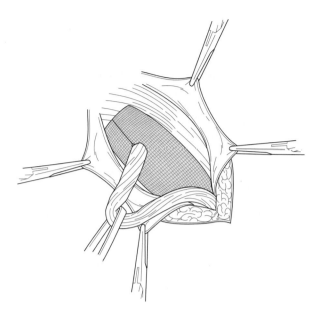

Figure 11-5 • Plug and patch inguinal hernia repair. Patch. From Blackbourne LH. *Advanced Surgical Recall.* 2nd ed. Baltimore: Lippincott Williams & Wilkins, 2004.

When a hernia is not reducible with gentle pressure, a trial of Trendelenburg position, sedation, and more forceful pressure can be attempted. If the hernia is thought to be strangulated, then reduction is contraindicated, because reducing necrotic bowel into the abdomen may produce bowel perforation and subsequent lethal sepsis. Emergency surgery is indicated in this situation. A sample operative note for an inguinal hernia is provided in the Appendix.

UMBILICAL HERNIAS

Umbilical hernias occur at the umbilicus and are congenital. They result from incomplete closure of the fetal umbilical defect. Most resolve spontaneously by the age of 4 years.

EPIDEMIOLOGY

The incidence is 10% of Caucasians and 40% to 90% of African Americans.

HISTORY

The patient may have a bulge at the umbilicus.

TREATMENT

Indications for operation include incarceration, strangulation, or cosmetic concerns.

OTHER HERNIAS

Femoral hernias occur through the femoral canal, located below the inguinal ligament and defined by the femoral vein laterally, the inguinal ligament superiorly, the lacunar ligament medially, and Cooper ligament inferiorly.

Incisional hernias occur through a previous surgical incision. Ventral hernias occur in the midline along the linea alba, usually between the xiphoid and umbilicus. The herniation is through a weakness of the decussating fibers of the linea alba. Spigelian hernias are found at or below the junction between the vertically oriented semilunar line lateral to the rectus abdominus muscle and the transversely oriented arcuate line (linea semicircularis). A pantaloon hernia is a combined direct and indirect inguinal hernia where both hernias straddle each side of the inferior epigastric vessels and protrude like pant legs (pantaloon). Richter hernia occurs when a knuckle of bowel protrudes into a hernia defect, but only a portion of the circumference is involved and the bowel lumen remains patent. Typically, the result is gangrenous necrosis of the herniated tissue. A sliding hernia is any hernia that contains intra-abdominal organs. Internal hernias may occur in patients after abdominal operations when bowel gets trapped as a result of new anatomic relationships. Obturator hernias are typically found in thin, older adult women who present with bowel obstruction caused by small bowel herniation into the obturator canal. Obturator nerve compression by the hernia can result in paresthesias or pain radiating down the medial thigh (the Howship-Romberg sign). Littre hernia is any groin hernia that contains a Meckel's diverticulum.

Something that is not a hernia but is often confused as one is diastasis recti. An upper midline bulge develops when the patient performs a Valsalva maneuver, and herniation is suspected. On close physical examination, however, no actual defect or "hole" in the fascia is found. Rather, the linea alba has become attenuated and weak, resulting in widening of the distance between the rectus muscles. It is this thin, stretched linea alba that bulges out and mimics a large hernia. Surgical repair is not indicated.

KEY POINTS

- Hernias are extremely common. Inguinal hernias are the most common, and 5% of people require repair during their lifetime.
- Indirect inguinal hernias arising from a patent processus vaginalis are more common than direct hernias from abdominal wall weakness.
- Hernias that become incarcerated should be operated on urgently.
- Hernias that become strangulated are a surgical emergency.
- Umbilical hernias are congenital, more common in African Americans, and frequently resolve spontaneously.
- Diastasis recti is not a true herniation and does not require surgical repair.
- Modern hernioplasty is based on the principle of tension-free repair using an implantable biocompatible prosthesis to reconstruct the fascial hernia defect.

Part III

Endocrine

12 Thyroid Gland

Surgical thyroid disease encompasses those conditions in which partial or complete removal of the thyroid gland is required as a result of goiter and hyperthyroid conditions that are unresponsive to medical management or benign and malignant neoplastic disease.

ANATOMY

The thyroid gland develops embryologically from the first and second pharyngeal pouches, migrating caudally to form a butterfly-like structure anterior to the trachea at the level of the second tracheal ring. The thyroglossal duct is the remnant of the tract. Neural crest cells, which are the source of the C cells that produce calcitonin, are also involved in the process of thyroid formation. The normal thyroid gland is bilobed, weighing 15 to 25 g. There is usually an isthmus connecting the two lobes, as well as a pyramidal lobe, which is superior to the isthmus. The thyroid gland receives its main blood supply from the superior and inferior thyroidal arteries, the latter of which is shared with its neighboring parathyroid glands (Figs. 12-1 and 12-2).

In close proximity to the thyroid are the paired recurrent laryngeal nerves (RLNs), which control the cricopharyngeus muscle as well as the vocal cords. The RLNs originate from the vagus nerves in the chest. The right RLN runs behind the subclavian artery at the base of the neck more lateral than the left RLN at this level. Occasionally the right RLN may be nonrecurrent. The right RLN tends to course lateral to medial as it approaches the inferior thyroidal artery from the base of the neck, whereas the left RLN courses with less angulation, running parallel to the

tracheoesophageal groove. The RLN enters the larynx at the level of the inferior constrictor muscles.

The superior laryngeal nerves originate from the vagus nerves as well. It is the external branch of the superior laryngeal nerves which holds significance, given its motor innervation to the cricothyroid muscle. This latter structure controls the high pitch of voice. It lies within the superior pole vessels, and care must be taken when the superior pole of the thyroid is being removed.

PHYSIOLOGY

The purpose of the thyroid gland is to maintain the body's metabolism via the hormone thyroxine (T4) or triiodothyronine (T3), produced by the follicular cells. A negative feedback loop with the hypothalamus and pituitary controls the state of the gland via thyroid-stimulating hormone (TSH; Fig. 12-3).

GRAVE'S DISEASE AND TOXIC NODULAR GOITER

Grave's disease and toxic nodular goiter (TNG) encompass the majority of hyperthyroidism cases. TNG has also been referred to as Plummer's disease. Whereas Grave's disease is an autoimmune process in which the body's own antibodies stimulate the TSH receptor, causing excess T4 and T3 in addition to gland growth, the mechanism of action of TNG is through autoproduction of thyroid hormones regardless of TSH control.

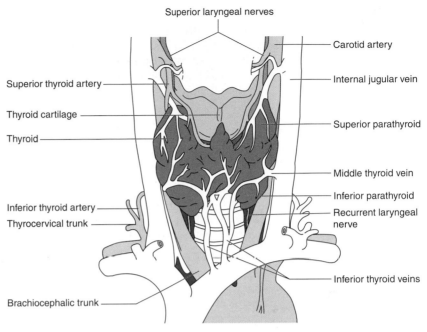

Figure 12-1 • Anatomy of the thyroid gland.

HISTORY AND PHYSICAL EXAMINATION

Both diseases clinically can lead to similar symptoms and signs, such as anxiety, heat sensitivity, nervousness, weight loss, fatigue, palpitations, tachycardia, and palpable goiter, but findings unique to Grave's disease are eye proptosis, which is irreversible, and pretibial myxedema (see Color Plate 9).

DIAGNOSTIC EVALUATION

Laboratory tests consist of TSH and free T4. One finds the TSH to be suppressed to near zero, with elevated free T4. Radioactive iodine uptake testing will differentiate thyroiditis from Grave's disease but is not necessary for confirmation if the clinical picture is consistent with Grave's disease. In TNG, diffuse areas of uptake will be seen.

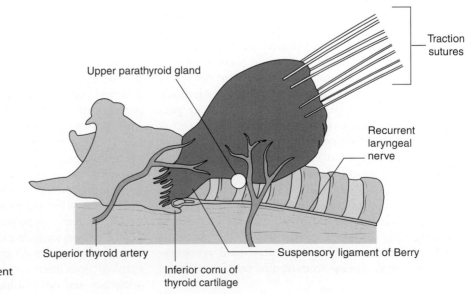

Figure 12-2 • Course of the recurrent laryngeal nerve.

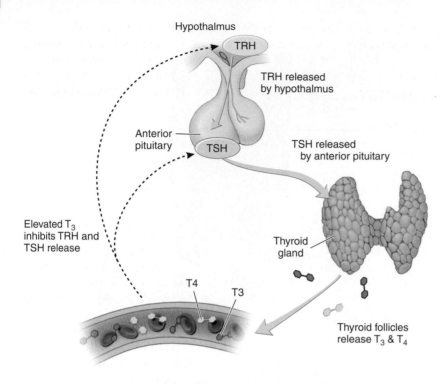

Hypothalmus

TRH

TRH released
by hypothalmus

Anterior
pituitary

TSH

TSH released
by anterior pituitary

Elevated T_3
inhibits TRH and
TSH release

Thyroid
gland

T4

T3

Thyroid follicles
release T_3 & T_4

Figure 12-3 • Regulation of thyroid gland secretion. TRH, thyroid-releasing hormone; TSH, thyroid-stimulating hormone. From Premkumar K. *The Massage Connection Anatomy and Physiology*. Baltimore: Lippincott Williams & Wilkins, 2004.

TREATMENT

Hyperthyroidism treatment can be medical, with use of radioactive iodine or, in the case of Grave's disease, drugs that inhibit synthesis of thyroid hormones, such as methimazole and propylthiouracil. In addition, beta-blockers can be used for symptomatic relief in Grave's disease as well. Surgery is the best option when patients are symptomatic from their goiters (e.g., dysphagia or pressure-like sensations in the neck), when malignancy cannot be excluded in the enlarged thyroid, and when radioactive iodine is not a suitable option (children, pregnant women, resistant cases, and patients not agreeable to risks of radioactive iodine). Specifically, bilateral subtotal thyroidectomy is performed to minimize risk of hyperthyroidism recurrence. However, surgery also puts the patient at risk for long-term hypothyroidism, particularly in Grave's disease, where a euthyroid state rarely is achieved after surgery alone. All patients preoperatively must be made euthyroid using methimazole or propylthiouracil. Iodide preparations are avoided in patients preoperatively as they may worsen the patient's condition, whereas iodides are often used preoperatively in Grave's disease to minimize vascularity of the thyroid.

THYROID NODULE

Evaluation of the thyroid nodule is what leads a patient eventually to surgery. Although thyroid nodules are common in the general population, with a higher incidence in women than in men, only a small portion are clinically evident, and within this group, nearly 90% of the nodules are benign, with the rest being malignant. However, risk factors that would lead one to suspect malignancy include history of head/neck radiation, family history of thyroid cancer (familial medullary thyroid carcinoma, multiple endocrine neoplasia syndrome), male sex (because more female patients present with benign thyroid nodules than male patients), very young age (<20 years) and old age (>60 years), rapid enlargement of the nodule, voice changes, and presence of thyroid disease. The palpable nodule on examination or, as is now being seen more often, incidental nodules on radiologic studies for other purposes, can be definitively tested with fine-needle aspiration (FNA). The technique of FNA involves sampling the contents of the nodule in several planes via a 25-gauge needle on a syringe. The cytologic specimen can be evaluated immediately for adequacy and morphology, determining whether the lesion is benign, malignant, or indeterminate. Light microscopy remains the gold standard, although molecular markers, microarrays, and associated gene mutations are coming into play. These latter tools may further differentiate the numerous classification of thyroid cancers involved in a continuum from well differentiated to poorly differentiated, allowing appropriate treatment.

ALGORITHM

After taking an adequate history and conducting a physical examination, the patient's TSH level should be checked, after which point an ultrasound should be performed. The ultrasound can characterize the nodule by echogenicity, borders, vascularity, and calcifications. In addition, ultrasound evaluation of any nearby lymphadenopathy can further predict risk of malignancy. Nodules 1 to 1.5 cm are considered biologically significant and should undergo FNA.

Repeat FNA is recommended in the event of an inadequate specimen. Presence of follicular or Hürthle cells without malignancy is an indication for surgical intervention, because cytological examination alone is insufficient for determining presence of malignancy. Presence of capsular invasion or angioinvasion can only be seen on histological examination where the thyroid architecture is intact. In addition, frozen section of the thyroid specimen will not necessarily confirm the diagnosis, as multiple sections must be investigated. Thus in many instances, the diagnosis will be deferred to review of permanent sections on pathological examination.

GOITERS

In most parts of the world, enlarged thyroid gland, or goiter, is due to iodine deficiency; however, in the United States, it is most likely due to Hashimoto thyroiditis. Classically, the mechanism of action has been TSH stimulation, but now consideration is given to nodular growth that occurs with age and is made worse with other exposures, such as excess iodine, Hashimoto thyroiditis, environmental goitrogens, Grave's, and lithium.

Indications for surgery include neck compression syndromes affecting swallowing, breathing, and speaking, where malignancy cannot be excluded; hyperthyroidism and progressive growth in the presence of suppression medically; and cosmesis (see Color Plate 10).

Rather than classify goiters by size or weight criteria, the World Health Organization in 1960 developed a grading system for clinical evaluation, with grade 0 representing no enlargement and grade 3 representing enlargement that is evident from a distance (Color Plate 10). The majority of goiters remain in the neck; however, a minority have substernal extension into the anterior mediastinum.

THYROID CANCER

Thyroid cancer incidence is greater in women than men (3% versus 1%, respectively) for unknown reasons. Compared with other cancers with greater incidence, such as breast, lung, and prostate, thyroid cancer mortality is favorable overall. Multiple types of thyroid tumors exist, which can be distinguished by cell origin. Most common are the follicular cell neoplasms, which include papillary and its variants; follicular and Hürthle cell; poorly differentiated; and anaplastic. These occur on a spectrum ranging from well differentiated to poorly differentiated, determining biologic behavior and subsequent treatment. Other cancers include medullary cancer derived from C cells and lymphoma. Papillary and follicular cancers tend to have a more favorable prognosis than the medullary and anaplastic variants.

STAGING

Staging for thyroid cancer is according to the TNM classification (Table 12-1).

TREATMENT

Papillary

Surgery is the mainstay of treatment for papillary carcinoma and its variants. There has been much discussion regarding extent of surgery, which can range from lobectomy and isthmectomy to total thyroidectomy. Papillary cancer can be multicentric, spreading into nearby lymph nodes. Lymph node dissection is performed selectively. In selected patients where the cancer is confined to one lobe and is <1.5 cm without extracapsular involvement, minimal lobectomy with isthmectomy may be sufficient. However, total thyroidectomy is advocated to minimize risk of local recurrence if injury to the parathyroids and recurrent laryngeal nerves are minimal. Postoperatively, TSH is suppressed with thyroidal hormone replacement, and radioactive iodine may be used to ablate any residual thyroidal tissue. Measurement of serum thyroglobulin, which is a tumor marker for well-differentiated thyroid

■ TABLE 12-1 American Joint Committee on Cancer (AJCC) TNM Classification of Thyroid Carcinoma

Primary Tumor (T)

Note: All categories may be subdivided: (a) solitary tumor, (b) multifocal tumor (the largest determines the classification).	
TX	Primary tumor cannot be assessed
T0	No evidence of primary tumor
T1	Tumor 2 cm or less in greatest dimension limited to the thyroid
T2	Tumor >2 cm but not >4 cm in greatest dimension limited to the thyroid
T3	Tumor >4 cm in greatest dimension limited to the thyroid or any tumor with minimal extrathyroid extension (e.g., extension to sternothyroid muscle or perithyroid soft tissues)
T4a	Tumor of any size extending beyond the thyroid capsule to invade subcutaneous soft tissues, larynx, trachea, esophagus, or recurrent laryngeal nerve
T4b	Tumor invades prevertebral fascia or encases carotid artery or mediastinal vessels
All anaplastic carcinomas are considered T4 tumors.	
T4a	Intrathyroidal anaplastic carcinoma—surgically resectable
T4b	Extrathyroidal anaplastic carcinoma—surgically unresectable

Regional Lymph Nodes (N)

Regional lymph nodes are the central compartment, lateral cervical, and upper mediastinal lymph nodes.	
NX	Regional lymph node(s) cannot be assessed
N0	No regional lymph node metastasis
N1	Regional lymph nodes metastasis
N1a	Metastasis to level VI (pretracheal, paratracheal, and prelaryngeal/Delphian lymph nodes)
N1b	Metastasis to unilateral, bilateral, or contralateral cervical or superior mediastinal lymph nodes

Distant Metastasis (M)

MX	Distant metastasis cannot be assessed
M0	No distant metastasis
M1	Distant metastasis

Stage Grouping

Separate stage groupings are recommended for follicular, medullary, and anaplastic (undifferentiated) carcinoma.

Papillary or Follicular

Under 45 years

Stage I	Any T	Any N	M0
Stage II	Any T	Any N	M1

Papillary or Follicular

45 years and older

Stage I	T1	N0	M0
Stage II	T2	N0	M0
Stage III	T3	N0	M0
	T1	N1a	M0
	T2	N1a	M0
	T3	N1a	M0

(Continued)

■ TABLE 12-1 American Joint Committee on Cancer (AJCC) TNM Classification of Thyroid Carcinoma (*continued*)

Stage IVA	T4a	N0	M0
	T4a	N1a	M0
	T1	N1b	M0
	T2	N1b	M0
	T3	N1b	M0
	T4a	N1b	M0
Stage IVB	T4b	Any N	M0
Stage IVC	Any T	Any N	M1

Medullary carcinoma

Stage I	T1	N0	M0
Stage II	T2	N0	M0
Stage III	T3	N0	M0
	T1	N1a	M0
	T2	N1a	M0
	T3	N1a	M0
Stage IVA	T4a	N0	M0
	T4a	N1a	M0
	T1	N1b	M0
	T2	N1b	M0
	T3	N1b	M0
	T4a	N1b	M0
Stage IVB	T4b	Any N	M0
Stage IVC	Any T	Any N	M1

Anaplastic Carcinoma

All anaplastic carcinomas are considered stage IV.

Stage IVA	T4a	Any N	M0
Stage IVB	T4b	Any N	M0
Stage IVC	Any T	Any N	M1

Histopathologic Type

There are four major histopathologic types:

- Papillary carcinoma (including follicular variant of papillary carcinoma)
- Follicular carcinoma (including Hürthle cell carcinoma)
- Medullary carcinoma
- Undifferentiated (anaplastic) carcinoma

Stage 0	Tis	N0	M0
Stage IA	T1	N0	M0
Stage IB	T1	N1	M0
	T2a/b	N0	M0
	T3	N0	M0

(*Continued*)

■ **TABLE 12-1** American Joint Committee on Cancer (AJCC) TNM Classification of Thyroid Carcinoma (*continued*)

Stage II	T1	N2	M0
	T2a/b	N1	M0
	T3	N0	M0
Stage IIIA	T2a/b	N2	M0
	T3	N1	M0
	T4	N0	M0
Stage IIIB	T3	N2	M0
Stage IV	T4	N1-3	M0
	T1-3	N1-3	M0
	Any T	Any N	M1

Used with permission of the American Joint Committee on Cancer (AJCC), Chicago, Ill. Original source: *AJCC Cancer Staging Manual*. 6th ed. New York, NY: Springer-Verlag, 2002.

cancers, can be performed after total thyroidectomy and at follow-up to monitor signs of recurrence.

Follicular

A follicular lesion on FNA is not definitive in distinguishing benign from malignant, because the components of the capsule and blood vessels must be evaluated via histological examination. The minimal approach is to perform lobectomy and await permanent pathology reading. Obtaining frozen section of a follicular lesion usually is not meaningful or cost effective. However, if one highly suspects follicular carcinoma based on size (>4 cm), selective frozen section may be helpful or one may proceed with total thyroidectomy. Also, evaluation of the contralateral lobe at the time of surgery is important in deciding extent of surgery. After lobectomy with pathology showing minimally invasive follicular carcinoma, completion thyroidectomy is not necessarily indicated in low-risk patients. Follicular cancer does not metastasize to lymph nodes as much as papillary cancer. Thus elective nodal dissection is not performed in the absence of adenopathy. In contrast to papillary cancer, follicular cancer tends to metastasize via the bloodstream. Radioactive iodine may be used in patients with unresectable, gross disease.

Medullary

In the familial form of the disease, whether isolated or associated with multiple endocrine neoplasia 2A or 2B, medullary thyroid cancer is known to metastasize

early to surrounding lymph nodes. Patients should be genetically tested given their risk profile and undergo total thyroidectomy with central neck dissection at an early age. Nearly 70% of medullary cancers are sporadic. These patients may present with a thyroid nodule associated with cervical adenopathy. Staining of FNA for calcitonin and absence of thyroglobulin is diagnostic. As with the familial forms, total thyroidectomy with central neck dissection is performed (see Color Plate 11).

Anaplastic/Lymphoma

Rarely are anaplastic thyroid cancer and lymphoma treated surgically. Both processes present with a rapidly enlarging neck mass. The undifferentiated anaplastic cancer is considered lethal with a short survival time of months, whereas the prognosis for lymphoma is better. FNA with appropriate immunohistochemical staining is used for appropriate diagnosis, but sometimes open biopsy for tissue histology is confirmatory. Non-Hodgkin B-cell type is the most common lymphoma pathology for thyroid. Airway management rather than thyroidectomy is the surgical intervention of choice.

COMPLICATIONS OF THYROID SURGERY

There are unique risks involved in thyroid surgery that increase with extent of surgery. The most important is injury to the recurrent laryngeal nerve, which not only controls voice but airway function. The best prevention is identification of the nerve by visualization and assistance with use of intraoperative nerve monitoring. Even if the nerve is not known to be injured, vocal cord paresis can occur postoperatively. Temporary paresis/paralysis of the nerve can last up to 3 months. Symptoms include voice changes and aspiration of liquids. Bilateral vocal cord paralysis requires tracheostomy. Long-term paralysis may be treated with synthetic injection such as Teflon, gel foam, or collagen; this technique is known as laryngoplasty.

Injury to the external branch of the superior laryngeal nerve can occur during the takedown of the superior pole of the thyroid. The result is minimization of high pitch, which may not be apparent except when singing and yelling.

Calcium balance disruption occurs postoperatively from parathyroid manipulation and devascularization. It is not uncommon to see hypocalcemia immediately after surgery, which can be supplemented with oral as well as intravenous calcium. Vitamin D is added if calcium addition alone is insufficient. This condition is temporary. However, if the parathyroids are known to be removed or permanently devascularized and no reimplantation occurs, permanent hypoparathyroidism is likely to occur. These patients will need lifelong calcium and Vitamin D supplementation.

Postoperative bleeding in the wound bed given the location is life-threatening. The expanding hematoma causes compression on the airway, and this surgical emergency should be addressed in the operating room.

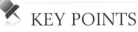 KEY POINTS

- The thyroid gland is a bilobed structure connected by an isthmus and derived from the migration of the first and second pharyngeal pouches from the base of the tongue.
- Grave's disease and toxic nodular goiter are the most common causes of hyperthyroidism.
- Grave's disease is an autoimmune disorder where the body's own immune system stimulates the thyroid-stimulating hormone receptor, whereas autoproduction of thyroid hormone not responding to thyroid-stimulating hormone is the mechanism of action in toxic nodular goiter.
- Patients must be made euthyroid before surgery.
- Evaluation of the thyroid nodule includes ultrasound and fine-needle aspiration.
- Fine-needle aspiration can be used to determine whether the lesion is benign, malignant, or indeterminate.
- Follicular lesions on fine-needle aspiration require minimal lobectomy for definitive classification. Elements of capsular or angioinvasion determine malignancy, which can only be seen on histology.
- Goiters are classified by a grading system developed by the World Health Organization. Patients with disease that is symptomatic or for which malignancy cannot be excluded, causes hyperthyroidism, or is progressively enlarging or cosmetically deforming are candidates for thyroidectomy.
- Thyroid cancer has a spectrum of well-differentiated to poorly differentiated cell types, with follicular cell origin being the most common. In descending order of incidence: papillary and its variants, follicular, and anaplastic. Medullary is from the C cells and has isolated familial form as well as association with multiple endocrine neoplasia 2A and 2B. Papillary and follicular cancers tend to have more favorable outcomes than medullary and anaplastic cancers.
- Surgical treatment is the mainstay for differentiated thyroid cancers but is rarely effective for aggressive anaplastic and lymphoma.
- Complications of surgery are related to the extent of surgery. These include injuries to the recurrent laryngeal nerve, external branch of superior laryngeal nerve, and parathyroids. Postoperative bleeding in the wound bed can be life-threatening.

13 Parathyroid Gland

The surgical treatment of parathyroid disease relates mainly to hyperparathyroidism.

ANATOMY

Parathyroid glands are normally small, yellowish-brown tissues measuring $2 \times 3 \times 5$ mm. Each gland on average weighs 30 to 40 mg. Pathologic glands, whether they are parathyroid adenomas or hyperplasia, appear grossly enlarged and reddish-brown. Both are hypercellular microscopically.

At least four parathyroid glands are present in all individuals, residing posterior to the thyroid. Embryologically, the upper or superior paired glands arise from the fourth branchial pouch, located in a plane posterior to the recurrent laryngeal nerve (RLN), usually within 1 cm where the RLN and inferior thyroidal artery cross. The lower or inferior paired glands along with the thymus arise from the third branchial pouch, located in a plane anterior to the RLN within 2 cm of the lower thyroid pole. Superior glands can also be found more lateral than inferior glands. All four glands receive their blood supply from the inferior thyroidal artery, sharing it with the thyroid gland (Figs. 13-1, 13-2, and 13-3).

Ectopic locations of parathyroid glands are based on embryology and are the key to localization. Aberrant lower glands rarely are intrathyroidal but can be found undescended, with thymic tissue high in the neck near the hyoid bone (Fig. 13-4).

PHYSIOLOGY

Parathyroid glands are endocrine organs regulating calcium and phosphate metabolism. The parathyroid hormone (PTH), which can be biochemically detected in its intact 84 amino acid form, works on bone as well as kidney tubules to increase blood calcium. PTH is regulated through a feedback system.

Hyperparathyroidism exists in several forms. Primary hyperparathyroidism (HPT) results from excess PTH, which causes mobilization of calcium deposits from bone, inhibition of renal phosphate reabsorption, and stimulation of renal tubular absorption of calcium. Overall, both total body calcium and phosphate wasting occur, leading to osteoporosis and bony mineral loss.

Secondary HPT is from hyperplasia of the parathyroid glands, occurring in those with chronic hypocalcemia, as is usually seen in patients with renal disease. The hyperphosphatemia suppresses calcium levels, leading to excess PTH production.

Tertiary HPT is the consequence of secondary HPT becoming autonomous. Long after a renal dialysis patient undergoes successful renal transplantation, the hyperplastic parathyroid glands will eventually function normally. Therefore, it is rare to intervene surgically.

Pseudohyperparathyroidism or humoral hypercalcemia of malignancy leads to hypercalcemia as well as hypophosphatemia similar to primary HPT; however, it is PTH-related protein that is the cause. This latter molecule is not detected in the assays for PTH. The malignancy causes hypercalcemia as a result of these mechanisms: PTH-related protein, lytic bone metastases, and ectopic calcitriol secretion.

EPIDEMIOLOGY

HPT is the most common cause of hypercalcemia, followed by malignant disease. The majority of HPT cases occur sporadically or in a nonfamilial form, often from a single hyperfunctioning gland or adenoma.

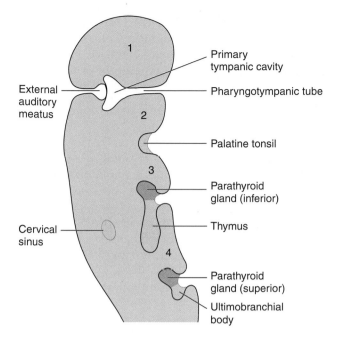

Figure 13-1 • The pharyngeal pouches. The inferior parathyroid arises from the third pouch and the superior arises from the fourth.

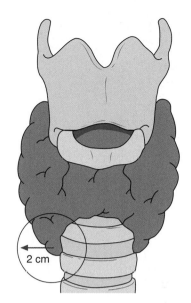

Figure 13-3 • Normal siting of the lower parathyroid glands.

Patients with multiple endocrine neoplasia 1 (involvement of the three Ps: parathyroid, pituitary, pancreas) and multiple endocrine neoplasia 2A (hyperparathyroidism, pheochromocytoma, and medullary cancer of the thyroid) have HPT involving multigland hyperplasia of the parathyroids.

PATHOLOGY

Solitary parathyroid adenoma accounts for 80% of primary HPT. Nearly 15% of cases are due to hyperplasia, where up to all four glands are involved. It is thought that single-gland disease and multigland disease lie within a spectrum. Double adenoma lies between solitary adenoma and hyperplasia. Parathyroid carcinoma is rare, occurring in fewer than 2% of cases. Typically the hypercalcemia is more

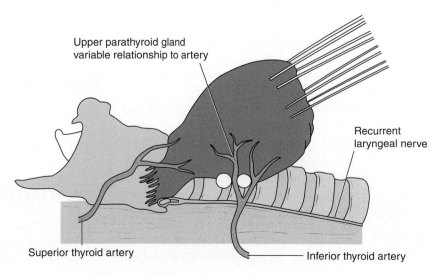

Figure 13-2 • Normal siting of the upper parathyroid glands.

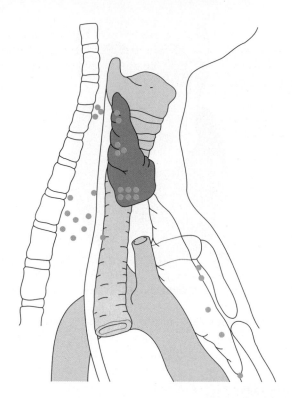

Figure 13-4 • Ectopic parathyroid gland locations secondary to aberrant migration.

pronounced in value and presentation. The lesions can be encapsulated like their benign counterparts but tend to be more ill defined, possibly invading the thyroid or nearby structures.

HISTORY

Historically, patients presented with long-term complications related to "stones, bones, groans, and moans."

- Renal stones/nephrocalcinosis
- Bones: aches and arthralgias
- Groans: abdominal pain from constipation, pancreatitis, or peptic ulcer disease
- Psychic moans: mood swings, fatigue, anxiety, or memory loss

Today's surgical treatment of parathyroid disease is seen more in asymptomatic individuals rather than those sustaining long-term complications. Presently it is not uncommon to see postmenopausal women who have abnormal bone mineral densitometry to detect osteoporosis be screened on calcium blood tests and are found to be normal or hypercalcemic. This then prompts a workup for hypercalcemia where the

PTH is elevated. The 2002 updated National Institutes of Health Consensus Development Conference on the Management of Asymptomatic Primary Hyperparathyroidism issued guidelines for surgery of the hyperparathyroid patient:

- Serum calcium >1.0 mg/mL above upper limit of normal
- >400 mg/d hypercalciuria
- Sequelae of hypercalcemia resulting from primary hyperparathyroidism, such as nephrolithiasis, osteitis fibrosa cystica, classic neuromuscular disease, severe psychoneurologic disorder
- Cortical bone density reduction with T score <2.5 standard deviation (SD) of lumbar spine, hip, or wrist
- <30% reduction of renal function in the absence of other cause
- Inability to have appropriate follow-up
- Age <50 years

PHYSICAL EXAMINATION

Rarely will any abnormalities be found on the physical examination, as the early diagnosis is captured biochemically. Should a palpable neck mass be associated with HPT, one would then suspect parathyroid carcinoma.

DIFFERENTIAL DIAGNOSIS

In addition to medical conditions associated with hypercalcemia that must be excluded, it is important to distinguish benign familial hypocalciuric hypercalcemia (BFHH) from HPT, as the former is not treated. Thus surgical intervention will be of no benefit. BFHH can present with hypercalcemia associated with mildly elevated PTH levels. The test of choice for exclusion of BFHH is presence of low urinary calcium (Table 13-1).

DIAGNOSTIC EVALUATION

A combination of elevated calcium and PTH levels is highly suggestive of primary HPT. Again, BFHH can be ruled out by presence of low urinary calcium.

TREATMENT

Primary HPT is a surgical disease, and only parathyroidectomy can successfully treat the disease. The success of the operation is measured by the return of

■ TABLE 13-1 Disease and Factors Causing Hypercalcemia

Hyperparathyroidism
Multiple myeloma
Sarcoid and other granulomatous diseases
Milk-alkali syndrome
Vitamin D intoxication
Vitamin A intoxication
Paget disease
Immobilization
Thiazide diuretics
Addisonian crisis
Familial hypocalciuric hypercalcemia

calcium to normal limits. Those with hypercalcemic crisis such as coma, delirium, anorexia, vomiting, and abdominal pain must be initially stabilized with vigorous intravenous hydration and forced diuresis with furosemide. Associated hypokalemia and hyponatremia must also be corrected.

Once HPT is confirmed, preoperative localization of the suspecting gland may be performed in an attempt to perform minimally invasive surgery or assist in determining whether the source is from adenoma versus hyperplasia. Moreover, localization studies are indicated in those undergoing reoperative surgery for persistent or recurrent HPT. The preferred modality is technetium (Tc)-sestamibi scanning, including oblique and single photon emission computed tomography scans, but ultrasound and computed tomography may also be complementary

To maximize the success of surgery, preoperative Tc-sestamibi scanning and intraoperative rapid PTH assay are recommended. The intraoperative rapid PTH assay is a means to monitor adequate removal of the abnormal parathyroid gland. Once the tumor is removed, PTH levels should decrease to <50% of the baseline value in as short as 10 minutes. These two modalities also allow for a minimally invasive approach, decreasing operative time and length of stay.

SURGERY

Traditionally, the four gland bilateral neck exploration has been implemented without prior localization studies. Recently, with the assistance of preoperative Tc-sestamibi where a single adenoma is localized, a patient may undergo minimally invasive surgery, during which the gland of concern is targeted via a smaller incision, sometimes under regional anesthesia and as an outpatient procedure under experienced hands. If level of experience is sufficient, endoscopic parathyroidectomy is also used.

If there is no localization preoperatively and ultrasound is also nonrevealing, the likely finding is hyperplasia. Four-gland exploration should be used. All four glands are identified in their usual locations before any removal; their size, appearance, and color will usually determine presence of abnormality without resorting to biopsy and pathologic confirmation. If all glands are hyperplastic, a subtotal parathyroidectomy, which is the equivalent to 3.5-gland removal, or total parathyroidectomy with autotransplantation is performed.

If a missing gland is not identified in its usual location, the search for ectopic sites should be performed. These ectopic sites are related to the embryologic development. Thymic and thyroidal tissues may need to be encompassed as well.

After surgery, although calcium levels may return to normal, the patient may still develop symptoms of hypocalcemia, such as perioral numbness/tingling, distal extremity paresthesias, and signs of a positive Chvostek, where the facial muscle twitches with tapping of the facial nerve. Calcium should be replenished, even if normal, in these instances.

KEY POINTS

- Hyperparathyroidism is the most common cause of hypercalcemia for which surgical intervention can successfully treat the disease.
- There are many forms of hyperparathyroidism; however, primary HPT is usually due to single-gland adenoma.
- Embryologic migration of parathyroid tissue determines resting location as well as ectopic sites.
- Hyperparathyroidism is diagnosed biochemically using blood studies as well as urine tests.
- Minimally invasive surgery is possible as a result of localization studies and rapid parathyroid hormone assay availability.

ANATOMY AND PHYSIOLOGY

The breast extends from the clavicle (approximately the second rib) to the sixth rib and from the sternum to the mid axillary line. Approximately 10 to 100 alveoli (secretory units) form lobules that drain into ducts, which eventually lead to the nipple. The breast is surrounded by fascia connected by the suspensory ligaments of Cooper.

The blood supply to the breast is mostly from anterior perforating branches of the internal mammary artery, various branches of the axillary artery, and posterior intercostal arteries. The lymphatic drainage is primarily to axillary lymph nodes, internal mammary lymph nodes, and interpectoral nodes of Rotter. Axillary lymph nodes are stratified into three levels depending on their location relative to the pectoralis minor muscle. Level I lymph nodes are lateral to the muscle. Level II lymph nodes are deep to (behind) the muscle, and level III lymph nodes are medial to the muscle (Fig. 14-1).

The nipple is innervated by T4, no matter how pendulous the breast. Although they do not innervate the breast, the long thoracic and thoracodorsal nerves are important because of their proximity to axillary lymph nodes. Injury to the long thoracic and thoracodorsal nerves during axillary nodal dissection may result in winged scapula or weakness in shoulder adduction, respectively. Additionally, the intercostal brachial cutaneous nerves pierce the tail of the breast parenchyma and, when divided, will cause paresthesias of the medial aspect of the upper arm.

Cyclic hormonal changes affect the breast. The breasts may feel lumpy and tender before menses. Pregnancy causes marked hypertrophy of the alveoli, lobules, and ducts in preparation for lactation. With menopause, the lobules become atrophic.

PATHOLOGY

Benign conditions of the breast include fibrocystic changes, fibroadenomas, simple cysts, intraductal papillomas, and gynecomastia. Phyllodes tumors can be benign, borderline, or malignant. High-risk and premalignant lesions include atypical ductal and lobular hyperplasia and lobular carcinoma in situ (LCIS). The most common malignancies are intraductal carcinoma (also known as ductal carcinoma in situ [DCIS], which is noninvasive because it does not penetrate the basement membrane), invasive ductal carcinoma, and invasive lobular carcinoma. Inflammatory breast cancer is characterized by skin involvement (invasion of the subdermal lymphatics). Paget disease of the nipple is an intraepithelial neoplasm that may be associated with an underlying breast cancer (invasive or in situ).

EPIDEMIOLOGY

Lifetime risk of American women for developing breast cancer is one in eight (12%). It is the most frequently diagnosed cancer in women and the second most frequent cause of cancer-related death among women. Incidence increases with age and varies among various ethnic groups: incidence of breast cancer in Hawaiians is greater than that in Whites, which is greater than that in Blacks, which is greater than that in Asians and Hispanics, which is greater than that in American Indians. Significant risk factors are female

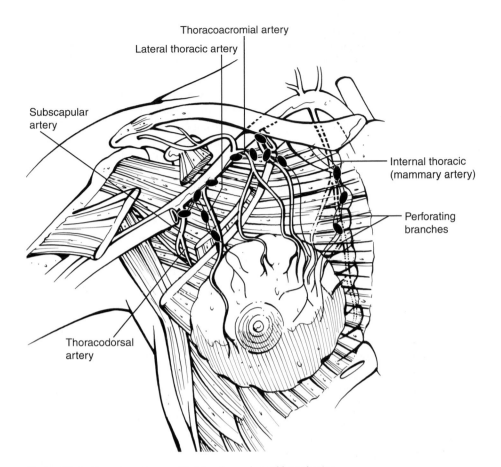

Figure 14-1 • Breast anatomy with blood supply and lymphatics.

sex, age, *BRCA* gene mutations, hormone replacement therapy, personal history of breast cancer, radiation to the chest at age younger than 40 years, first-degree relative with breast cancer (higher if the relative was premenopausal), and prior biopsy-proven LCIS or atypical hyperplasia (ductal or lobular). The incidence of breast cancer in men is 1%. The most common tumor in young women is fibroadenoma.

HISTORY

Most women report finding a breast lump while showering or with breast self-examination. Breast pain is usually associated with benign lesions, but may occasionally be present with malignant lesions. Lumps that increase before menses and decrease after menses are usually benign simple cysts or fibrocystic changes. Spontaneous or bloody nipple discharge is associated with intraductal papillomas. Malignant lesions do not vary in size with the menstrual cycle.

Patients with advanced stages may have weight loss, odor from ulcerating or fungating lesions, pain from bone metastasis (back, chest, or extremities), nausea or abdominal pain from liver metastasis, or headaches from brain metastasis.

PHYSICAL EXAMINATION

When examining the breasts, one looks for skin changes, asymmetry (visible bulge or dimpling of skin), nipple retraction, palpable masses, and lymphadenopathy in the axilla and supraclavicular fossa. Well-circumscribed, mobile, nontender lumps in young women are usually fibroadenomas or phyllodes tumors. Breast tenderness is associated with fibrocystic changes or simple cysts. Vague masses or firm lumps with indistinct borders are suggestive of malignancy. With advanced stages, there may be skin changes such as dimpling, peau d'orange (edema of the skin, making it look like an orange peel), ulceration, erythema, or fixation to the skin or chest wall. Enlarged or matted lymph nodes may indicate metastasis. Paget disease usually presents with nipple or areolar rash or excoriation. Inflammatory breast cancer may have erythema, peau d'orange, or skin thickening.

DIAGNOSTIC EVALUATION

With the increase in breast cancer awareness, screening mammograms initially led to an increase in breast cancer diagnoses. This increased incidence has subsequently reached a plateau. Screening mammograms have resulted in diagnosing breast cancer at an earlier stage, with improved survival and decreased mortality.

Mammograms miss 15% of palpable breast cancers and should be done in conjunction with clinical breast examination. Mammographic signs that suggest malignancy include a density with indistinct margins, spiculated mass (Fig 14-2), and clusters of or linear/branching microcalcifications. Lesions not seen on prior mammograms need further work up. Also, if the patient reports a palpable lump, then a diagnostic mammogram (additional views to magnify and/or compress the breast are obtained to identify or characterize the lesion) and breast ultrasound are performed.

Ultrasound can differentiate between solid and cystic masses (Fig. 14-3). It is not optimal for screening because it rarely detects microcalcifications and is extremely dependent on the experience of the person performing the examination.

Breast magnetic resonance imaging (MRI) is rapidly increasing in popularity. Current indications include identifying occult primary cancer with axillary metastasis in women with no clinical breast mass and normal mammogram, screening women at very high risk (>25%) for developing breast cancer, determining

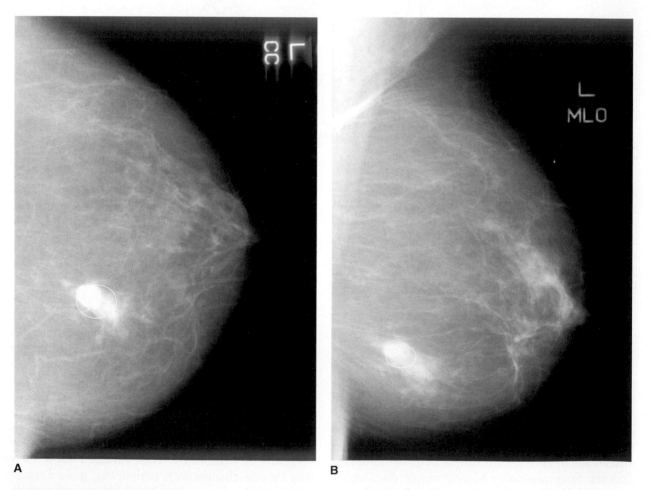

Figure 14-2 • Craniocaudal (CC) **(A)** and oblique (MLO) **(B)** views of mammogram showing a breast cancer (circle). Image courtesy of Rhona Chen, MD.

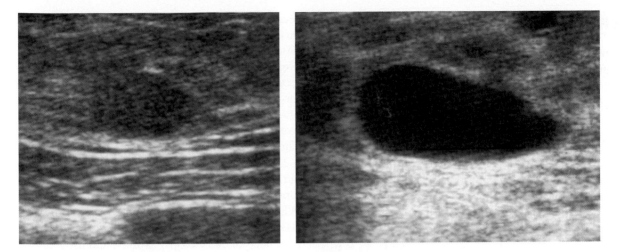

Figure 14-3 • Solid (fibroadenoma) and cystic (simple cyst) lesions on ultrasound.
Image courtesy of Rhona Chen, MD.

extent of breast cancer to help with surgical planning, and measuring response to neoadjuvant therapy. Advantages of breast MRI include creation of three-dimensional images, minimal or no breast compression, effectiveness in women with dense breasts, and high sensitivity for detecting breast cancer. Disadvantages are moderate to low specificity (false-positive results lead to unnecessary biopsies and patient anxiety), expensive cost, long time to perform examination (30 to 40 minutes, as compared with 5 to 10 minutes for mammogram), requirement of contrast, and inability to demonstrate microcalcifications.

Table 14-1 includes the American Cancer Society recommendations for breast cancer screening.

Lesions suggestive of malignancy on diagnostic examination are biopsied with image guidance: mammographic, ultrasonographic, or MRI guided core needle biopsy. Palpable masses not seen with imaging can be biopsied with fine-needle aspiration (FNA), core needle biopsy, excisional open biopsy, or incisional biopsy. A benign lesion can be observed radiographically and clinically. Malignant lesions require surgical consultation. If the pathology report shows atypia or LCIS or is discordant with radiologic or clinical findings, then an open biopsy should be performed. This may require wire localization by the radiologist. If the patient presents with skin changes over the breast mass, an incisional biopsy should be considered, taking an ellipse of skin with the mass to check for cancer involvement of dermal lymphatics.

If DCIS or invasive breast cancer is diagnosed pathologically, additional pathologic tests are performed. The tumor is checked for hormone receptors, HER-2/neu receptor, and, occasionally, various other biologic markers. Tumors with better prognostic indicators are well differentiated (low-grade cancer), have overexpression of estrogen receptors or progesterone receptors, and do not overexpress HER-2/neu receptor. The Oncogene DX test helps determine whether a woman will benefit from chemotherapy in borderline situations.

■ **TABLE 14-1** American Cancer Society Guidelines for Breast Cancer Screening
Yearly mammograms starting at the age of 40 years and continuing for as long as a woman is in good health.
Clinical breast examination should be part of a periodic health examination, about every 3 years for women in their 20s and 30s and every year for women 40 years and older.
Women should know how their breasts normally feel and report any breast change promptly to their health care providers. Breast self-examination is an option for women starting in their 20s.
Women at high risk (greater than 20% lifetime risk) should have magnetic resonance imaging (MRI) and a mammogram every year. Women at moderately increased risk (15%–20% lifetime risk) should talk with their doctors about the benefits and limitations of adding MRI screening to their yearly mammogram. Yearly MRI screening is not recommended for women whose lifetime risk of breast cancer is less than 15%.
Adapted from the American Cancer Society (www.cancer.org).

TREATMENT

Simple cysts may be aspirated if large or symptomatic. If the fluid is bloody, it should be sent for cytology to check for malignancy. If the cyst does not resolve completely after aspiration or recurs after three aspirations, it should be excised to rule out malignancy.

Solid lumps should be excised if enlarging or symptomatic or if other diagnostic studies have been inconclusive (pathology from image-guided biopsy is discordant with radiographic or clinical findings).

Treatment recommendations for LCIS have evolved from bilateral mastectomies to the current recommendation of close observation with annual mammogram and frequent clinical breast examination. LCIS is usually an incidental finding on a biopsy performed for other reasons. Although it does increase the risk for developing subsequent cancer in either breast, it is no longer thought to be a precursor of breast cancer.

For intraductal (noninvasive, in situ) or invasive breast cancers, surgical treatment options are breast-conserving therapy (lumpectomy with or without radiation therapy) or mastectomy. Lumpectomy is the removal of the cancer with a rim of normal breast tissue to obtain clear or negative margins to ensure the cancer has been completely removed. If there is cancer at the surgical margin, the patient should undergo re-excision to obtain clear margins or consider mastectomy. Mastectomy is the removal of the breast and nipple/areolar complex (from clavicle to rectus muscle and sternum to latissimus dorsi, taking pectoralis fascia with the breast tissue). Statistically, long-term survival is approximately the same, but local recurrence is slightly higher with breast-conserving therapy (BCT): 7% to 10% with radiation and up to 25% without radiation, as compared with mastectomy (3%). If the patient elects BCT and develops a recurrent cancer in the same breast, then mastectomy is usually recommended, especially if the breast has been previously irradiated.

Although BCT is being performed more often as a result of earlier stage at diagnosis, there are still some circumstances when mastectomy should be recommended: multicentric cancers (cancer in more than one quadrant of the breast), extensive high-grade DCIS, large tumor relative to size of breast where lumpectomy would result in poor cosmetic outcome, and when clear margins have not been obtained after re-excision.

In addition, lymph nodes should be checked for metastasis for staging purposes. Sentinel lymph node (SLN) biopsy is rapidly replacing the complete axillary lymph node dissection (CALND) for stage I and II breast cancer as the standard of care. SLN biopsy involves injection of a radioactive isotope and/or a vital blue dye (isosulfan blue or methylene blue) into the breast (subareolar, intradermal or intraparenchymal) to locate the first few draining lymph nodes the cancer is most likely to involve. The "hot" (radioactive) and/or blue lymph nodes are removed. The axilla is also palpated and any enlarged lymph nodes are also removed. The average number of sentinel lymph nodes removed is 2.8. The procedure is 97% accurate. If no SLN is found or if the SLN has metastasis, then CALND is performed, removing level I and II axillary lymph nodes. When CALND is performed with mastectomy, the procedure is called a modified radical mastectomy. The advantage of SLN biopsy is more intensive pathologic evaluation of fewer lymph nodes for more accurate staging and avoidance of lymphedema, which occurs in approximately 15% of patients who undergo CALND.

Radiation therapy is most commonly performed with external-beam irradiation to the breast and may include the axillary and supraclavicular nodal regions. Whole-breast radiation usually involves daily treatments over 4 to 6 weeks. Sometimes a boost dose is given to the lumpectomy site. Interest in partial breast irradiation has re-emerged with the advent of the Mammosite balloon. The balloon is inserted into the lumpectomy cavity and radioactive beads are implanted into the balloon (similar to brachytherapy). This permits high doses of radiation to be administered to the adjacent breast tissue in a shorter period of time (usually 4 to 5 days). The balloon is subsequently removed as a minor procedure.

Antiestrogen hormonal therapy is given to patients if breast cancer is estrogen or progesterone receptor positive. It can reduce the risk of recurrence by approximately 50%. Tamoxifen is given to premenopausal women. Aromatase inhibitors (e.g., anastrozole, letrozole, and exemestane) are now the recommended hormonal therapy for postmenopausal women because of the lower incidence of endometrial cancer and thromboembolic events. However, there is a higher incidence of osteoporosis and fractures. Ongoing clinical trials will determine whether premenopausal women will benefit from aromatase inhibitors. Sometimes premenopausal women are treated with chemical or surgical oophorectomy.

Chemotherapeutic options have also evolved. Doxorubicin (Adriamycin) and cyclophosphamide is used predominantly over the combination of cyclophosphamide, methotrexate, and fluorouracil. In addition, taxanes (taxoids) or anthracyclines may be added to the regimen. Trastuzumab (Herceptin), a monoclonal antibody, has been shown to improve survival in patients whose tumors test positive for the HER-2/neu receptor. Other monoclonal antibody drugs are currently being evaluated in clinical trials.

For patients who have mastectomy, reconstruction can be done immediately (at the same operation as the mastectomy) or delayed (requiring a second or third anesthetic). Reconstructive options include saline or silicone implants and a wide assortment of flaps. Flaps composed of muscle, subcutaneous fat, and skin can be transferred to the chest to recreate the breast mound. These can be pedicle flaps or free flaps. Latissimus

dorsi muscle or rectus muscle flaps are the most common. The nipple/areolar complex can also be recreated and tattooed, resulting in excellent cosmesis. If the patient is not interested in reconstruction, then an external prosthesis should be prescribed. This prevents neck, shoulder, and upper back pain from the body compensating for the uneven weight on the chest from the remaining breast.

Surgery and radiation therapy are performed for local control of breast cancer, whereas chemotherapy and hormonal therapy are initiated for systemic control. A select group of patients with small, low-grade DCIS may be treated by lumpectomy without radiation. Stage 0, I, and II breast cancers are usually treated with surgery first. The resulting pathology then guides subsequent adjuvant therapy (chemotherapy, hormonal therapy, radiation therapy, or a combination). Stage III and IV breast cancers are usually treated with neoadjuvant chemotherapy (and sometimes hormonal and/or radiation therapy) followed by surgery and radiation. Sometimes an advanced-stage breast cancer can be reduced in size to permit breast-conserving surgery. If the patient is a candidate, hormonal therapy may also be given preoperatively (neoadjuvant) or postoperatively once the chemotherapy and/or radiation therapy has finished.

Tables 14-2 and 14-3 show TNM Staging and American Joint Committee on Cancer Classification for Breast Cancer, respectively.

■ TABLE 14-2 TMN Staging for Breast Cancer

Stage	Description
Tumor	
TX	Primary tumor not assessable
T0	No evidence of primary tumor
Tis	Carcinoma in situ
T1	Tumor ≤2 cm in greatest dimension
T2	Tumor >2 cm but not >5 cm in greatest dimension
T3	Tumor >5 cm in greatest dimension
T4	Tumor of any size with direct extension into chest wall (not including pectoral muscles) or skin edema or skin ulceration or satellite skin nodules confined to the same breast or inflammatory carcinoma
Regional Lymph Nodes	
NX	Regional lymph nodes not assessable
N0	No regional lymph node involvement
N1	Metastasis to movable ipsilateral axillary lymph node(s)
N2	Metastasis to ipsilateral axillary lymph node(s) fixed to one another or to other structures
N3	Metastasis to ipsilateral internal mammary lymph nodes
Distant Metastasis	
MX	Presence of distant metastasis cannot be assessed
M0	No distant metastasis
M1	Distant metastasis present (including ipsilateral supraclavicular lymph nodes)

■ TABLE 14-3 AJCC Classification for Breast Cancer Based on TNM Criteria

Stage	Tumor	Nodes	Metastases
0	Tis	N0	M0
I	T1	N0	M0
IIA	T0, 1	N1	M0
	T2	N0	M0
IIB	T2	N1	M0
	T3	N0	M0
IIIA	T0, 1, 2	N2	M0
	T3	N1, 2	M0
IIIB	T4	N1, 2	M0
	Any T	N3	M0
IV	Any T	Any N	M1

AJCC, American Joint Committee on Cancer.
Adapted from *AJCC Cancer Staging Manual*. 6th ed. New York: Springer-Verlag, 2002.

■ TABLE 14-4 2004 Breast Cancer Prognosis Based on Stage

Stage	5 Years	10 Years
Localized	97%	94%
Regional	80%	66%
Distant	25%	<15%

From National Cancer Institute web site (www.cancer.gov), Surveillance, Epidemiology and End Results (SEER) fast stat results: SEER relative survival rates by stage at diagnosis for breast cancer, SEER 9 registries for 1988–2003.

As mentioned earlier, screening mammography has resulted in the diagnosis and treatment of earlier-staged breast cancers. In addition, improved understanding of molecular biology of breast cancer has resulted in the development and use of new hormonal and chemotherapeutic agents. All of this has resulted in longer survival rates and lower mortality (Table 14-4).

PROPHYLAXIS

In women with breast atypia and LCIS, clinical trials have shown that tamoxifen decreases the risk of developing breast cancer. Tamoxifen is usually administered for 5 years. Some experts postulate that it should be given longer. The Study of Tamoxifen and Raloxifene (STAR) trial showed that raloxifene is as effective as tamoxifen and is associated with 30% fewer thromboembolic events and 36% fewer uterine cancers.

For high-risk women who do not want to take drugs to reduce the risk of breast cancer, an alternative is prophylactic mastectomy. This reduces the risk of breast cancer by 97%.

KEY POINTS

- Breast cancer is the most frequently diagnosed cancer in women and the second most frequent cause of cancer death among women.

- Significant risk factors are female sex, age, *BRCA* gene mutations, hormone replacement therapy, personal history of breast cancer, radiation to the chest at age <40 years, first-degree relative with breast cancer (higher if the relative was premenopausal), and prior biopsy-proven LCIS or atypical hyperplasia (ductal or lobular).

- Screening mammography has resulted in earlier detection and treatment, improved survival, and decreased mortality. Screening magnetic resonance imaging is recommended in very high-risk women with mammography.

- Even if the mammogram is normal, a palpable abnormality should be evaluated further.

- Treatment options for breast cancer are lumpectomy and radiation (breast-conserving therapy) or mastectomy. Sentinel lymph node biopsy is rapidly replacing the axillary dissection for evaluation of lymph nodes.

- Chemoprophylaxis may be used in high-risk women to decrease the risk of breast cancer.

Pituitary, Adrenal, and Multiple Endocrine Neoplasias

PITUITARY

Anatomy and Pathophysiology

The pituitary gland is located at the base of the skull within the sella turcica, a hollow in the sphenoid bone. The optic chiasm lies anterior, the hypothalamus lies above, and cranial nerves III, IV, V, and VI and the carotid arteries lie in proximity. These structures are all at risk for compression or invasion from a pituitary tumor. Visual field defects can occur when a tumor encroaches on the optic chiasm. This most commonly presents as a bitemporal hemianopsia (Fig. 15-1). The gland weighs less than 1 g and is divided into an anterior lobe, or adenohypophysis (anterior-adeno), and a posterior lobe, or neurohypophysis. The anterior pituitary produces its own hormones—prolactin, growth hormone (GH), follicle-stimulating hormone (FSH), luteinizing hormone, adrenocorticotropin (ACTH), and thyrotropin—all under the control of hypothalamic hormones that travel directly from the hypothalamus through a portal circulation to the anterior pituitary (Fig. 15-2). The hormones of the posterior pituitary, vasopressin and oxytocin, are produced in the hypothalamus and are transported to the posterior lobe (Fig. 15-3).

PROLACTINOMA

Pathology

Most prolactin-secreting tumors are not malignant. Prolactin-secreting tumors are divided into macroadenomas (size >10 mm) and microadenomas (size <10 mm). Macroadenomas are characterized by gland enlargement, whereas microadenomas do not cause gland enlargement.

Epidemiology

Prolactinoma is the most common type of pituitary neoplasm. Macroadenomas are more common in men, whereas microadenomas are 10 times more common in women.

History

Macroadenomas usually produce headache as the tumor enlarges. Women may describe irregular menses, amenorrhea, or galactorrhea.

Physical Examination

Defects of extraocular movements occur in 5% to 10% of patients and reflect compromise of cranial nerves III, IV, or VI. Women may have galactorrhea, whereas only 15% of men have sexual dysfunction or gynecomastia.

Diagnostic Evaluation

A serum prolactin level of >300 µg/L establishes a diagnosis of pituitary adenoma, whereas a level >100 µg/L is suggestive. Magnetic resonance imaging (MRI) differentiates microadenomas from macroadenomas and allows characterization of local tumor growth (Fig. 15-4).

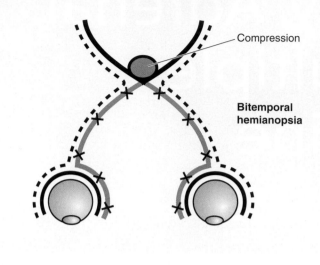

Bitemporal hemianopsia

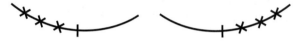

Figure 15-1 • Visual disturbances from compressive pituitary lesions.

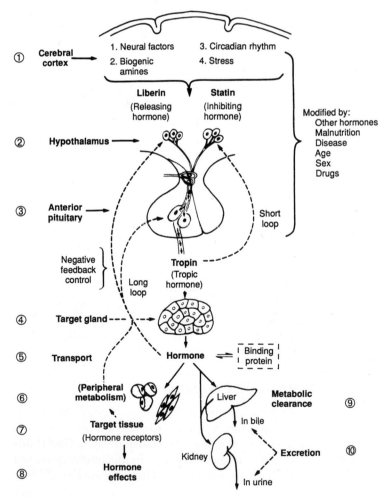

Anterior

Prolactin
Growth hormone
Follicle-stimulating hormone
Luteinizing hormone
Adrenocorticotropin
Thyrotropin

Posterior

Oxytocin
Vasopressin

Figure 15-2 • Pituitary hormones.

Figure 15-3 • Stimulation, production, control, and metabolism of hormones. (1) Stimulation of the cerebral cortex resulting in (2) stimulation of the hypothalamus to release tropic hormones from the anterior pituitary (3). The hormone circulates to a target gland (4), where a second hormone can be produced. This hormone is bound to transport or binding proteins (5) and can undergo peripheral metabolism (6) or bind to receptors in target tissues (7), which results in the specific hormone effect (8). Hormones can then be cleared metabolically (9) or excreted from the system (10). If the tropin acts on the hypothalamus, this is an example of the short-loop feedback, whereas if the hormone or peripheral metabolic products circulate to act on the hypothalamus, the control is termed long-loop negative feedback.
From Gornall AG, Luxton AW. Endocrine disorders. In: Gornall AG, ed. *Applied Biochemistry of Clinical Disorders.* 2nd ed. Philadelphia: Lippincott, 1986.

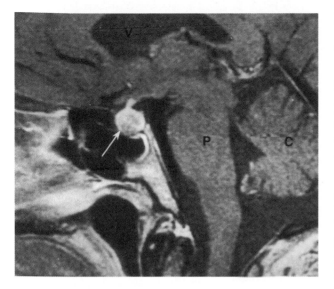

Figure 15-4 • Pituitary adenoma. A magnetic resonance sagittal view of the brain shows a distinct pituitary tumor (arrow). V, lateral ventricle; P, pons; C, cerebellum.
From Rubin E, Farber JL. *Pathology.* 3rd ed. Philadelphia: Lippincott Williams & Wilkins, 1999.

Treatment

Asymptomatic patients with microadenomas can be observed without treatment. When symptoms of hyperprolactinemia occur, a trial of bromocriptine or cabergoline should be initiated. In the event of failure, transsphenoidal resection provides an 80% short-term cure rate, although long-term relapse rate may be as high as 40%. For patients who desire children, transsphenoidal resection provides a 40% success rate for childbearing.

Management options for macroadenomas with compressive symptoms include bromocriptine, which may decrease the size of the tumor, and surgical resection, often in combination. Resection is associated with high recurrence rates. Radiation therapy is effective for long-term control but is associated with panhypopituitarism.

GROWTH HORMONE HYPERSECRETION

Pathogenesis

GH stimulates production of growth-promoting hormones, including somatomedins and insulin-like GH. Overproduction results in acromegaly, which is almost exclusively due to a pituitary adenoma, although abnormalities in hypothalamic production of GH-releasing hormone can also occur.

Epidemiology

Acromegaly has a prevalence of 40 per million.

History

Patients may complain of sweating, fatigue, headaches, voice changes, arthralgias, and jaw malocclusion. Symptoms usually develop over a period of years. The patient may have a history of kidney stones.

Physical Examination

The hallmark of the disease is bony overgrowth of the face and hands, with roughened facial features and increased size of the nose, lips, and tongue (Fig. 15-5). Signs of left ventricular hypertrophy occur in more than half of all patients, and hypertension is common.

Diagnostic Evaluation

Serum GH levels are elevated, and GH is not suppressed by insulin challenge. Insulin resistance may be present. An MRI should be obtained to delineate the extent of the lesion.

Treatment

Treatment options include resection, radiation, and bromocriptine. Surgical cure rates are approximately 75% in patients with lower preoperative GH levels but

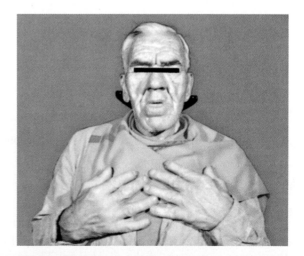

Figure 15-5 • Acromegaly is characterized by enlargement of the facial features (nose, ears) and the hands and feet.
From Weber J, Kelley J. *Health Assessment in Nursing.* 2nd ed. Philadelphia: Lippincott Williams & Wilkins; 2003:D10.1a.

only 35% in patients with high preoperative GH levels. Radiation is effective but slow and may result in panhypopituitarism. Bromocriptine can suppress GH production in combination with other treatment modalities; it is not usually effective as a single therapy.

FOLLICLE-STIMULATING HORMONE AND LUTEINIZING HORMONE HYPERSECRETION

Epidemiology

These tumors comprise approximately 4% of all pituitary adenomas.

History

Patients usually complain of headache or visual field changes from compression. Symptoms of panhypopituitarism may be present, as the tumors often grow to large size. Women have no symptoms that are attributable to oversecretion of FSH or LH. Men with FSH-secreting tumors may complain of depressed libido.

Physical Examination

The patient may have signs of compression of the structures surrounding the sella turcica.

Diagnostic Evaluation

Hormone levels are elevated.

Treatment

Surgery is necessary to relieve compression if it occurs.

THYROTROPIN AND ADRENOCORTICOTROPIN EXCESS

These diseases are discussed in their respective sections.

ADRENAL HYPERSECRETION

ANATOMY AND PHYSIOLOGY

The adrenal glands lie just above the kidneys, anterior to the posterior portion of the diaphragm. The right gland is lateral and just posterior to the inferior vena cava, whereas the left gland is inferior to the stomach and near the tail of the pancreas. The blood supply

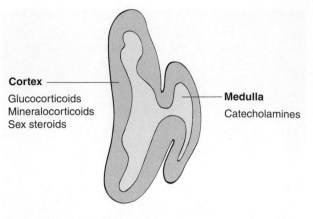

Cortex
Glucocorticoids
Mineralocorticoids
Sex steroids

Medulla
Catecholamines

Figure 15-6 • Adrenal hormones.

derives from the superior supra-adrenal, the middle supra-adrenal, and the inferior supra-adrenal coming from the inferior phrenic artery, the aorta, and the renal artery, respectively. Venous drainage on the right is to the inferior vena cava and on the left is to the renal vein.

The gland is divided into cortex and medulla. The cortex secretes glucocorticoids (cortisol), mineralocorticoids (aldosterone), and sex steroids, whereas the medulla secretes catecholamines (epinephrine, norepinephrine, and dopamine; Fig. 15-6). Cholesterol is the precursor for both glucocorticoids and mineralocorticoids through a variety of pathways, beginning with the formation of pregnenolone, the rate-limiting step for corticoid synthesis.

Cortisol is secreted in response to ACTH from the pituitary, which is, in turn, controlled by corticotropin-releasing factor secretion from the hypothalamus. Hypovolemia, hypoxia, hypothermia, and hypoglycemia stimulate cortisol production. Cortisol has many actions, including stimulation of glucagon release and inhibition of insulin release.

Exogenous glucocorticoids suppress the immune system and impair wound healing. They block inflammatory cell migration and inhibit antibody production, histamine release, collagen formation, and fibroblast function. These effects are significant causes of morbidity in patients maintained on corticosteroid therapy.

Aldosterone secretion is controlled by the renin-angiotensin system. In response to decreased renal blood flow or hyponatremia, juxtaglomerular cells secrete renin. This causes cleavage of angiotensinogen to angiotensin I, which in turn is cleaved to angiotensin II. Angiotensin II causes vasoconstriction and stimulates

CUSHING'S SYNDROME

Pathogenesis

Cushing's syndrome is due to overproduction of cortisol. In approximately 80% of patients, cortisol overproduction is secondary to ACTH hypersecretion. A pituitary adenoma is the cause in 80% of these patients (strictly termed "Cushing's disease"), whereas the remainder derive from other tumors, including small-cell carcinoma of the lung and carcinoid tumors of the bronchi and gut. Adrenal adenoma is the cause of cortisol hypersecretion in 10% to 20% of patients, whereas adrenal carcinoma and excess corticotropin-releasing factor production from the hypothalamus are unusual sources for increased cortisol production.

History

Patients may complain of weight gain, easy bruising, lethargy, and weakness.

Physical Examination

Patients have a typical appearance, with truncal obesity, striae, hirsutism, buffalo hump (accumulation of fat at the base of the neck), and moon facies (full, rounded face; Fig. 15-7). Hypertension, proximal muscle weakness, impotence or amenorrhea, osteoporosis, glucose intolerance, and ankle edema may be present.

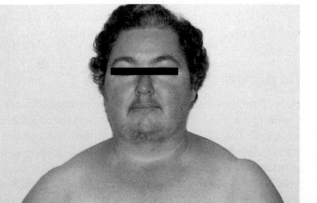

Figure 15-7 • Cushing's syndrome demonstrating hirsutism, moon facies, and a buffalo hump.

Diagnostic Evaluation

Increased cortisol production is most reliably demonstrated by 24-hour urine collection. Low ACTH levels suggest an adrenal source, as the autonomously secreted cortisol suppresses ACTH production. The dexamethasone suppression test is useful in differentiating among pituitary microadenomas, macroadenomas, and ectopic sources of ACTH. Dexamethasone is a potent inhibitor of ACTH release. In patients with pituitary microadenomas, dexamethasone is able to suppress ACTH production, whereas in other patient groups, this effect is not seen. Response to corticotropin-releasing hormone stimulation is accentuated when the source is pituitary but not when the source is adrenal or ectopic.

Treatment

Therapy is directed toward removing the source of increased cortisol production. For pituitary sources, resection is preferred. For an adrenal source, adrenalectomy is curative if the lesion is an adenoma. Resection should be attempted for adrenal carcinoma.

HYPERALDOSTERONISM (CONN'S SYNDROME)

Pathogenesis

Causes of excess secretion of aldosterone include adrenal adenoma (80%), idiopathic bilateral hyperplasia (15%), adrenal carcinoma (rare), or ectopic production (rare).

Epidemiology

The prevalence among patients with diastolic hypertension is one in 200.

History

Symptoms are usually mild and include fatigue and nocturia.

Physical Examination

Hypertension is the most common finding.

Diagnostic Evaluation

Hypokalemia occurs as sodium is preferentially reabsorbed in the distal tubule, causing kaliuresis. Aldosterone levels in serum and urine are increased, and serum renin levels are decreased. If hyperaldosteronism is demonstrated, computed tomography (CT) or MRI is used to evaluate the adrenals. In this setting, the presence of a unilateral adrenal mass >1 cm strongly suggests the diagnosis of adrenal neoplasm.

Treatment

Surgical excision is indicated for adenoma, whereas excision or debulking, or both, and chemotherapy are the treatments of choice for carcinoma. Pharmacologic therapy for patients with idiopathic bilateral hyperplasia usually includes a trial of potassium-sparing diuretics and dexamethasone.

EXCESS SEX STEROID PRODUCTION

Adrenal neoplasms can secrete excess sex steroids. Virilization suggests the lesion is malignant. Treatment is surgical removal.

ADRENAL INSUFFICIENCY

Pathogenesis

Long-term corticosteroid use can lead to suppression of the adrenal cortex. In the setting of surgical stress, the cortex may not be able to respond with the appropriate release of glucocorticoids and mineralocorticoids. These patients are at risk for Addison's disease or acute adrenal insufficiency, which is life-threatening.

History

Patients complain of abdominal pain and vomiting.

Physical Examination

Obtundation may occur. Hypotension, hypovolemia, and hyperkalemia can lead to shock and cardiac arrhythmias.

Treatment

Preoperative identification of patients at risk for adrenal suppression is critical, and perioperative corticosteroids are necessary. The corticosteroids should be continued if the patient is in critical condition.

PHEOCHROMOCYTOMA

Pathophysiology

This tumor produces an excess of catecholamines.

Epidemiology

Pheochromocytoma is a rare tumor. It occurs most commonly in the third and fourth decades, with a slight female predominance. Approximately 5% to 10% occur in association with syndromes, including the multiple endocrine neoplasias types IIa and IIb. Approximately 10% are malignant. Pheochromocytoma is the cause of hypertension in fewer than 0.2% of patients. The catecholamine source is most commonly the adrenals but can occur elsewhere in the abdomen (10%) or outside the abdomen (2%).

History

Patients may complain of headaches, tachycardia or palpitations, anxiety, sweating, chest or abdominal pain, and nausea either in paroxysms or constant in nature. Physical exertion, tyramine-containing foods, nicotine, succinylcholine, and propranolol can precipitate attacks.

Diagnostic Evaluation

Systolic blood pressure can be marked by peaks approaching 300 mm Hg but may be normal on a single reading. Diagnosis is established by elevated urinary epinephrine and norepinephrine, as well as their metabolites, metanephrine, normetanephrine, and vanillylmandelic acid. CT or MRI yields information about tumor size and location (Fig. 15-8). Nuclear medicine scan using radioactive metaiodobenzylguanidine is especially useful for finding extra-adrenal tumors.

Treatment

Pheochromocytomas are removed surgically (see Color Plate 12). Preoperative preparation is critical to ensure that the patient does not have a hypertensive crisis in the operating room. Alpha blockade with phenoxybenzamine or phentolamine is usually combined with beta blockade. It is important to establish alpha blockade first. Isolated beta blockade in the setting of catecholamine surge can produce shock, as cardiac function is prevented from increasing while systemic vascular resistance increases.

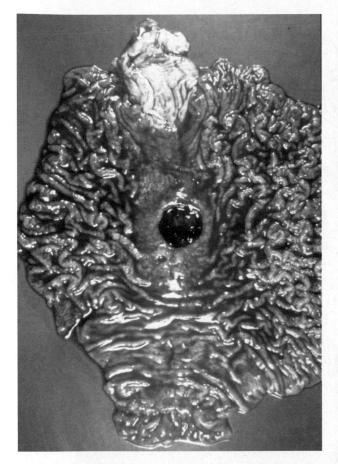

Color Plate 1 • Gastric ulcer. The stomach has been opened to reveal a sharply demarcated, deep peptic ulcer on the lesser curvature.
From Rubin E, Farber JL. *Pathology*. 3rd ed. Philadelphia, PA: Lippincott Williams & Wilkins, 1999.

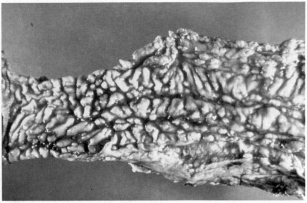

Color Plate 2 • Crohn's disease. The mucosal surface of the colon displays a "cobblestone" appearance owing to the presence of linear ulcerations and edema and inflammation of the intervening tissue.
From Rubin E, Farber JL. *Pathology*. 3rd ed. Philadelphia, PA: Lippincott Williams & Wilkins, 1999.

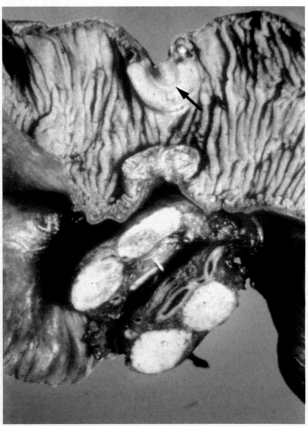

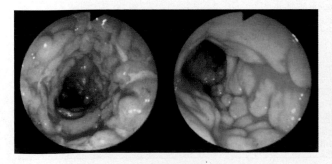

Color Plate 3 • Crohn's disease. Active phase of Crohn's disease shows cobblestoning, caused by interconnecting ulcerations (left). An area of cobblestoning after therapy is shown on the right.
From Yamada T, Alpers DH, Kaplowitz N, et al. *Atlas of Gastroenterology*. 3rd ed. Philadelphia, PA: Lippincott Williams & Wilkins, 2003.

Color Plate 4 • Carcinoid tumor of the small intestine. A bisected annular carcinoid tumor (arrows) constricts the lumen of the small intestine. Lymph node metastases are evident.
From Rubin E, Farber JL. *Pathology*. 3rd ed. Philadelphia, PA: Lippincott Williams & Wilkins, 1999.

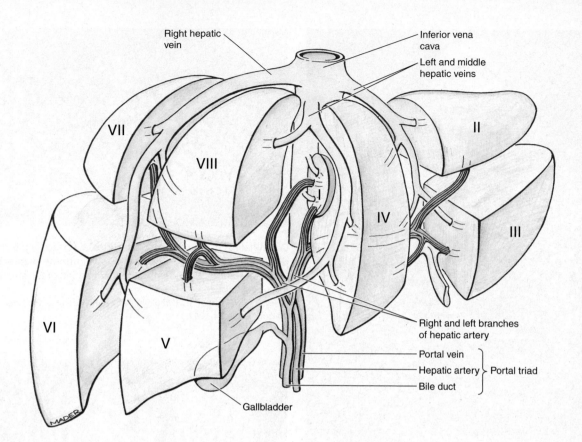

Right hepatic vein

Inferior vena cava

Left and middle hepatic veins

Right and left branches of hepatic artery

Portal vein ⎱
Hepatic artery ⎰ Portal triad
Bile duct ⎰

Gallbladder

VII VIII I II IV III VI V

Schema of Terminology for Subdivisions of the Liver

Anatomical Term	Right Lobe				Left Lobe	Caudate Lobe	
Functional/ Surgical Term**	Right (part of) Liver [Right portal lobe*]		Left (part of) Liver [Left portal lobe⁺]			Posterior (part of) Liver	
	Right lateral division	Right medial division	Left medial division	Left lateral division		[Right caudate lobe*]	[Left caudate lobe⁺]
	Posterior lateral segment **Segment VII** [Posterior superior area]	Posterior medial segment **Segment VIII** [Anterior superior area]	[Medial superior area]

Left medial segment **Segment IV**

[Medial inferior area = quadrate lobe] | Lateral segment **Segment II** [Lateral superior area] | | Posterior segment **Segment I** | |
| | Right anterior lateral segment **Segment VI** [Posterior inferior area] | Anterior medial segment **Segment V** [Anterior inferior area] | | Left lateral anterior segment **Segment III** [Lateral inferior area] | | | |

** The labels in the table and figure above reflect the new *Terminologia Anatomica: International Anatomical Terminology*.
Previous terminology is in brackets.

*⁺ Under the schema of the previous terminology, the caudate lobe was divided into right and left halves.

* The right half of the caudate lobe was considered a subdivision of the right portal lobe.

⁺ The left half of the caudate lobe was considered a subdivision of the left portal lobe.

Color Plate 5 • Hepatic segmentation. **A.** The segmental anatomy of the liver is based on the blood supply. Segment I is the caudate lobe. Segments II, III, and IV are part of the left lobe, and segments V, VI, VII, and VIII are part of the right lobe.
From Moore KL, Dalley AF. *Clinically Oriented Anatomy*. 4th ed. Baltimore, MD: Lippincott Williams & Wilkins, 1999.

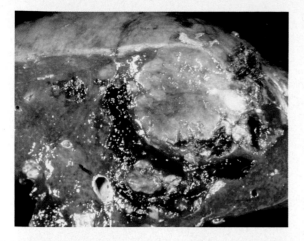

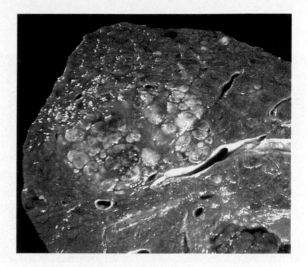

Color Plate 6 • Hepatic adenoma. A surgically resected portion of liver shows a tan, lobulated mass beneath the liver capsule. Hemorrhage into the tumor has broken through the capsule and also into the surrounding liver parenchyma. The patient was a woman who had taken birth control pills for a number of years and presented with sudden intraperitoneal hemorrhage.
From Rubin E, Farber JL. *Pathology.* 3rd ed. Philadelphia, PA: Lippincott Williams & Wilkins, 1999.

Color Plate 7 • Hepatocellular carcinoma. Cross-section of a cirrhotic liver shows a poorly circumscribed, nodular area of yellow, partially hemorrhagic hepatocellular carcinoma.
From Rubin E, Farber JL. *Pathology.* 3rd ed. Philadelphia, PA: Lippincott Williams & Wilkins, 1999.

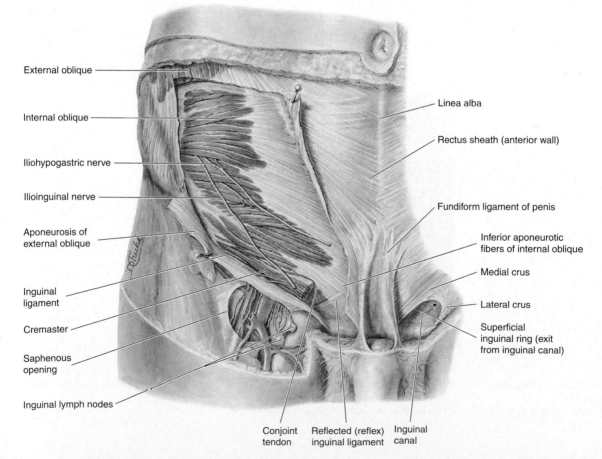

Color Plate 8 • Inguinal region of a male. The aponeurosis of the external oblique is partly cut away and the spermatic cord has been cut and removed from the inguinal canal. The reflected (reflex) inguinal ligament is formed by aponeurotic fibers of the external oblique. Observe the iliohypogastric and ilioinguinal nerves (branches of the first lumbar nerve) passing between the external and internal oblique muscles. The ilioinguinal nerve is vulnerable during repair of an inguinal hernia.
From Moore KL, Dalley AF. *Clinically Oriented Anatomy.* 4th ed. Baltimore, MD: Lippincott Williams & Wilkins 1999.

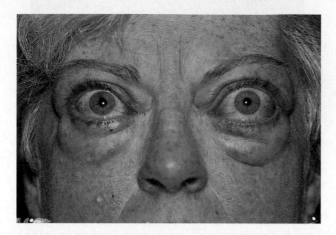

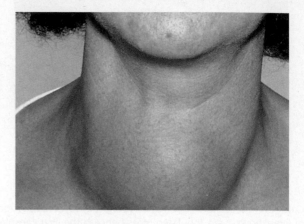

Color Plate 9 • Thyroid-related ophthalmopathy with proptosis, lid retraction, and limited motility.

From Tasman W, Jaeger E. *The Wills Eye Hospital Atlas of Clinical Ophthalmology.* 2nd ed. Philadelphia, PA: Lippincott Williams & Wilkins, 2001.

Color Plate 10 • Diffuse enlargement of the thyroid gland.

From Weber J, Kelley J. *Health Assessment in Nursing.* 2nd ed. Philadelphia, PA: Lippincott Williams & Wilkins, 2003.

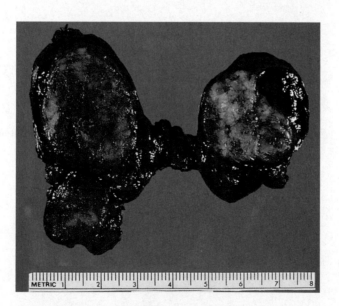

Color Plate 11 • Medullary thyroid carcinoma. Coronal section of a total thyroid resection shows bilateral involvement by a firm, pale tumor.

From Rubin E, Farber JL. *Pathology.* 3rd ed. Philadelphia, PA: Lippincott Williams & Wilkins, 1999.

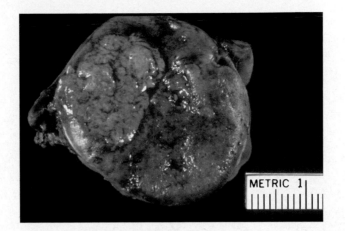

Color Plate 12 • Pheochromocytoma. The cut surface of an adrenal tumor from a patient with episodic hypertension is reddish brown with a prominent area of fibrosis. Foci of hemorrhage and cystic degeneration are evident.
From Rubin E, Farber JL. *Pathology*. 3rd ed. Philadelphia, PA: Lippincott Williams & Wilkins, 1999.

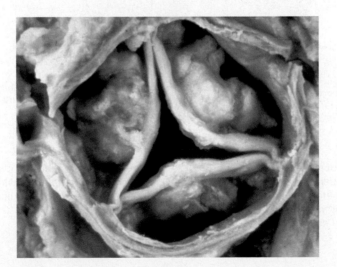

Color Plate 13 • Calcific aortic stenosis. Large deposits of calcium salts are evident in the cusps and the free margins of the thickened aortic valve, viewed from above.
From Rubin E, Farber JL. *Pathology*. 3rd ed. Philadelphia, PA: Lippincott Williams & Wilkins, 1999.

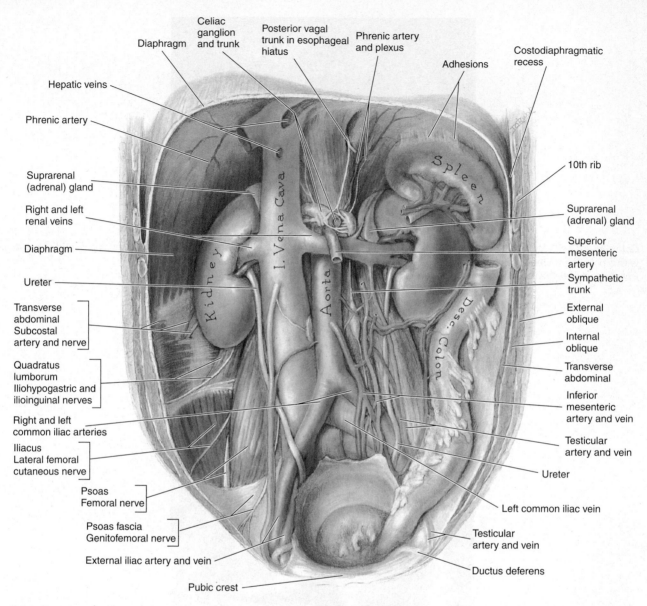

Diaphragm

Celiac ganglion and trunk

Posterior vagal trunk in esophageal hiatus

Phrenic artery and plexus

Adhesions

Costodiaphragmatic recess

Hepatic veins

Phrenic artery

Suprarenal (adrenal) gland

Right and left renal veins

Diaphragm

Ureter

Transverse abdominal Subcostal artery and nerve

Quadratus lumborum Iliohypogastric and ilioinguinal nerves

Right and left common iliac arteries

Iliacus Lateral femoral cutaneous nerve

Psoas Femoral nerve

Psoas fascia Genitofemoral nerve

External iliac artery and vein

Pubic crest

Spleen

Kidney

I. Vena Cava

Aorta

Desc. Colon

10th rib

Suprarenal (adrenal) gland

Superior mesenteric artery

Sympathetic trunk

External oblique

Internal oblique

Transverse abdominal

Inferior mesenteric artery and vein

Testicular artery and vein

Ureter

Left common iliac vein

Testicular artery and vein

Ductus deferens

Color Plate 14 • Posterior abdominal wall showing great vessels, kidneys, and suprarenal glands. Most of the fascia has been removed. Observe that the ureter crosses the external iliac artery just beyond the common iliac bifurcation and that the testicular vessels cross anterior to the ureter and join the ductus deferens (vas deferens) to enter the inguinal canal. Renal arteries are not seen because they lie posterior to the renal veins.

From Moore KL, Dalley AF. *Clinically Oriented Anatomy.* 4th ed. Baltimore, MD: Lippincott Williams & Wilkins, 1999.

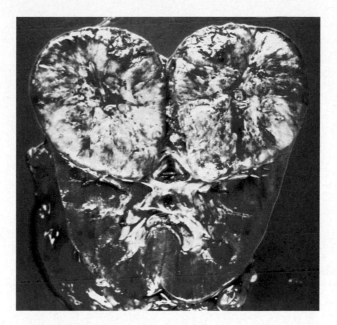

Color Plate 15 • Renal cell carcinoma. The kidney contains a large irregular neoplasm with a variegated cut surface, including yellow areas that correspond to lipid-containing cells.
From Rubin E, Farber JL. *Pathology*. 3rd ed. Philadelphia, PA: Lippincott Williams & Wilkins, 1999.

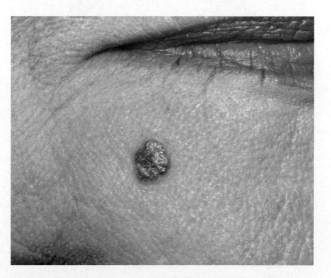

Color Plate 16 • Pigmented basal cell carcinoma. Note the pearly, waxy surface.
From Goodheart HP. *Goodheart's Photoguide of Common Skin Disorders*. 2nd ed. Philadelphia, PA: Lippincott Williams & Wilkins, 2003.

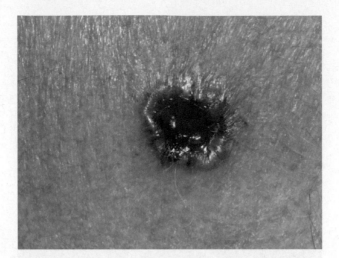

Color Plate 17 • Nodular basal cell carcinoma. Note the rolled borders with telangiectasia.
From Goodheart HP. *Goodheart's Photoguide of Common Skin Disorders.* 2nd ed. Philadelphia, PA: Lippincott Williams & Wilkins, 2003.

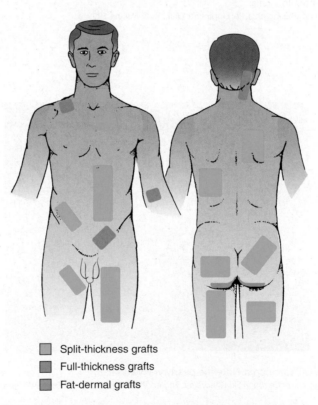

Split-thickness grafts
Full-thickness grafts
Fat-dermal grafts

Color Plate 18 • Common donor skin graft sites. Blue skin areas are appropriate for full-thickness grafts; green areas are used for split-thickness grafts and rose sites are used for fat-dermal grafts.
From Smeltzer SC, Bare BG. *Textbook of Medical-Surgical Nursing.* 9th ed. Philadelphia, PA: Lippincott Williams & Wilkins, 2000.

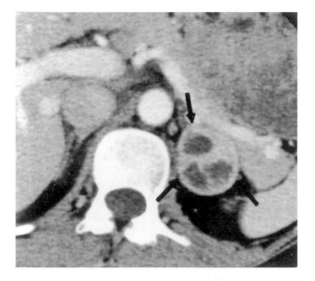

Figure 15-8 • Computed tomography scan demonstrating a pheochromocytoma.

INCIDENTAL ADRENAL MASS

Approximately 1% of CT scans obtained for any reason reveal an adrenal mass, making the incidental adrenal mass a common clinical scenario. Workup includes a thorough history to find symptoms of Cushing's syndrome, hyperaldosteronism, or pheochromocytoma. Laboratory evaluation includes urine for 24-hour urinary-free cortisol, dexamethasone suppression test, serum sodium and potassium, and epinephrine, norepinephrine, and their metabolites. Resection is recommended for evidence of metabolite activity either by symptoms or by laboratory evaluation or if the mass is larger than 4 cm.

MULTIPLE ENDOCRINE NEOPLASIAS

Multiple endocrine neoplasia (MEN) I consists of the three P's: parathyroid hyperplasia, pancreatic islet cell tumors, and anterior pituitary adenomas. It is a rare genetic disorder, inherited in an autosomal dominant manner, affecting approximately 20 people per million. Parathyroid hyperplasia is the most common manifestation of the syndrome and occurs in 90% of cases. Pancreatic neoplasms occur in 50%. These are most commonly gastrinoma, but tumors of cells producing insulin, glucagon, somatostatin, and vasoactive intestinal peptide can also occur. The anterior pituitary tumor is most commonly prolactin-secreting and occurs in approximately 25% of patients.

A consensus panel established the diagnosis as the presence of at least two of these tumor types. When one relative exhibits at least one of the tumor types the diagnosis of familial MEN I is made. The syndrome is caused by a defect in the *MENI* gene, also called menin, which resides on the long end of chromosome 11. The exact pathogenesis is unknown.

Compared with sporadic hyperparathyroidism, in these patients, this aspect of the disease generally presents earlier and with no female predilection. The defect driving hyperparathyroidism seems to be persistent and diffuse, causing multifocality and high recurrence rates after parathyroidectomy.

Patients generally present with hypercalcemia, and most commonly complain of gastrointestinal symptoms, including constipation and vague abdominal discomfort. Renal colic may be caused by nephrolithiasis. Psychiatric complaints of depression, anxiety, or cognitive defects may occur. Gout, pseudogout, and chondrocalcinosis may also be present. Hypertension and accelerated atherosclerosis are common. Diagnosis is based on hypercalcemia in the presence of elevated parathyroid hormone levels.

Pituitary adenomas in these patients are most commonly prolactinomas, but different kindreds may have other tumors that predominate. When associated with MEN I, these tumors tend to be larger and more aggressive than sporadic cases.

Because treatments for hyperparathyroidism and pituitary adenomas are well established, pancreatic tumors are the major threat to long-term survival for these patients. Major tumor types are gastrinoma, insulinoma, and other nonfunctioning pancreatic tumors. These lesions are discussed in their respective sections in Chapter 9, Pancreas.

Treatment of MENI generally follows treatment recommendations for the individual tumors. Subtotal parathyroidectomy should be performed for marked hypercalcemia, nephrolithiasis, or decreased bone density. Pituitary tumors are treated as described for sporadic cases. Survival with gastrinoma may not be improved with resection; medical therapy only may be appropriate in select patients. Patients with insulinoma should generally be offered resection depending on tumor location; options include local resection of pancreatic head tumors and subtotal distal pancreatectomy.

MEN II is a rare disease, with a prevalence of approximately 25 people per million. It is divided into MEN IIa, IIb, and familial medullary thyroid cancer. The syndrome is inherited in an autosomal dominant fashion and is due to a defect in a protein on chromosome 10 that codes for a *RET* proto-oncogene. This is a

■ **TABLE 15-1** Multiple Endocrine Neoplasias (MEN)

MEN I
Parathyroid hyperplasia
Pancreatic islet cell tumors
Anterior pituitary adenoma
MEN IIa
MTC
Pheochromocytoma
Parathyroid hyperplasia
MEN IIb
MTC
Pheochromocytoma
Mucosal neuromas
MTC, medullary thyroid carcinoma.

receptor tyrosine kinase that is involved in cell growth and differentiation. Because the hallmark of this disease is medullary thyroid carcinoma (MTC), a potentially fatal lesion that can be prevented by early thyroidectomy when the patient is still a child, screening is essential in high-risk populations to make the diagnosis early.

MEN IIa consists of MTC, pheochromocytoma, and parathyroid hyperplasia. MTC occurs in almost all affected patients. Diagnosis is often started with a thyroid nodule or cervical lymphadenopathy, although it is also commonly found as a result of screening in patients with the appropriate family history. Pheochromocytoma occurs in 40% of patients with MEN IIa. This entity should be treated first because it can complicate treating other aspects of this syndrome, although it is unusual for this to occur before the onset of MTC.

MEN IIb consists of MTC, pheochromocytoma, and mucosal neuromas, with characteristic body habitus, including thick lips, kyphosis, and pectus excavatum. Diagnosis and treatment follow treatment for the individual lesions (Table 15-1).

KEY POINTS

- Prolactinoma is the most common pituitary tumor and is usually not malignant.
- The diagnosis of acromegaly is based on characteristic appearance and elevated growth hormone levels; treatment options include surgery, radiation, and bromocriptine.
- Cushing's syndrome results from overproduction of cortisol, most commonly due to adrenocorticotropin overproduction from a pituitary tumor.
- Adrenal adenoma is the most common cause of hyperaldosteronism.
- Patients on corticosteroids preoperatively must be identified and perioperative corticosteroids considered to avoid life-threatening adrenal insufficiency.
- Patients with pheochromocytoma may present with paroxysms of headache, flushing, and anxiety. Diagnosis is made on urine examination for catecholamines and catecholamine metabolites.
- Establishing alpha blockade before beta blockade is imperative to prevent cardiovascular collapse.
- Incidental adrenal masses should be excised if they have symptomatic or biochemical evidence of activity or if they are >4 cm in diameter.
- Multiple endocrine neoplasia (MEN) I consists of parathyroid hyperplasia, pancreatic islet cell tumors, and anterior pituitary adenomas. MEN IIa consists of medullary thyroid carcinoma, pheochromocytoma, and parathyroid hyperplasia. MEN IIb consists of medullary thyroid carcinoma, pheochromocytoma, and mucosal neuromas.

Part IV

Cardiac, Thoracic, and Vascular

Vascular Surgery

ANEURYSMS AND DISSECTIONS

An aneurysm is an abnormal dilation of an artery. Saccular aneurysms occur when a portion of the artery forms an outpouching, or "mushroom." Fusiform aneurysms occur when the entire arterial diameter grows. True aneurysms involve all layers of the arterial wall: intima, media, and adventitia. An artery is considered aneurysmal if the diameter is >1.5 times its normal size. Otherwise, an enlarged artery is considered ectatic.

In contrast, a dissection occurs when a defect in the intima allows blood to enter between layers of the wall (Fig. 16-1). Blood pressure then causes the layers of the wall to separate from one another. The serious nature of aneurysms and dissections is due to the weakened vessel wall and the potential for catastrophic events. In the case of an aneurysm, this includes rupture or vascular compromise; dissections can result in the occlusion of the ostia of visceral arteries or progress into the heart and can affect the coronary circulation or lead to tamponade.

ABDOMINAL AORTIC ANEURYSM

Anatomy

The abdominal aorta lies below the diaphragm and above the iliac arteries. Branches include the celiac trunk, superior mesenteric artery, inferior mesenteric artery, renal arteries, and gonadal arteries. Approximately 95% of abdominal aneurysms begin distal to the takeoff of the renal arteries.

Etiology

Ninety-five percent of aneurysms of the abdominal aorta are associated with atherosclerosis. Other causes include trauma, infection, syphilis, and Marfan's syndrome. Protease activity in the vessel wall is commonly increased.

Epidemiology

Abdominal aortic aneurysms are responsible for 15,000 deaths per year. The incidence is approximately 0.05%, but in selected high-risk populations, the incidence increases to 5%. Men are affected 10 times more frequently than women, with an age of onset usually between 50 and 70 years. Risk factors include atherosclerosis, hypertension, hypercholesterolemia, smoking, and obesity. The disease is associated with peripheral vascular disease, heart disease, and carotid artery disease.

History

Most aneurysms are asymptomatic. Pain usually signifies a change in the aneurysm—commonly enlargement, rupture, or compromise of vascular supply—and should therefore be considered an ominous symptom. Pain may occur in the abdomen, back, or flank. The legs could be involved if the aneurysm includes the iliac arteries or if an embolic event occurs. The pain is usually sudden in onset and does not remit.

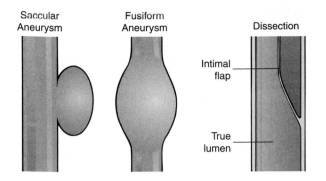

Saccular Aneurysm | Fusiform Aneurysm | Dissection

Intimal flap

True lumen

Figure 16-1 • Aneurysms and dissections.

■ **TABLE 16-1** Ankle-Brachial Index	
Aneurysm Size	**Risk of Rupture per Year**
<5 cm	4%
5–7 cm	7%
>7 cm	19%

Physical Examination

Abdominal examination may reveal a pulsatile abdominal mass. Enlargement, rupture, or compromise of vascular supply may manifest by tenderness, hypotension, tachycardia, or a change in the location or intensity of pain. In addition, the lower extremities may have pallor, cool temperature or pulses that are diminished or unequal.

Diagnostic Evaluation

Ultrasound is an accurate, noninvasive method to assess the size of the aneurysm and the presence of clot within the arterial lumen. Computed tomography (CT) or magnetic resonance imaging provides anatomic detail and precise localization of the aneurysm. An aortogram may be helpful in planning surgical intervention to demonstrate involvement of other vessels, specifically the renal, mesenteric, and iliac arteries.

Treatment

If the patient is asymptomatic, workup can proceed electively. Treatment of asymptomatic abdominal aortic aneurysms depends on the size of the lesion, which is directly proportional to its propensity to grow, leak, or rupture. Aneurysms <4 cm in diameter are unlikely to rupture, and medical management with antihypertensives, preferably beta-blockers, is advocated. When the aneurysm reaches approximately 4 to 5 cm, two options are available: early operation or close follow-up. A recent randomized trial suggests that mortality is the same in both options. When the aneurysm reaches 5 cm in diameter, the incidence of rupture is >25% at 5 years, and repair is recommended, unless the patient is at prohibitive operative risk. Table 16-1 lists rupture rates per year based on aneurysm size. Treatment options have recently expanded with the advent of stent grafts that can be placed through the femoral artery. In selected patients, these stents carry less morbidity than traditional operative repair. Concerns include stent migration and leaks around the prosthesis, but in general, these complications can be managed effectively. Technologic advances and clinical experience are widening the versatility of these stents, allowing the placement of fenestrated stents with orifices for visceral vessels and stents with limbs that can be placed at arterial bifurcations.

Any patient presenting on physical examination with symptoms that suggest a catastrophic aortic event should undergo emergent diagnostic workup or intervention. Once the diagnosis of ruptured or leaking abdominal aortic aneurysm is determined, arrangements should be made for fluid resuscitation and immediate operative intervention.

Repair of Abdominal Aortic Aneurysm: The Operation

Consistent with the size of the operation, preoperative preparation includes large-bore intravenous lines, central monitoring, and intravenous antibiotics. Blood, either autologous or cross-matched, should be available. Abdominal aortic aneurysms can be approached via either a midline incision or an oblique incision over the left 11th intercostal space. Using a midline incision requires mobilization of the small bowel to the patient's right. Incision of the posterior peritoneum to the left of the aorta allows exposure of the entire aorta. The oblique incision is reserved for a retroperitoneal approach, in which the entire contents of the peritoneal cavity are mobilized to the right, allowing exposure of the aorta. Proximal and distal control around the aneurysm is obtained, and heparin is administered before clamping. A graft is placed using permanent sutures. If a transabdominal

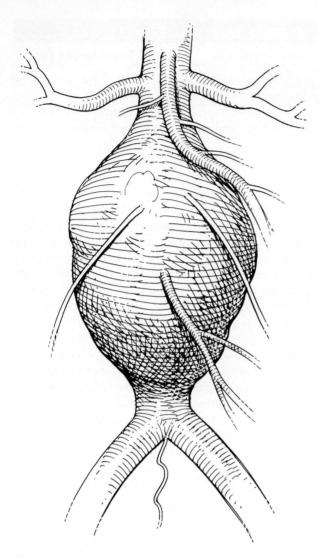

Figure 16-2 • Aneurysm, aortic: abdominal aneurysm of the descending aorta.

approach is used, the peritoneum is closed over the graft if possible (Fig. 16-2).

THORACIC AORTIC ANEURYSM

Anatomy

The thoracic aorta lies between the heart and the diaphragm. It gives rise to the brachiocephalic, left common carotid, left subclavian, bronchial, esophageal, and intercostal arteries.

Etiology

Thoracic aortic aneurysms are caused by cystic medial necrosis, atherosclerosis, or, less commonly, trauma, dissection, or infection.

Epidemiology

Males are affected three times as often as females. Risk factors include atherosclerosis, smoking, hypertension, and family history.

History

Most aneurysms are asymptomatic. Rupture usually presents with chest pain or pressure. Expansion of the aneurysm can compress the trachea, leading to cough, or erode into the trachea or bronchus, causing massive hemoptysis. An aneurysm close to the aortic valve can cause dilation of the annulus, resulting in aortic valve insufficiency and chest pain, dyspnea, or syncope.

Physical Examination

Hypotension and tachycardia may be present. If the aneurysm involves the aortic annulus, it can lead to aortic regurgitation and congestive heart failure. Pulse examination may be abnormal if distal embolization occurs.

Diagnostic Evaluation

Chest radiography may show a widened thoracic aorta. Electrocardiography may demonstrate myocardial ischemia, especially if the aneurysm compromises the coronary supply. In the asymptomatic patient with a thoracic aneurysm, CT or echocardiography is helpful in establishing the diagnosis. Echocardiography can also determine the extent of involvement of the aortic valve and possible cardiac tamponade. Aortography may be useful for planning operative intervention, because it defines the aneurysm's relation to a number of critical structures.

Treatment

As with abdominal aortic aneurysms, operative repair should be considered when the maximum diameter approaches 5 cm. Symptomatic presentation is an indication for immediate operative intervention. As with abdominal aortic aneurysms, the indications for stent grafts for thoracic aortic aneurysms are being carefully evaluated.

AORTIC DISSECTION

Pathogenesis

Dissections can be caused by hypertension, trauma, Marfan syndrome, or aortic coarctation.

Epidemiology

Aortic dissections are more common than either thoracic or abdominal aneurysms. Incidence increases with age, and men are more commonly affected than women.

History

Patients usually complain of the immediate onset of severe pain, often described as tearing, usually in the chest, back, or abdomen. Nausea or light-headedness may also be present.

Physical Examination

Patients may be hypotensive. Rales on chest auscultation or a new murmur suggest that the dissection continues retrograde into the aortic root. Peripheral pulses are diminished if distal blood flow is compromised. If the dissection continues into the visceral arteries, compromise of mesenteric vessels can produce abdominal pain, compromise of renal arteries can cause oliguria, and compromise of spinal blood supply can produce neurologic deficits.

Diagnostic Evaluation

A chest radiograph may show a widened mediastinum. CT may show the dissection or clot in the arterial lumen. Diagnosis can be made with transesophageal ultrasound, magnetic resonance imaging, or aortogram. Dissections are classified according to the DeBakey classification: type I involves both the ascending and the descending aorta, type II involves only the ascending aorta, and type III involves only the descending aorta.

Treatment

Dissection of the ascending thoracic aorta usually requires surgery, because of the potential for retrograde progression into the aortic root and subsequent compromise of the coronary circulation or tamponade from rupture into the pericardium. Eighty percent of patients with involvement of the ascending aorta die without treatment. Antihypertensive therapy is used preoperatively in an attempt to halt the progression of the dissection.

In contrast, dissections limited to the descending aorta are best managed medically, with antihypertensives, including sodium nitroprusside and beta blockade. Invasive monitoring with fluid resuscitation should be instituted immediately. Surgery is reserved for lesions that progress or cause distal ischemia. Stent grafts have been shown to be safe in selected patients. Determination of who should receive a stent graft is being studied.

CAROTID ARTERY DISEASE

ANATOMY

The common carotid artery on the right arises from the brachiocephalic artery, and on the left, from the aorta. The common carotid then bifurcates into internal and external branches. The internal carotid gives off the ophthalmic artery before continuing to the circle of Willis to supply the brain. The area around the bifurcation is clearly "high-rent" territory, which contains a number of vital structures which can be injured during surgery. The marginal mandibular branch of the facial nerve lies deep and inferior to the horizontal ramus of the mandible. Injury to this nerve during dissection results in lower lip paralysis. Branches of the cervical plexus, including the greater auricular nerve, may be at the cranial aspect of the incision and should be avoided to preserve sensation to the ear and the angle of the mandible. Posterolateral to the carotid artery in the carotid sheath lies the vagus nerve. Injury results in vocal cord paralysis. One or two centimeters above the carotid bifurcation is the hypoglossal nerve; injury results in dysphagia and tongue deviation. In contrast, the ansa cervicalis, which courses inferiorly from the hypoglossal to innervate the strap muscles, can be sacrificed as needed for exposure. Laterally and deep to the carotid artery lies the jugular vein, a branch of which, the facial vein, is generally divided to facilitate exposure of the carotid.

PATHOGENESIS

Symptoms are the result of atherosclerosis. Mechanisms of morbidity include plaque rupture, ulceration, hemorrhage, thrombosis, and low flow states. Because of the rich collateralization of the cerebral circulation through the circle of Willis, thrombosis and low flow states may be asymptomatic.

EPIDEMIOLOGY

Atherosclerotic occlusive disease of the carotid artery is a major cause of stroke. In the United States, 400,000 people are hospitalized for stroke each year, and cerebrovascular events are the third most common cause of death. The incidence of stroke increases with age. Other risk factors include hypertension, diabetes, smoking, and hypercholesterolemia. Markers for carotid disease include evidence of other atherosclerotic disease and prior neurologic events.

HISTORY

Patients often relate previous neurologic events, including focal motor deficits, weakness, clumsiness, and expressive or cognitive aphasia. These could occur as a transient ischemic attack, which resolves in 24 hours; a reversible ischemic neurologic deficit, which resolves in greater than 24 hours; or a fixed neurologic deficit. One characteristic presentation for carotid disease is amaurosis fugax, or transient monocular blindness, usually described as a shade being pulled down in front of the patient's eye. This is due to occlusion of a branch of the ophthalmic artery.

PHYSICAL EXAMINATION

Patients may exhibit a fixed neurologic deficit. Hollenhorst plaques on retinal examination are evidence of previous emboli. A carotid bruit is evidence of turbulence in carotid blood flow, but the presence of a bruit does not unequivocally translate into a hemodynamically significant lesion, and the absence of a bruit does not unequivocally indicate the absence of significant disease.

DIAGNOSTIC EVALUATION

Carotid duplex scanning is both sensitive and specific for carotid disease. Conventional or magnetic resonance angiography is more accurate for assessing the degree of stenosis.

TREATMENT

Treatment depends on the history, degree of stenosis, and characteristics of the plaque. Antiplatelet therapy with aspirin is effective in preventing neurologic events. When dealing with an acute event, heparin should be considered after head CT determines that the event is not hemorrhagic. Indications for carotid endarterectomy are controversial. Results of two large randomized controlled trials—the Asymptomatic Carotid Atherosclerosis Study (ACAS) and the North American Symptomatic Carotid Endarterectomy Trial (NASCET)—suggest surgery is best reserved for the following patients: those with >75% stenosis, those with 70% stenosis and symptoms, those with bilateral disease and symptoms, or those with >50% stenosis and recurring transient ischemic attacks despite aspirin therapy. The role of stenting is controversial. Despite the Systolic and Pulse Pressure Hemodynamic Improvement by Restoring Elasticity (SAPPHIRE) trial, which suggested stenting is not inferior to endarterectomy in high-risk patients, there were problems with the study design, and the procedure is still being evaluated as an alternative to open surgery, which has low morbidity and mortality in large centers.

CAROTID ENDARTERECTOMY: THE OPERATION

Perioperative monitoring is surgeon-dependent. Techniques include keeping the patient awake through the procedure, using local or regional anesthesia, using continuous electroencephalogram monitoring, or using no monitoring at all. Administration of intravenous antibiotics, usually a first-generation cephalosporin, precedes the incision. After site verification, the neck is extended, and an incision is made over the anterior border of the sternocleidomastoid muscle. Dissection continues through the platysma and along the sternocleidomastoid. Ligation of the facial vein allows complete exposure of the carotid, which lies just medial to the jugular vein. Care is taken not to injure the hypoglossal nerve at the superior aspect of the dissection or the spinal accessory nerve (Fig. 16-3). Proximal and distal control of the carotid is obtained, the patient

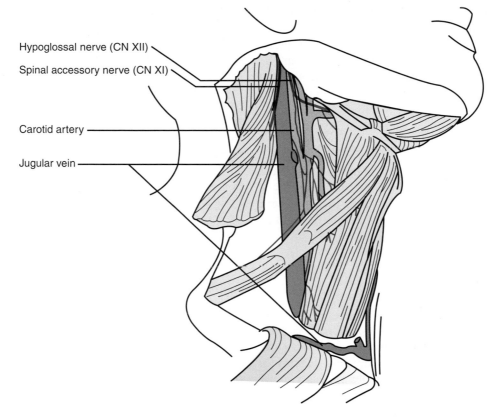

Hypoglossal nerve (CN XII)

Spinal accessory nerve (CN XI)

Carotid artery

Jugular vein

Figure 16-3 • Carotid endarterectomy: pertinent anatomical structures.

is heparinized, and the artery is opened after clamps are applied. Use of a stent may provide cerebral protection. Plaque is carefully dissected out of the artery, and the artery is usually closed with a patch.

ACUTE AND CHRONIC MESENTERIC VASCULAR DISEASE

ANATOMY

Acute and chronic mesenteric vascular disease includes disease of the celiac axis, which is the arterial supply to the liver, spleen, pancreas, and stomach; the superior mesenteric artery, which supplies the pancreas, small bowel, and proximal colon; and inferior mesenteric artery, which supplies the distal colon and rectum. In addition, thrombosis of the superior mesenteric vein can cause visceral ischemia.

The celiac axis arises from the aorta below the crus of the diaphragm. It travels ventrally and is surrounded by a dense network of nerves and connective tissue. After a short distance, it gives rise to the splenic

artery, which travels to the left behind the pancreas to the spleen; the common hepatic artery, which travels to the right toward the hepatic hilum; and the smaller left gastric artery, which travels cranial and toward the left. The superior mesenteric artery courses below the pancreas and slightly to the right toward the mesentery of the bowel. The inferior mesenteric artery arises below the renal arteries and above the aortic bifurcation and travels to the left toward the bowel. The superior mesenteric vein runs above and to the right of the superior mesenteric artery. Its location can be determined by palpating the artery at the root of the mesentery in thin patients. The vein then joins the splenic and inferior mesenteric veins to form the portal vein.

PATHOGENESIS

Acute ischemia is caused by embolization, thrombosis, nonocclusive ischemia, and mesenteric vein thrombosis. Embolization is associated with atherosclerotic disease or mural cardiac thrombus. Acute thrombosis is associated with atherosclerosis and hypercoagulable states. Vasopressor agents can produce acute ischemia. Chronic ischemia usually requires severe atherosclerotic disease in at least two major arterial trunks among the superior and inferior mesenteric arteries and the celiac axis, because of the extensive collateralization.

EPIDEMIOLOGY

The incidence of acute mesenteric ischemia is estimated at one in 1,000 hospital admissions, and mortality is >50%. Prevalence of chronic ischemia increases with age, and risk factors include hypertension, smoking, hypercholesterolemia, and diabetes.

HISTORY

Patients with acute ischemia may have a history of previous embolic events, atrial fibrillation, or congestive failure. Abdominal pain is usually sudden in onset and is severe, with diarrhea or vomiting. History in chronic mesenteric ischemia usually reveals crampy abdominal pain after eating. This results in decreased oral intake and weight loss. Nausea, vomiting, constipation, or diarrhea may occur. The disease can be mistaken for malignant disease or cholelithiasis.

PHYSICAL EXAMINATION

In episodes of acute ischemia, the classic finding is "pain out of proportion to physical examination." The abdomen may be distended. Rectal examination often reveals guaiac-positive stool. Atrial fibrillation may be present. Physical findings in chronic ischemia include abdominal bruits, guaiac-positive stool, and evidence of peripheral vascular disease or coronary artery disease.

DIAGNOSTIC EVALUATION

In acute ischemia, there could be an elevated white blood cell count, metabolic acidosis, or an elevated hematocrit as fluid is sequestered in the infarcting bowel. Abdominal radiographs are often normal in the early phase of the disease, but as the intestine becomes edematous, "thumbprinting" of the bowel wall occurs. Evaluation in chronic ischemia includes selective visceral angiography to identify the site of the lesion.

TREATMENT

Once the diagnosis of acute ischemia is made, laparotomy with examination and resection of any infarcted bowel should be considered. In selected cases, angiography can be therapeutic, as well as diagnostic, with catheter-based therapies. Aggressive surgical intervention should not be delayed if there is evidence suggestive of dead bowel. Despite aggressive intervention, mortality is extremely high. For chronic ischemia, angiography can define the lesion and allow consideration of surgical options. Acute mesenteric vein thrombosis is treated with anticoagulation and laparotomy if necrotic bowel is suspected.

PERIPHERAL VASCULAR DISEASE

ANATOMY

Lesions may occur in the iliac, common and superficial femoral, popliteal, peroneal, anterior tibial, and posterior tibial arteries. The common iliac arteries arise at approximately the level of the umbilicus. They course in the retroperitoneal space and give rise to the internal iliac artery, which runs to the pelvis, and the external, which becomes the femoral artery in the femoral canal as it passes under the inguinal ligament. It enters the adductor canal, below the Sartorius, and continues through the adductor hiatus, where is becomes the popliteal artery. Below the knee, the popliteal artery branches into the anterior tibial, the posterior tibial, and dorsalis pedis arteries, which supply the distal leg. In general, of the three vessels that supply the distal ankle and foot, a single direct arterial supply is adequate to prevent limb loss and rest pain.

PATHOGENESIS

In acute disease, the most common cause is an embolus that causes a sudden decrease in blood flow. The most common sources are the aorta and the heart. Rarer causes include acute arterial thrombosis, acute venous thrombosis, and arterial spasm. In chronic disease, progressive atherosclerotic disease causes narrowing of the arterial lumen and decreased blood flow. Pain occurs as decreased blood flow is unable to meet the metabolic and waste-removal demand of the tissue.

EPIDEMIOLOGY

Acute disease occurs in patients with cardiac thrombus, atrial fibrillation, or atherosclerosis. Risk factors for chronic disease include atherosclerosis, smoking, diabetes, hypertension, and advanced age.

HISTORY

Acute ischemia causes sudden and severe lower-extremity pain and paresthesias. Patients with chronic ischemia typically present with claudication, defined as reproducible pain on exercise relieved by rest. The site of claudication provides a clue to the level of disease. Buttock claudication usually indicates aortoiliac disease, whereas calf claudication suggests femoral atherosclerosis. Pain at rest is indicative of severe disease and a threatened limb. Slow or nonhealing ulcers may be present.

PHYSICAL EXAMINATION

In acute disease, the patient may exhibit pulselessness, pallor, and poikilothermia (coolness). Taken together with pain and paresthesia, these form the five P's of acute vascular compromise (Fig. 16-4). In chronic disease, the lower extremity may reveal loss of hair, pallor on elevation, rubor on placing the extremity in a dependent position, wasting of musculature, thick nails, and thin skin. The extremity may be cool to the touch, and pulses may be diminished or absent. Ulcers or frank necrosis may be present.

DIAGNOSTIC EVALUATION

Angiography is necessary in cases of acute ischemia to identify the lesion. Evaluation for chronic ischemia includes Doppler flow measurement of distal pulses. The normal signal is triphasic; as disease progresses, the signal becomes biphasic, monophasic, and then absent. Ankle-brachial indices are calculated as the systolic blood pressure at the ankle divided by the systolic pressure in the brachial artery. A value of <0.5 is indicative of significant disease (Table 16-1). Arteriography is the gold standard for defining the level and extent of disease and for planning surgery.

TREATMENT

Acute ischemic embolus can be treated with heparin, thrombolysis, or embolectomy. For chronic ischemia, patients with claudication have a low rate of limb loss, and initial therapy is based on smoking cessation and a graded exercise program. Success rates with nonoperative therapy are good. In patients with disabling

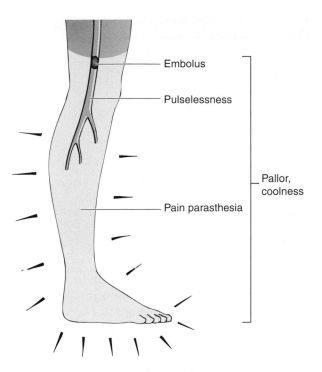

Figure 16-4 • Signs and symptoms of acute embolus.

claudication, threatened limbs, nonhealing ulcers, or gangrene, angioplasty or revascularization should be considered (Table 16-2). It is always prudent to consider amputation in selected patients with long-standing acute ischemia or chronic ischemia, though this decision is often a difficult one and requires experience and careful discussions with the patient.

PERIPHERAL BYPASS: THE OPERATION

Patients usually have concurrent coronary artery disease, and preoperative evaluation and intraoperative beta blockade should be considered. The entire leg is usually prepped. Intravenous antibiotics are often a first-generation cephalosporin, and central monitoring should be considered. The most common techniques for anesthesia include general and regional. If the proximal vessels are open, inflow is usually from the femoral artery, which is dissected via an infrainguinal incision directly over the artery. If the target is the popliteal, it is isolated via an incision over the medial aspect of the knee, at the level where the outflow will be targeted. If the target is the dorsalis pedis, tibialis anterior, or peroneal, the incision is made directly over the target. Above-knee popliteal reconstruction can be accomplished with synthetic grafts, but infrapopliteal reconstructions should use either in situ or reversed saphenous vein.

■ TABLE 16-2 Progression of Peripheral Vascular Disease

	Claudication	Rest Pain	Gangrene
Blood flow	Decreased	Markedly decreased	Minimal
ABI	~0.5	0.3–0.5	<0.3
Treatment	Smoking cessation	Revascularization	Amputation
	Graded exercise	Angioplasty	Revascularization
			Angioplasty

VENOUS DISEASE

DEEP VENOUS THROMBOSIS

First-line therapy for patients with deep venous thrombosis or pulmonary embolism is systemic anticoagulation. In patients for whom this therapy is contraindicated (e.g., patients requiring a planned major surgery, those with active bleeding, or those facing significant complication of anticoagulation), filter placement in the inferior vena cava may decrease the short-term risk of pulmonary embolism. The use of filters, though common, is generally not well supported by randomized controlled trials. They have not been shown to decrease mortality and are associated with significant complications, including inferior vena cava thrombosis, recurrent deep venous thrombosis, and postphlebitic syndrome. Recently, removable filters increasingly are being used to try to decrease the risk of long-term complications, but their use is still being studied.

VARICOSE VEINS

This is an extremely common lesion, affecting up to 15% of men and 25% of women. Over time, the pressure of gravity in the lower extremity may cause enlargement of the veins in the leg as valves fail. In most cases, the lesions are of cosmetic concern only, though they can become large and painful and cause ulcers. In deep veins this can lead to venous thrombosis. Treatment options include sclerotherapy, laser or catheter-based ablation, and vein stripping.

KEY POINTS

- Aneurysms and dissections can be rapidly fatal.
- Repair via open operation or stent graft should be considered for asymptomatic aneurysms with diameter >4 or 5 cm.
- Symptomatic aneurysms or dissections require emergency diagnosis and treatment.
- Dissections that involve the ascending aorta usually require surgery, whereas dissections that involve the descending aorta are best managed medically.
- Carotid artery disease is a major cause of stroke in the United States.
- Indications for operation include 75% stenosis, 70% stenosis and symptoms, bilateral disease and symptoms, or >50% stenosis and recurring transient ischemic attacks despite aspirin therapy.
- Stenting is an option for selected patients.
- Patients with acute mesenteric ischemia present with "pain out of proportion to examination," and a mechanism for embolic disease is usually present.
- Chronic mesenteric ischemia results in weight loss and abdominal pain and is frequently mistaken for malignant disease.
- Acute peripheral embolus is marked by the five P's: pulselessness, pallor, poikilothermia, pain, and paresthesia.
- Symptoms of chronic peripheral vascular disease usually follow a well-defined progression.
- Operation should be considered only in patients with severe chronic peripheral vascular disease.

Heart

ANATOMY

Coronary circulation begins at the sinus of Valsalva, where the right and left coronary arteries (RCA, LCA) arise. The left main artery branches into the left anterior descending and the left circumflex arteries. The left anterior descending artery supplies the anterior of the left ventricle, the apex of the heart, the intraventricular septum, and the portion of the right ventricle that borders the intraventricular septum (Fig. 17-1). The left circumflex artery travels in the groove separating the left atrium and ventricle and gives off marginal branches to the left ventricle. The RCA travels between the right atrium and ventricle to supply the lateral portion of the right ventricle (Fig. 17-2). The posterior descending artery (PDA) comes from the RCA in 90% of patients and supplies the arteriovenous node. Patients whose PDA arises from the RCA are termed right dominant. If the PDA arises from the left circumflex, the system is left dominant.

The aortic valve is located between the left ventricle and the aorta. It usually has three leaflets, which form three sinuses. One sinus gives rise to the RCA, another to the LCA, and the third forms the noncoronary sinus. The mitral valve is located between the left atrium and ventricle. It normally has two leaflets, with the anterior protruding farther across the valve. Chordae tendineae attach the leaflets to the papillary muscles, which in turn serve to tether the leaflets to the ventricular wall.

CONGENITAL HEART DISEASE

Approximately 0.6% of live births will be complicated by congenital heart defects. This risk more than doubles in subsequent siblings. Most cases are sporadic, although there are well-known associations of genetic syndromes and congenital heart defects. These include atrioventricular canal defects in children with Down syndrome, coarctation of the aorta in children with Turner's syndrome, and supravalvular aortic stenosis in children with William's syndrome.

Congenital heart defects are best understood by the pathophysiology they cause, either congestive heart failure or cyanosis. Most anomalies fit into one of these categories.

Congestive heart failure can be caused either by a left-to-right shunt or an obstructive lesion. Left-to-right shunts result in a certain fraction of blood leaving the left side of the heart to the right side, increasing pulmonary pressure and necessitating large volume of left ventricular output to satisfy peripheral demands. Among these lesions are patent ductus arteriosus, in which the normal fetal connection between the pulmonary artery and aorta is not obliterated at birth. Depending on the size of the communication, it can cause severe failure. Premature infants with pulmonary compromise and/or children with an audible murmur should undergo closure, which can be achieved via catheter-based therapies.

Atrial and ventricular septal defects also result in left-to-right shunting. Patients with atrial septal defects classically have a second heart sound in which the split is of fixed duration. Over time such patients can develop pulmonary hypertension, right and left ventricular failure, and atrial arrhythmias. Most atrial septal defects can be closed using percutaneous methods. Ventricular septal defects may present in a similar fashion with pulmonary hypertension and congestive heart failure, culminating in Eisenmenger syndrome when the shunt reverses to a right-to-left shunt, causing cyanosis. These lesions should be fixed.

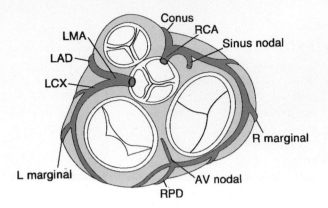

Figure 17-1 • Schematic showing the origin of the coronary circulation. LMA, left main artery; LAD, left anterior descending; RCA, right coronary artery; RPD, right posterior descending; LCX, left circumflex; AV, aortic valve; L, left; R, right.
LifeART image copyright © 2009 Lippincott Williams & Wilkins. All rights reserved.

Atrioventricular canal defects are complicated lesions involving the atrial and ventricular septae and the atrioventricular valves. When diagnosed, these lesions should be fixed. In its extreme form, a single arterial trunk arises from a joined ventricular chamber; this is termed a truncus arteriosus.

Obstructive lesions can also cause congestive heart failure. Aortic stenosis most commonly occurs as a result of a bicuspid aortic valve, but can also occur at the supravalvular or subvalvular location, or as a result of subvalvular ventricular hypertrophy, termed hypertrophic muscular subaortic stenosis. Although many procedures may be used to treat this condition,

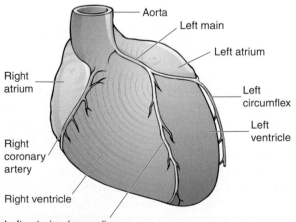

Figure 17-2 • Schematic showing the path of the coronary circulation. The left main artery gives rise to the left anterior descending and left circumflex arteries.

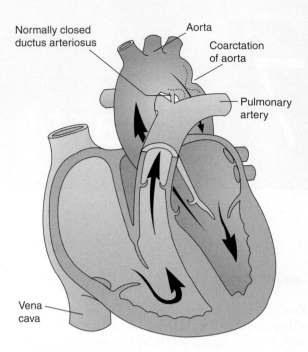

Figure 17-3 • Coarctation of the aorta. The aorta is narrowed distal to the takeoff of the left subclavian artery. The increased pressure caused by this lesion frequently causes the ductus arteriosus to remain open.
From Pillitteri A. *Maternal and Child Nursing*. 4th ed. Philadelphia, PA: Lippincott Williams & Wilkins, 2003.

of particular interest is the Ross operation, which involves transposing the pulmonary valve to the aortic position and using a prosthetic graft for a new pulmonary valve.

Mitral stenosis commonly occurs in association with other congenital heart defects. Pulmonic stenosis is often mildly symptomatic and is generally treated with percutaneous methods.

The most common obstructive lesion in children is coarctation of the aorta. This occurs when the aorta becomes narrowed, usually just after the takeoff of the left subclavian artery (Fig. 17-3). Often, blood flow to the lower extremities will depend on a patent ductus arteriosus, closure of which can cause severe heart failure. Because of the risk of endocarditis, severe hypertension, congestive heart failure, and stroke, these lesions are repaired.

Right-to-left shunts occur when deoxygenated blood makes its way into the peripheral circulation; this is also referred to as cyanotic heart disease. The most common cause is Tetralogy of Fallot (Fig. 17-4). This abnormality has four components: ventricular septal defect, pulmonic stenosis, right ventricular hypertrophy, and an overriding aorta.

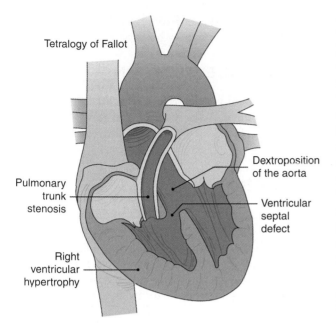

Tetralogy of Fallot

Pulmonary trunk stenosis

Dextroposition of the aorta

Ventricular septal defect

Right ventricular hypertrophy

Figure 17-4 • Tetralogy of Fallot. Coronal view of heart in tetralogy of Fallot. Characteristics include pulmonary trunk stenosis, right ventricular hypertrophy, dextroposition of the aorta, and ventricular septal defect.
LifeART image copyright (c) 2009 Lippincott Williams & Wilkins. All rights reserved.

Tricuspid atresia prevents flow from the right atrium to the right ventricle, and instead, deoxygenated blood traverses an atrial septal defect into the left atrium. Other lesions that can cause a right-to-left shunt include pulmonic atresia, transposition of the great arteries, and total anomalous pulmonary venous connection.

CORONARY ARTERY DISEASE

EPIDEMIOLOGY

Atherosclerosis of the coronary arteries is the most common cause of mortality in the United States, responsible for one third of all deaths. Approximately 5 million Americans have coronary artery disease, which is five times more prevalent in men than in women. Risk factors include hypertension, family history, hypercholesterolemia, smoking, obesity, diabetes, and physical inactivity.

PATHOPHYSIOLOGY

Coronary artery stenosis is a gradual process that begins in the second decade. When the lumen decreases to 75% of the native area, the lesion becomes hemodynamically significant.

HISTORY

Patients with ischemic heart disease usually complain of substernal chest pain or pressure that may radiate down the arms or into the jaw, teeth, or back. Typically, the pain occurs during periods of physical exertion or emotional stress. Episodes that are reproducible and resolve with rest are termed stable angina. If the pain occurs at rest or does not improve with rest, is new and severe, or is progressive, it is termed unstable angina and suggests impending infarction. Presentation can be variable, with patients complaining of indigestion, nausea, vomiting, diaphoresis, cough, new onset arrhythmia, syncope, and, in older adult patients, confusion or delirium. Ischemic heart disease can also be asymptomatic, classically in patients with diabetes.

PHYSICAL EXAMINATION

The patient may have evidence of peripheral vascular disease, including diminished pulses. Signs of ventricular failure, including cardiomegaly, congestive heart failure, an S3 or S4, or murmur of mitral regurgitation (MR), may occur.

DIAGNOSTIC EVALUATION

Electrocardiogram (ECG) may show signs of ischemia or an old infarct. A chest radiograph may show an enlarged heart or pulmonary congestion. An exercise stress test is sensitive in identifying myocardium at risk. These areas can be localized using nuclear medicine scans, including thallium imaging. Echocardiography is extremely useful in evaluating myocardial function and valvular competence. Angiography is the gold standard for identifying lesions in the coronary arteries, assessing their severity, and planning operative intervention.

TREATMENT

Patients with severe disease of the left main artery or with severe disease in the three major coronary arteries have decreased mortality after coronary artery bypass surgery. Pain is reliably relieved in >85% of patients. Surgical options include bypass using the internal mammary arteries or saphenous veins. Internal mammary bypass is preferred because of higher patency rates.

Percutaneous coronary interventions include balloon angioplasty and stent placement. Despite the tremendous volume of procedures performed in the United States, the exact indications for interventions are not well known. A large study in 2005 in the *New England Journal of Medicine* by Hannon et al. demonstrated that in patients with two or more diseased vessels, stents were associated with an increased need for further procedures and increased mortality compared with bypass grafting. Because early mortality was higher with bypass grafting, care must be individualized to the patient.

One common problem with coronary stents is in-stent restenosis. Benefits of drug-eluting stents, which elaborate various substances including sirolimus and paclitaxel, remain unclear.

It is important to note that nearly all risk factors for coronary artery disease are modifiable before and after an event. Preventive medicine used to aggressively lower blood pressure and cholesterol, combined with diet and exercise regimens, is critical.

AORTIC STENOSIS

ETIOLOGY

Aortic stenosis (AS) can present early in life—for example, when the valve is unicuspid—but more commonly occurs in the older population. A congenitally bicuspid valve usually causes AS by the time the patient reaches 70 years of age. Other causes include rheumatic fever, which results in commissural fusion and subsequent calcification, and degenerative stenosis, in which calcification occurs in the native valve (see Color Plate 13).

PATHOPHYSIOLOGY

The initial physiologic response to AS is left ventricular hypertrophy to preserve stroke volume and cardiac output. Left ventricular hypertrophy and increasing resistance at the level of the valve result in decreased cardiac output, pulmonary hypertension, and myocardial ischemia.

HISTORY

Patients often complain of angina, syncope, and dyspnea, with dyspnea being the worst prognostic indicator.

PHYSICAL EXAMINATION

A midsystolic ejection murmur, as well as cardiomegaly and other signs of congestive heart failure, may be present. Pulsus tardus et parvus, a delayed, diminished impulse at the carotid, may be apparent.

DIAGNOSTIC EVALUATION

Echocardiography or cardiac catheterization reliably studies the valve. A decrease in the aortic valve area from the normal 3 or 4 cm to <1 cm signifies severe disease.

TREATMENT

Patients who are symptomatic should undergo aortic valve replacement unless other medical conditions make it unlikely that the patient could survive the operation. In asymptomatic individuals, progressive cardiomegaly is an indication for operation, because surgical therapy is superior to medical therapy.

AORTIC INSUFFICIENCY

ETIOLOGY

Aortic insufficiency can be caused by rheumatic fever, connective tissue disorders including Marfan and Ehlers-Danlos syndromes, endocarditis, aortic dissection, and trauma.

PATHOPHYSIOLOGY

The incompetent valve causes a decrease in cardiac output, and left ventricular dilatation occurs. The larger ventricle is subject to higher wall stress, which increases myocardial oxygen demand.

HISTORY

Patients complain of angina or symptoms of systolic dysfunction.

PHYSICAL EXAMINATION

Typically, there is a crescendo-decrescendo diastolic murmur and a wide pulse pressure with a water hammer quality. The point of maximal impulse may be displaced or diffuse.

DIAGNOSTIC EVALUATION

Echocardiography is a sensitive and specific means of making the diagnosis.

TREATMENT

Symptomatic patients should undergo replacement surgery if their medical condition allows them to tolerate a major procedure.

MITRAL STENOSIS

ETIOLOGY

Mitral stenosis (MS) develops in 40% of patients with rheumatic heart disease. Rheumatic heart disease occurs after pharyngitis caused by group A streptococcus. A likely autoimmune phenomenon causes pancarditis, resulting in fibrosis of valve leaflets. Histologic findings include Aschoff nodules. MS may also be caused by malignant carcinoid and systemic lupus erythematosus.

PATHOPHYSIOLOGY

Fibrosis progresses over a period of two or three decades, causing fusion of the leaflets, which take on a characteristic "fish mouth" appearance, significantly impeding blood flow through the valve. Increased left atrial pressures lead to left atrial hypertrophy, which in turn may cause atrial fibrillation or pulmonary hypertension. Pulmonary hypertension can further progress to right ventricular hypertrophy and right-sided heart failure.

EPIDEMIOLOGY

MS has a female predominance of 2:1.

HISTORY

Characteristic complaints include dyspnea and fatigability. Occasionally, pulmonary hypertension leads to hemoptysis.

PHYSICAL EXAMINATION

Cachexia or symptoms of congestive heart failure may be present, with pulmonary rales and tachypnea. Jugular venous distention, peripheral edema, ascites, and a sternal heave of right ventricular hypertrophy may be appreciable. Heart sounds are usually characteristic, consisting of an opening snap followed by a low rumbling murmur. The splitting of the second heart sound is decreased, and the pulmonary component is louder. The heart rate may demonstrate the irregular pattern of atrial fibrillation.

DIAGNOSTIC EVALUATION

Chest x-ray may show cardiomegaly, including signs of left atrial hypertrophy. Pulmonary edema may be present. ECG may show atrial fibrillation. Broad, notched P waves are an indication of left atrial hypertrophy. Right axis deviation is evidence of right ventricular hypertrophy. Echocardiography with Doppler flow measurement is extremely useful for demonstrating MS, estimating flow, and assessing the presence of thrombi. Cardiac catheterization gives a direct measurement of transvalvular pressure gradient, from which the area of the mitral annulus can be calculated.

THERAPY

Surgical options include valvulotomy or replacement. Therapy is indicated for symptomatic patients.

MITRAL REGURGITATION

ETIOLOGY

Approximately 40% of cases are caused by rheumatic fever; other causes include idiopathic calcification associated with hypertension, diabetes, AS, and renal failure. Mitral valve prolapse progresses to MR in 5% of affected individuals. Less common causes include myocardial ischemia, trauma, endocarditis, and hypertrophic cardiomyopathy.

PATHOPHYSIOLOGY

As regurgitation becomes hemodynamically significant, the left ventricle dilates to preserve cardiac output. A significant volume is ejected retrograde, increasing cardiac work, left atrial volumes, and pulmonary venous pressure. This, in turn, may lead to left atrial enlargement and fibrillation or cause pulmonary hypertension, which could result in right ventricular failure.

EPIDEMIOLOGY

MR is more common than MS and has a male predominance.

HISTORY

Patients commonly complain of dyspnea, orthopnea, and fatigue.

PHYSICAL EXAMINATION

Patients may appear cachectic. Frequently, there is an irregular pulse, pulmonary rales, and a sternal heave. The pulse characteristically has a rapid upstroke, and v waves may be present. A holosystolic murmur that radiates to the axilla or back is common. The point of maximal impulse is often displaced.

DIAGNOSTIC EVALUATION

Chest x-ray may show cardiomegaly and pulmonary edema. ECG commonly demonstrates left ventricular or biventricular hypertrophy, left atrial enlargement, and P mitrale. Echocardiography is extremely useful in establishing the diagnosis and the underlying lesion. Cardiac catheterization is useful in establishing pulmonary pressures and cardiac output.

TREATMENT

Medical therapy consists of afterload reducing agents, such as angiotensin-converting enzyme inhibitors, nitroglycerin, and diuretics. Surgical intervention is indicated if congestive failure interferes with daily life, if pulmonary hypertension or left ventricular dilation worsens, or if atrial fibrillation develops. If life-threatening MR develops from endocarditis, ischemia, or trauma, aggressive treatment with afterload reduction, a balloon pump if necessary, and antibiotics if indicated should be used to convert an emergency operation to an elective one. Because of the severe hemodynamic instability that can occur, operative intervention involving repair or replacement may be necessary in the acute setting. These emergency operations carry >15% mortality rate.

AORTIC BALLOON PUMPS AND VENTRICULAR ASSIST DEVICES

In patients with markedly decreased cardiac output insufficient to sustain end organ perfusion, an intra-aortic balloon pump may be useful to decrease afterload, increase coronary perfusion, decrease myocardial oxygen demand, and increase cardiac output (Figs. 17-5 and 17-6). These are temporary devices, generally placed via a femoral approach. Correct placement is critical. Occlusion of the left subclavian artery during inflation must be avoided, and proximal location above the renal arteries is also critical. Vascular complications, including arterial thrombosis and embolism, must be

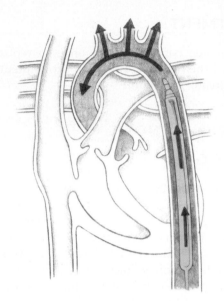

Figure 17-5 • How the intra-aortic balloon pump works: Balloon inflation. The balloon inflates as the aortic valve closes and diastole begins. Diastole increases perfusion to the coronary arteries.
From *Nursing Procedures.* 4th ed. Ambler, PA: Lippincott Williams & Wilkins, 2004.

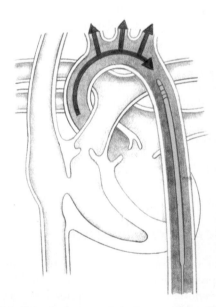

Figure 17-6 • How the intra-aortic balloon pump works: Balloon deflation. The balloon deflates before ventricular ejection, when the aortic valve opens. This permits ejection of blood from the left ventricle against a lowered resistance. As a result, aortic end-diastolic pressure and afterload decrease and cardiac output increases.
From *Nursing Procedures.* 4th ed. Ambler, PA: Lippincott Williams & Wilkins, 2004.

constantly checked for and may necessitate balloon removal.

When medical therapy and intra-aortic balloon pumps are insufficient to provide adequate cardiac output, left ventricular assist devices may be used. These are divided into pulsatile flow pumps and nonpulsatile flow pumps, which use axial or centrifugal flow. These pumps can be used in the short term, generally in patients with temporary heart failure. These patients are expected to improve, and a common indication is post-cardiotomy syndrome. Left ventricular assist devices can also be useful longer term as a bridge to transplantation. Thromboembolism, bleeding, and infection are common complications.

KEY POINTS

- Coronary artery disease is the leading cause of mortality in the United States.
- Risk factors include hypertension, smoking, obesity, diabetes, hypercholesterolemia, inactivity, and family history.
- Coronary artery disease is treated surgically if all three coronary arteries or the left main coronary artery are diseased or if patients have debilitating symptoms.
- Aortic stenosis can be caused by a congenital bicuspid valve or rheumatic fever; symptoms include angina, syncope, and dyspnea.
- Aortic insufficiency can be caused by rheumatic fever, endocarditis, connective tissue disorders, aortic dissection, and trauma; symptoms include angina and dyspnea.
- Mitral stenosis is most commonly caused by rheumatic fever; symptoms include fatigue and dyspnea.
- Mitral regurgitation is caused by rheumatic fever, idiopathic calcification, mitral valve prolapse, myocardial ischemia, trauma, endocarditis, and hypertrophic cardiomyopathy; symptoms include fatigue and dyspnea.
- Congenital heart disease can be broadly divided into lesions causing congestive heart failure or cyanosis.
- Tetralogy of Fallot has four components: ventricular septal defect, pulmonic stenosis, right ventricular hypertrophy, and an overriding aorta.

Chapter

18 Lung

In this chapter, common surgical diseases and disorders of the lung, tracheobronchial tree, and pleura are discussed. An important key point is to understand the scope of the "silent epidemic" of smoking-related deaths from lung cancer, as it is the leading cause of cancer-related deaths for both men and women in North America, killing more people annually than breast, prostate, and colorectal cancer combined. The reader should ponder why more societal and governmental efforts are not directed at combating the main cause of this lethal disease, namely, tobacco products.

ANATOMY

The lungs are divided into three lobes with 10 segments on the right and two lobes with nine segments on the left (Fig. 18-1). The decreased number of divisions on the left can be thought of as space taken up by the heart. The right mainstem bronchus forms a gentler curve with the trachea than does the left mainstem bronchus (Fig. 18-2). Therefore, aspirated foreign bodies are more likely to lodge in the right mainstem bronchus. In aspiration pneumonia, the aspirated material is most likely to deposit in the most dependent portions of the lungs. For a supine individual, these are the posterior segments of the upper lobes and the superior segments of the lower lobes. The arterial supply to the lungs is through the pulmonary arteries as well as the bronchial arteries, which arise from the aorta and intercostal vessels.

BENIGN TUMORS OF THE TRACHEA AND BRONCHI

PATHOLOGY

Types of benign tumors include squamous papilloma, angioma, fibroma, leiomyoma, and chondroma. Squamous papillomatosis is associated with human papilloma viruses 6 and 11.

EPIDEMIOLOGY

Truly benign neoplasms of the trachea and bronchi are rare.

HISTORY

Patients commonly present with recurrent pneumonias, cough, or hemoptysis.

PHYSICAL EXAMINATION

Patients may have decreased breath sounds on the affected side, with the additional signs and symptoms owing to postobstructive pneumonia.

DIAGNOSTIC EVALUATION

Chest radiography may demonstrate a mass, and there is often a postobstructive pneumonia if the lesion significantly narrows the bronchial lumen.

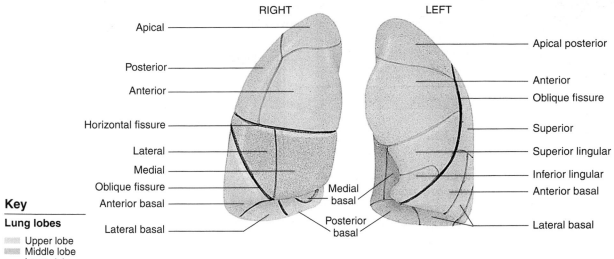

Figure 18-1 • Lung lobes. Anterior view.
From Anatomical Chart Company.

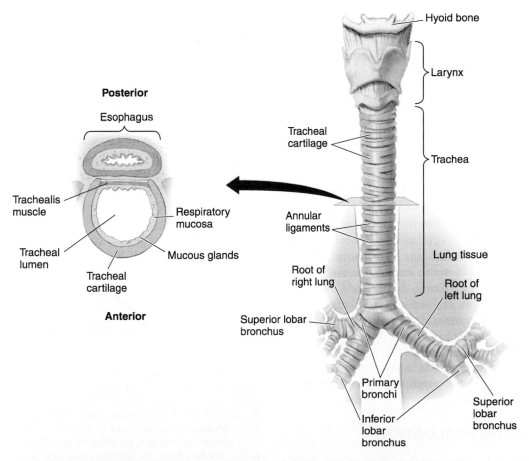

Figure 18-2 • Transverse section of the trachea and the esophagus and trachea (anterior views).
From Premkumar K. *The Massage Connection Anatomy and Physiology.* Baltimore, MD: Lippincott Williams & Wilkins, 2004.

TREATMENT

Angiomas frequently regress, and observation is recommended. Other lesions require surgical removal to relieve symptoms and establish a diagnosis. This may require partial lung resection or sleeve resection, where a segment of bronchus is removed and primarily reanastomosed. Squamous papillomatosis has a high recurrence rate.

TRACHEOBRONCHIAL TUMORS WITH MALIGNANT POTENTIAL

Tumors with malignant potential include bronchial carcinoids, adenoid cystic carcinoma, and mucoepidermoid tumors. Carcinoid tumors, which are malignant in approximately 10% of patients, may cause paraneoplastic syndromes through release of various substances, including histamine, serotonin, vasoactive intestinal peptide, gastrin, growth hormone, insulin, glucagon, and catecholamines.

EPIDEMIOLOGY

These tumors make up fewer than 5% of all pulmonary neoplasms and have no obvious age or sex predilection. Carcinoids make up approximately 1% of all lung tumors; adenoid cystic carcinoma, approximately 0.5%; and mucoepidermoid, approximately 0.2%.

HISTORY

Patients most commonly complain of cough, dyspnea, hemoptysis, or recurrent pneumonia. Less frequently, carcinoid tumors may produce carcinoid syndrome, with complaints of flushing and diarrhea, as well as manifestations of specific hormone excess. This syndrome only occurs in approximately 3% of patients with carcinoid tumors.

PHYSICAL EXAMINATION

The patient may have respiratory compromise or decreased breath sounds. Carcinoid tumors may cause valvular heart disease with signs of pulmonic stenosis or tricuspid regurgitation.

DIAGNOSTIC EVALUATION

Chest radiography may reveal a lesion or postobstructive pneumonia. Bronchoscopy is useful to obtain tissue diagnosis and define bronchial anatomy. Computed

tomography (CT) of the chest is routine for preoperative planning.

TREATMENT

These tumors should all be resected. Long-term survival for carcinoid tumors is 80%; for adenoid cystic carcinoma and mucoepidermoid tumors, the prognosis is also favorable.

LUNG CANCER

EPIDEMIOLOGY

Lung cancer is the leading cause of cancer-related death for both men and women in North America, responsible for >150,000 deaths each year in the United States and accounting for almost 30% of all cancer-related deaths. More than 80% of lung cancers are smoking-related (Fig. 18-3). In the United States, more people die each year from lung cancer than from breast, prostate, and colorectal cancers combined. Lung cancer kills more men than prostate cancer and more women

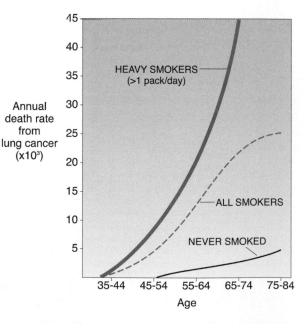

Figure 18-3 • Death rate from lung cancer among smokers and nonsmokers. Nonsmokers exhibit a small, linear increase in the death rate from lung cancer from the age of 50 years onwards. By contrast, those who smoke more than one pack per day show an exponential increase in the annual death rate from lung cancer starting at approximately age 35 years. By age 70, heavy smokers have an approximately 20-fold greater death rate from lung cancer than nonsmokers.
From Rubin E, Farber JL. *Pathology*. 3rd ed. Philadelphia, PA: Lippincott Williams & Wilkins, 1999.

than breast cancer. Lung cancer incidence rates among women continue to increase. Deaths from lung cancer in women have increased 400% between 1960 and 1990. Smoking cessation significantly reduces an individual's risk of developing lung cancer, although the level of risk remains greater than for nonsmokers. Asbestos, formaldehyde, radon gas, arsenic, uranium, chromates, and nickel have been identified as carcinogens, especially when combined with smoking.

PATHOLOGY

Lung cancer is divided into small-cell lung cancer (SCLC; 20% to 25%) and non–small-cell lung cancer (NSCLC; 75% to 80%). NSCLC is further divided into squamous cell carcinoma (30%), adenocarcinoma (35%), and large-cell carcinoma (10%). SCLC is usually centrally located and may be associated with paraneoplastic syndromes. Approximately 5% of patients have symptoms of inappropriate secretion of antidiuretic hormone, whereas 3% to 5% have Cushing's syndrome from adrenocorticotropin production. Squamous cell cancer usually occurs centrally and can be associated with symptoms of hypercalcemia secondary to production of a substance similar to parathyroid hormone. Adenocarcinoma typically occurs at the periphery.

HISTORY

Most patients come to seek medical attention as a result of signs and symptoms indicating advanced disease. Ninety percent of patients with lung cancer are symptomatic at the time of diagnosis. Worsening cough with increased sputum production and hemoptysis often indicates airway obstruction by tumor. A history of recurrent pneumonia requiring antibiotic therapy is common. Persistent chest, back, or shoulder pain is related to nerve involvement or direct tumor invasion. Bone pain indicates distant skeletal metastases, whereas neurologic symptoms indicate brain metastases. Systemic symptoms include fatigue, loss of appetite, and unintentional weight loss.

PHYSICAL EXAMINATION

Chest auscultation may reveal diminished breath sounds owing to pneumonia or malignant pleural effusion. Supraclavicular lymphadenopathy may be present. Recent onset of hoarseness indicates involvement of the recurrent laryngeal nerve. Horner syndrome (ptosis, myosis, and anhydrosis) results from a superior sulcus tumor causing neural invasion. Superior vena cava syndrome and Pancoast syndrome (shoulder and arm pain on the affected side) may occur. Paralysis of the diaphragm indicates phrenic nerve involvement. Patients with advanced disease are usually ill-appearing and exhibit significant weight loss.

DIAGNOSTIC EVALUATION

Chest x-ray is often the modality first used to diagnose a malignant pulmonary lesion. Chest CT including the liver and adrenal glands often follows to delineate tumor size, presence of lymphadenopathy and pleural effusion, and evidence of the likelihood of distant disease (Fig. 18-4).

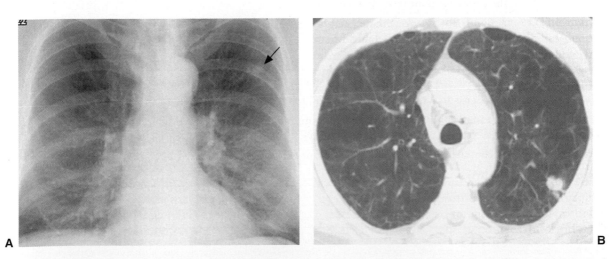

Figure 18-4 • Solitary pulmonary nodule evaluated by computed tomography (CT). **A.** Chest radiograph shows nodule in the left upper lobe (arrow). **B.** CT shows extensive emphysema and a noncalcified nodule in the posterior segment, left upper lobe, with a "tail" extending to the pleura. The nodule is noncalcified and was proven to be a non–small-cell lung cancer.
From Crapo JD, Glassroth JL, Karlinsky JB, et al. *Baum's Textbook of Pulmonary Diseases*. 7th ed. Philadelphia, PA: Lippincott Williams & Wilkins, 2004.

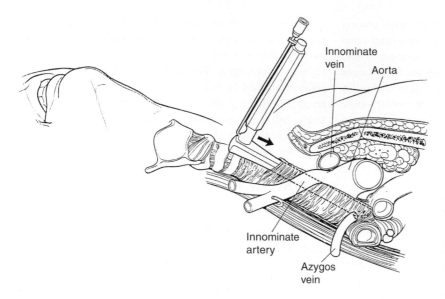

Figure 18-5 • Mediastinoscopy. The passive angle of the mediastinoscope within the pretracheal fascia aims the tip of the scope directly at the trachea or subcarinal space.
From Shields TW, LoCicero J III, Ponn RB, et al. *General Thoracic Surgery*. 6th ed. Philadelphia, PA: Lippincott Williams & Wilkins, 2004.

■ **TABLE 18-1** Current International Staging System for Non–Small-Cell Lung Cancer Staging	
Primary Tumor (T)	
T1	A tumor that is ≤3 cm in greatest dimension, surrounded by lung or visceral pleura, and without evidence of invasion proximal to a lobar bronchus at bronchoscopy.
T2	A tumor >3 cm in greatest dimension, or a tumor of any size that either invades the visceral pleura or has associated atelectasis or obstructive pneumonitis extending to the hilar bronchus or at least 2 cm distal to the carina. Any associated atelectasis or obstructive pneumonitis must involve less than an entire lung.
T3	A tumor of any size with direct extension into the chest wall (including superior sulcus tumors), diaphragm, or the mediastinal pleura or pericardium without involving the heart, great vessels, trachea, esophagus, or vertebral body, or a tumor in the main bronchus within 2 cm of the carina without involving the carina.
T4	A tumor of any size with invasion of the mediastinum or involving the heart, great vessels, trachea, esophagus, vertebral body, or carina or presence of malignant pleural effusion.*
Nodal Involvement (N)	
N0	No metastasis to regional lymph nodes
N1	Metastasis to lymph nodes in the peribronchial or the ipsilateral hilar region
N2	Metastasis to ipsilateral mediastinal lymph nodes and subcarinal lymph nodes
N3	Metastasis to contralateral mediastinal lymph nodes, contralateral hilar lymph nodes, ipsilateral or contralateral scalene lymph nodes, or supraclavicular lymph nodes
Distant Metastasis (M)	
M0	No distant metastasis
M1	Distant metastasis

*Most pleural effusions associated with lung cancer are due to tumor. There are, however, a few patients in whom cytopathologic examination of pleural fluid (on more than one specimen) is negative for tumor and in whom the fluid is nonbloody and is not an exudate. In cases in which these elements and clinical judgment dictate that the effusion is not related to the tumor, the patient should be staged T1, T2, or T3, excluding effusion as a staging element.

Bone scan and brain imaging may also be obtained, if necessary. Noninvasive functional testing for distant disease can be conducted via positron emission tomography scan. This information allows for clinical staging and decision making.

Invasive testing is usually required for definitive diagnosis. Diagnostic thoracentesis is used to evaluate for malignant pleural effusion. Flexible bronchoscopy allows for tissue biopsy and bronchial washings. Transthoracic CT-guided fine-needle biopsy can also provide diagnostic tissue sampling. Mediastinoscopy with lymph node biopsy can be diagnostic while also providing information for accurate nodal staging (Fig. 18-5).

STAGING

The TNM system is used for staging of lung cancer (Tables 18-1 and 18-2). T1 lesions are <3 cm; T2 lesions are >3 cm or involve the main bronchus >2 cm from the carina or involve the visceral pleura. T3 lesions invade the chest wall, diaphragm, mediastinal pleura, or pericardium or involve the main bronchus within 2 cm of the carina. T4 lesions invade the heart, great vessels, mediastinum, trachea, esophagus, vertebral bodies, or carina or have malignant effusions or satellite tumors.

N1 lesions have positive nodes in the ipsilateral peribronchial or hilar region. N2 lesions have positive nodes in the ipsilateral mediastinal or subcarinal region. N3 lesions have metastases either to contralateral nodes or ipsilateral scalene or supraclavicular regions.

Stage IA lesions are T1N0M0 lesions. Stage IB lesions are T2N0M0 lesions. Stage IIA lesions are T1N1M0 lesions. Stage IIB lesions are T2N1M0 or T3N0M0 lesions. Stage IIIA lesions are T3N1M0, T1N2M0, T2N2M0, or T3N2M0 lesions. Stage IIIB lesions are tumors without distant metastases, including primary tumors to T4 and N3 regional lymph node metastases. Stage IV patients have evidence of distant metastases.

TREATMENT

Since the first successful pneumonectomy for lung cancer in 1933, surgical resection has been considered the standard therapy for patients with potentially curable disease. For patients with NSCLC, those with clinical stage I and II disease are referred for an attempt at curative surgical resection. For patients with stage III disease, some may be considered for resection as part of a multimodality therapeutic program usually involving neoadjuvant chemoradiotherapy. Patients with N3 disease and clinical stage IV are not typically candidates for surgical resection.

Standard surgical treatment of NSCLC consists of complete resection of the disease. In addition to parenchymal resection, the operation should also include either sampling or removal of all intrathoracic ipsilateral lymph node stations into which the tumor could potentially drain. For tumors confined to a single lung lobe, the most common surgical procedure performed is lobectomy. For tumors invading an adjacent lobe, a bilobectomy is required. If complete resection requires removal of all lobes on the effected side, then pneumonectomy is performed. For a patient with poor pulmonary function and limited pulmonary reserve, then segmentectomy or wedge resection may be performed. However, the decision to perform a smaller resection provides poorer overall survival because studies show higher locoregional recurrence rates after segmentectomy versus the more oncologically complete lobectomy (23% versus 5%).

■ TABLE 18-2 Lung Cancer Staging	
Stage 1A	T1, N0, M0
Stage 1B	T2, N0, M0
Stage IIA	T1, N1, M0
Stage IIB	T2, N1, M0
	T3, N0, M0
Stage IIIA	T3, N1, M0
	T1, N2, M0
	T2, N2, M0
	T3, N2, M0
Stage IIIB	T4, N0, M0
	T4, N1, M0
	T4, N2, M0
	T1, N3, M0
	T2, N3, M0
	T3, N3, M0
	T4, N3, M0
Stage IV	Any T, Any N, M1

Results of clinical trials now support the use of adjuvant platinum-based chemotherapy in patients with completely resected lung cancer (stage I, II, and IIIA). The use of adjuvant chemotherapy improves 5-year survival rates by approximately 5% to 15% when compared with surgical therapy alone. Standard chemotherapy regimens for NSCLC include a platinum agent (cisplatin or carboplatin) combined with a nonplatinum agent (etoposide, irinotecan, paclitaxel, gemcitabine, and others). Radiotherapy is often added if mediastinal lymph nodes are involved (stage III).

As opposed to NSCLC, SCLC is usually widely disseminated at the time of diagnosis, so surgery is rarely indicated. Only very early-stage small-cell tumors (T1 to T2, N0) are considered for potential resection. The standard treatment for this aggressive disease is combined chemotherapy and radiotherapy. Chemotherapy usually consists of combination therapy (including cyclophosphamide, doxorubicin, vincristine, cisplatin, carboplatin, or etoposide), with triplet combinations often used. Radiation therapy, usually in combination with chemotherapy, is an important modality for treating SCLC. Various radiation treatment plans exist, with differing doses, timing, and fractionation schedules. Elective whole-brain irradiation is used in many centers to minimize the risk of developing brain metastases. The principle of brain irradiation is to destroy any hidden tumor cells that may potentially lurk in the brain, because asymptomatic cerebral metastases are theoretically protected from systemic chemotherapy by the blood-brain barrier. By undergoing so-called prophylactic cranial irradiation, it is argued that survival rates are increased and symptomatic metastases are prevented, because approximately 25% to 50% of untreated patients will develop brain metastases.

PROGNOSIS

Lung cancer remains a lethal disease, despite recent advances. The 5-year survival rate for all patients is slightly >10%. For early-stage asymptomatic NSCLC (stage IA), usually detected incidentally on chest radiograph, the 5-year survival rate is approximately 80%. This figure rapidly decreases to 55% for stage IB and to 30% for stage II disease. Given the overall poor survival rates, there has been a resurgence of interest in screening tests using spiral CT scans for early detection of lung cancer. This is an active area of ongoing research. Long-term survival in SCLC is rare.

MESOTHELIOMA

PATHOLOGY

Mesothelioma is a malignant lesion derived most commonly from the visceral pleura.

EPIDEMIOLOGY

Mesothelioma is rare. Asbestos is the major risk factor. Cigarette smoking markedly increases the incidence of mesothelioma in patients exposed to asbestos.

HISTORY

Chest pain from local chest wall extension, dyspnea secondary to pleural effusion, and lung entrapment, weight loss, and unexplained night sweats may occur.

PHYSICAL EXAMINATION

The patient may have decreased breath sounds on the side of the tumor as a result of pleural effusion and lung entrapment.

DIAGNOSTIC EVALUATION

Chest radiography often demonstrates a pleural effusion. Thoracocentesis typically yields bloody fluid, and cytology is often negative for malignant disease. CT scan shows a chronic effusion with irregular thickened visceral pleura. Patients with a suggestive history and a recurrent pleural effusion with no clear cause should undergo thoracoscopy and pleural biopsy, even in the presence of negative fluid cytology.

TREATMENT

Overall prognosis is poor, with few survivors living beyond 2 years. Early-stage lesions may be resectable but require induction chemotherapy followed by extrapleural pneumonectomy, a significantly morbid procedure. Chemotherapy and radiotherapy are used for nonoperative patients.

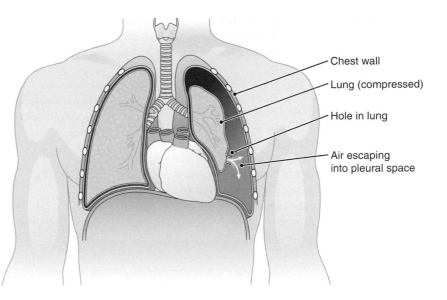

Figure 18-6 • Pneumothorax. Injury to lung tissue allows air to leak into the pleural space and put pressure on the lung.
From Cohen BJ. *Medical Terminology*. 4th ed. Baltimore, MD: Lippincott Williams & Wilkins, 2003.

PNEUMOTHORAX

The lung is covered by visceral pleura, and the inner chest wall is covered by parietal pleura. These two continuous surfaces form a potential space. Simple pneumothorax occurs when air enters this space and the lung falls away from the chest wall resulting in a "dropped" lung (Fig. 18-6). Open pneumothorax occurs when a defect in the chest wall allows continuous entry of air from the outside (Fig. 18-7). Tension pneumothorax occurs when air enters the potential space but cannot escape. A ball valve–like effect

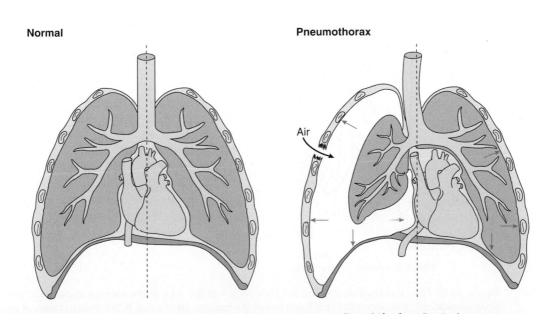

Figure 18-7 • Open pneumothorax with element of tension causing midline shift of mediastinal structures.
From Willis MC. *Medical Terminology: A Programmed Learning Approach to the Language of Health Care*. Baltimore, MD: Lippincott Williams & Wilkins, 2002.

allows pressure to increase within the hemithorax, thereby forcibly collapsing the ipsilateral lung and compressing mediastinal structures.

ETIOLOGY

Spontaneous pneumothorax is usual seen in young thin males with rupture of congenital apical blebs or in older patients with bullous emphysema from smoking. It can also occur in patients on mechanical ventilation, especially if high inspiratory pressures are required. Infection, specifically tuberculosis or *Pneumocystis carinii*, can cause pneumothorax, as can lung tumors on rare occasion. Placement of central venous catheters results in pneu-

mothorax in 1% of cases. The use of ultrasound guidance for central line placement in the internal jugular position reduces the chance of pneumothorax to nearly zero. Thoracocentesis, needle biopsy, and operative trauma are other iatrogenic causes. Open pneumothorax is caused by penetrating trauma, whereas tension pneumothorax can occur by any of the above mechanisms.

HISTORY

Patients can be entirely asymptomatic, or they may complain of dyspnea or pleuritic chest pain.

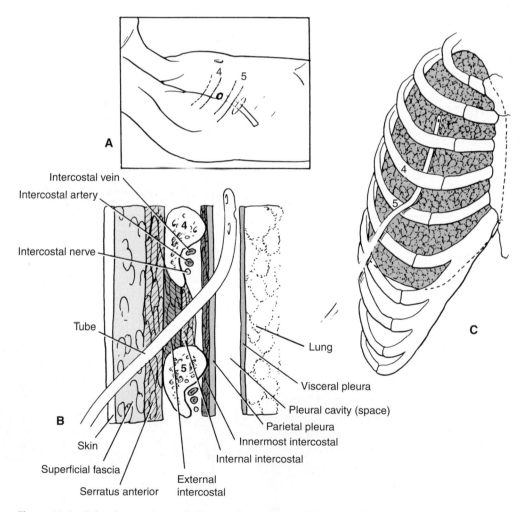

Figure 18-8 • Tube thoracostomy. **A.** The site for insertion of the tube at the anterior axillary line. The skin incision is usually made over the intercostal space one below the space to be pierced. **B.** The various layers of tissue penetrated by the scalpel and later the tube as they pass through the chest wall to enter the pleural cavity (space). The incision through the intercostal space is kept close to the upper border of the rib to avoid injuring the intercostal vessels and nerve. **C.** The tube advancing superiorly and posteriorly in the pleural space.
From Snell RS. *Clinical Anatomy.* 7th ed. Philadelphia, PA: Lippincott Williams & Wilkins, 2003.

PHYSICAL EXAMINATION

Simple pneumothorax may result in decreased breath sounds and hyperresonance on the affected side. Tension pneumothorax may cause tachycardia, hypotension, and hypoxia, and the trachea may be displaced away from the affected side.

DIAGNOSTIC EVALUATION

Chest radiography reveals absence of lung markings in the affected area, usually in the apex, in an upright film. A visible line corresponding to the visceral pleural surface of the lung is evident. Tracheal deviation or mediastinal shift suggests tension pneumothorax.

TREATMENT

Simple pneumothoraces of less than 20% can be observed if no increase in size is demonstrated on serial chest x-rays and the patient is hemodynamically stable. Indications for chest tube placement include size >20% or those that demonstrate increase in size during serial radiographic observation. Open pneumothorax requires repair of the defect and tube thoracostomy. Symptomatic tension pneumothorax is a surgical emergency and requires immediate needle thoracostomy, usually in the midclavicular line in the second intercostal space on the affected side. This will decompress the chest and allow normalization of hemodynamics and oxygenation. Tube thoracostomy should then follow (Fig. 18-8).

EMPYEMA

Empyema is an infection within the pleural space.

ETIOLOGY

Empyema is most commonly caused by pneumonia, lung abscess, recent thoracic surgery, or esophageal perforation. The most common organisms are those that cause primary lung infection, including *Staphylococcus, Streptococcus, Pseudomonas, Klebsiella, Escherichia coli, Proteus,* and *Bacteroides.*

HISTORY

The patient may have a history of previous pneumonia, thoracic surgery, or esophageal instrumentation. Fatigue, lethargy, and shaking chills may occur.

PHYSICAL EXAMINATION

The patient is often systemically ill. Fever and decreased breath sounds at the affected lung base are common.

DIAGNOSTIC EVALUATION

The serum white blood cell count is elevated. Chest radiography reveals a pleural effusion. Chest CT shows a defined fluid collection (Fig. 18-9). Aspiration of the pleural fluid by thoracentesis shows an exudative effusion, characterized by a high white blood cell count with predominantly polymorphonuclear cells, a low pH, a low glucose, and high lactate dehydrogenase. Bacteria on Gram stain and culture may be present.

TREATMENT

On rare occasions, antibiotics and needle aspiration alone are successful, but usually tube thoracostomy is required. For patients who have inadequate re-expansion owing to "trapped" lung after chest tube insertion, surgical decortication may be required to remove the restricting pleural peel and facilitate lung re-expansion.

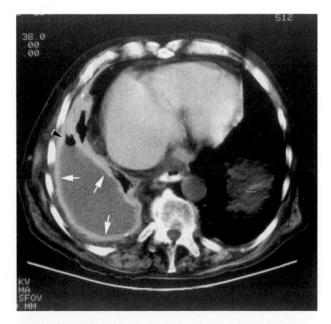

Figure 18-9 • Empyema. Air fluid level (arrowhead) in the pleural space in this patient with an empyema and bronchopleural fistula. An elliptical fluid collection is present, and the inner margin of the collection is smooth and thin. The inner margin also appears dense (straight arrows), indicating enhancement, with a split-pleura sign.
From Shields TW, LoCicero J III, Ponn RB, et al. *General Thoracic Surgery.* 6th ed. Philadelphia, PA: Lippincott Williams & Wilkins, 2004.

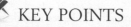 KEY POINTS

- Benign lesions of the trachea and bronchi are rare. Sleeve resection or partial lung resection may be required for treatment.

- Carcinoid tumors can release a variety of substances, causing paraneoplastic syndromes.

- Lung cancer is the leading cause of cancer-related death in North America. More than 80% of lung cancers are smoking-related. Most patients are symptomatic at the time of presentation and are not surgical candidates. Accurate preoperative staging is required to determine appropriate treatment.

- Early-stage lung cancer is treated with surgery and chemotherapy.

- Asbestos is the major risk factor for developing mesothelioma. Cigarette smoking greatly increases the risk of developing mesothelioma. Prognosis is poor.

- Tension pneumothorax is a surgical emergency and requires rapid decompression.

- Empyema is treated with tube thoracostomy and antibiotics. Surgical decortication may be required.

Chapter

19 Esophagus

ANATOMY AND PHYSIOLOGY

The esophagus is a muscular tube that functions primarily as a conduit for transporting ingested solids and liquids from the mouth into the intra-abdominal gastrointestinal tract. It extends from the pharynx to the stomach, traversing the posterior mediastinum, and is bounded posteriorly by the vertebral column and thoracic duct, anteriorly by the trachea, laterally by the pleura, and on the left by the aorta (Figs. 19-1 and 19-2). It begins at the cricoid cartilage in the neck and courses downward to the left, then to the right, and back to the left to pierce the diaphragm and join the cardia of the stomach. The intra-abdominal portion of the esophagus measures <3 cm. The upper one third of the esophageal musculature is skeletal, whereas the lower two thirds is smooth muscle. Unlike the intra-abdominally located stomach, small intestine, and colon, there is no true serosal layer covering the esophagus.

The vagus nerves form a plexus around the esophagus, which condenses distally to form two trunks on the lateral esophagus. These trunks, in turn, rotate so that the left trunk moves anteriorly, whereas the right trunk moves posteriorly.

The esophageal mucosa is lined by squamous epithelium that becomes columnar near the gastroesophageal junction. The next layer encountered moving radially outward is the submucosa, which contains the submucous (Meissner) plexus. Next are two muscular layers, the inner circular muscle layer and the outer longitudinal muscle layer. Sandwiched in between these two muscular layers is the myenteric (Auerbach) plexus.

The arterial supply of the esophagus involves vessels from the neck, chest, and abdomen. The superior and inferior thyroid arteries supply the upper esophagus, whereas the intercostals, left gastric, and phrenic arteries supply the lower esophagus. Venous drainage of the upper esophagus is into the inferior thyroid and vertebral veins, whereas the mid and lower esophagus drains into the azygous, hemiazygous, and left gastric veins. Submucosal veins can become engorged in patients with portal hypertension, causing varices and potentially life-threatening bleeding. Lymphatics drain into cervical, mediastinal, celiac, and gastric nodes. Innervation is from the vagus, cervical sympathetic ganglion, splanchnic ganglion, and celiac ganglion. These nerves are responsible for esophageal motility.

Peristasis conveys food into the stomach. Gastric reflux is prevented by increased tone in the lower portion of the esophagus; there is no true sphincter. Air ingestion is prevented by resting tone in the upper esophagus.

ESOPHAGEAL NEOPLASMS

PATHOLOGY

Esophageal neoplasms are almost always malignant. Benign tumors account for fewer than 1% of cases and are usually leiomyomas or congenital cysts. Symptomatic benign esophageal neoplasms are treated with local resection or enucleation. Most malignant esophageal neoplasms seen worldwide are of squamous cell histologic type, whereas adenocarcinoma histology predominates in the United States and other industrialized nations. Most cases of adenocarcinoma arise in the distal third or gastroesophageal junction (80%). Metastases are usually to liver, lungs, and bones, with at least 35% of patients with distant metastases at the

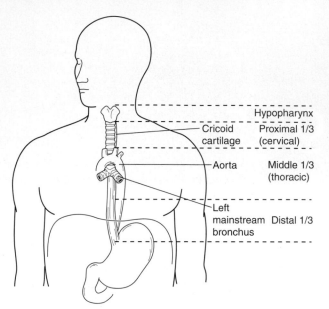

Figure 19-1 • Clinical divisions of the esophagus.
From Lawrence PF. *Essentials of General Surgery*. 4th ed. Philadelphia, PA: Lippincott Williams & Wilkins, 2006.

time of diagnosis. Early-stage cancers are usually diagnosed only incidentally or else discovered on screening studies. Prognosis is poor, with an overall 5-year survival rate of only 5%.

PATHOGENESIS

Mucosal insult seems to be a common pathway toward the genesis of esophageal cancer. Chronic ingestion of extremely hot liquids, esophageal burns from acid or base ingestions, radiation-induced esophagitis, and reflux esophagitis are all implicated in causing esophageal cancer. Alcohol, smoking, nitrosamines, and malnutrition/vitamin deficiency also play a role in cancer development. Barrett esophagus, which occurs when the normal squamous epithelium becomes columnar in response to injury from acid reflux, is considered a premalignant lesion. Approximately 10% of patients with Barrett esophagus will develop adenocarcinoma.

In patients with achalasia, approximately 6% will develop squamous cell carcinoma of the esophagus.

EPIDEMIOLOGY

The incidence of esophageal cancer varies according to the presence of the etiologic factors described previously. For example, in places with high soil nitrosamine content, the prevalence of esophageal cancer is almost

1% of adults. In the United States, the incidence of esophageal cancer is four in 100,000 White men and 12 in 100,000 Black men. It is most commonly a disease of men between 50 and 70 years of age.

HISTORY

At the time of diagnosis, most patients have advanced disease and are not surgical candidates for curative resection. The lack of a serosal lining and the rich submucosal lymphatic network of the esophagus allows early extension of tumor into adjacent mediastinal structures as well as early local lymph node spread. Approximately 75% of patients have mediastinal or extrathoracic lymph node metastases at the time of diagnosis.

The classic presentation of distal esophageal adenocarcinoma is an older man with a history of gastroesophageal reflux disease complaining of progressive dysphagia to solids initially, and then to liquids. Typically, patients feel well and have no other symptoms. Some report noting mild weight loss, more often related to diminished caloric intake resulting from obstructive symptoms than to cachexia from metastatic disease. Chest pain and odynophagia (pain with swallowing) may also occur. Invasion of a recurrent laryngeal nerve may cause hoarseness from vocal cord paralysis.

Patients with esophageal squamous cell carcinoma often have a history of heavy alcohol and tobacco use and present with more pronounced symptoms owing to more advanced disease.

PHYSICAL EXAMINATION

Signs are nonspecific, and patients appear well unless significant metastatic disease is present. Supraclavicular lymphadenopathy at presentation is rare.

DIAGNOSTIC EVALUATION

Barium esophagogram detects malignant lesions in 96% of patients. Findings range from small mucosal defects to "apple core" lesions to complete obstruction (Fig. 19-3). This is usually the initial study for the evaluation of new onset dysphagia. Definitive diagnosis of cancer requires confirmation by flexible endoscopy with tissue biopsy. If Barrett esophagitis alone is noted, the extent of disease can be determined and biopsies performed to look for dysplasia or carcinoma in situ.

To determine the stage of the primary tumor (T) and regional lymph node status (N), endoscopic ultrasound

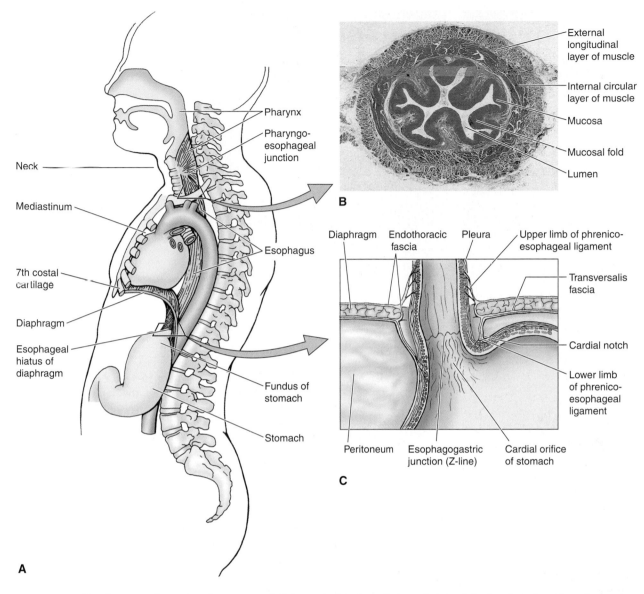

Figure 19-2 • Esophagus and associated structures. **A.** Schematic drawing of a lateral view of the head, neck, and trunk showing the esophagus and the structures associated with it. The esophagus descends posterior to the trachea and leaves the thorax through the esophageal hiatus in the diaphragm. **B.** Transverse section of the esophagus showing the muscular layers and microscopic structure of its wall. **C.** Coronal section of the esophagus, diaphragm, and stomach (superior part). Observe the phrenicoesophageal ligament that connects the esophagus flexibly to the diaphragm; it limits upward movement of the esophagus while permitting some movement during swallowing and respiration.
From Moore KL, Dalley AF II. *Clinically Oriented Anatomy.* 4th ed. Baltimore, MD: Lippincott Williams & Wilkins, 1999.

(EUS) is used. Ultrasound is best for evaluating local staging: the intramural extent of the tumor as well as assessing for lymph node enlargement or abnormality. Ultrasound depicts the normal five layers of the esophagus and can accurately determine the T status in 85% to 90% of patients. Fine-needle aspiration biopsy of abnormal-appearing lymph nodes under ultrasound guidance may be performed.

Evaluation of regional and distant disease is best done by computed tomography (CT) scan and positron emission tomography scan. CT scanning should be performed first after initial diagnosis, because lung and liver metastases are often detected. If CT is negative for metastases, then EUS is performed. Combined preoperative CT and EUS have an accuracy rate of 86% for TNM staging.

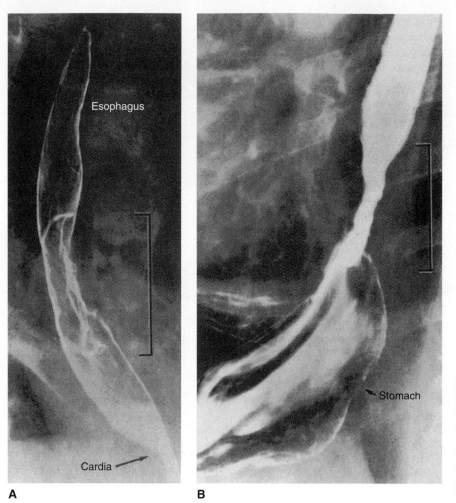

A   **B**

Figure 19-3 • **A.** Contrast radiograph showing the typical "apple core" lesion of carcinoma of the middle one third of esophagus. **B.** Ragged edge seen in carcinoma of the distal esophagus.

From Lawrence PF. *Essentials of General Surgery*. 4th ed. Philadelphia, PA: Lippincott Williams & Wilkins, 2006.

STAGING

The TNM system is used for staging esophageal cancer. Clinical stage (cTNM) is determined by evaluation of all information derived from physical examination, imaging studies, endoscopy, biopsy, and occasionally laparoscopy or thoracoscopy. Once the clinical stage is determined, rational treatment plans can be proposed to the patient (Table 19-1 and Fig. 19-4).

TREATMENT

Because there is no serosal layer covering the esophagus, disease is often locally advanced or metastatic on presentation, leading to poor overall survival statistics. Surgical cure rates are 20% to 30% at best. The goals of surgical treatment are removal of the tumor and regional lymph nodes followed by re-establishment of gastrointestinal tract continuity. For early-stage disease,

esophagectomy provides the possibility of cure. Preoperatively, induction chemoradiotherapy may be administered, especially to downstage patients with resectable bulky tumors. Some evidence has shown that induction chemotherapy and radiotherapy preoperatively, followed by surgery, can improve long-term survival, but this remains an area of controversy. The extent of lymphadenectomy is also an area of ongoing controversy.

Various operations with varying degrees of invasiveness have been developed for treating esophageal cancer. In deciding which procedure to perform, the surgeon must take into consideration the location of the tumor, the proposed esophageal substitute, and the physical condition and body habitus of the patient. Generally, the most common surgical approaches are transthoracic (thoracotomy) and transhiatal without thoracotomy. Incisions may be required in the neck, chest, and abdomen.

TABLE 19-1	AJCC TNM Classification of the Esophagus
Primary Tumor (T)	
Tis	Carcinoma in situ
T1	Tumor invades lamina propria or submucosa
T2	Tumor invades muscularis propria
T3	Tumor invades adventitia
T4	Tumor invades adjacent structures
Regional Lymph Nodes (N)	
T0	No regional lymph node metastasis
T1	Regional lymph node metastasis
Distant Metastasis (M)	
M0	No distant metastasis
M1	Distant metastasis
Stage Grouping	
Stage 0	Tis N0 M0
I	T1 N0 M0
IIA	T2 N0 M0, T3 N0 M0
IIB	T1 N1 M0, T2 N1 M0
III	T3 N1 M0, T4 Any N M0
IV	Any T Any N M1

Used with permission of the American Joint Committee on Cancer (AJCC), Chicago, IL. Original source: AJCC Cancer Staging Manual, 6th ed. New York, NY: Springer-Verlag, 2002.

The most common transthoracic esophagectomy is one called the Ivor Lewis esophagectomy, named after the distinguished Welsh surgeon who developed the approach. In brief, it involves upper midline laparot-omy with mobilization of the stomach and is followed by right thoracotomy with esophageal resection and anasto-mosis. It is useful for patients with tumors of the middle and lower esophagus. For tumors of the upper esophagus, many surgeons use a modified approach, called the McKeown modification, which involves additional intrathoracic esophageal mobilization and anastomosis in the right neck through a separate cervical incision (three-hole technique). The tubularized stomach is used as the esophageal substitute in most cases. Other possible sub-stitutes are the colon and small bowel (Fig. 19-5).

Esophagectomy without thoracotomy is termed the transhiatal approach. This technique uses laparot-omy for gastric and esophageal mobilization, fol-lowed by left cervical incision for the anastomosis. The major benefit of this approach is avoiding the complications that arise from thoracotomy.

Although open surgical approaches remain the standard for esophagectomy, recent advances in mini-mally invasive surgery have allowed esophagectomy to be performed using laparoscopic and thoracoscopic techniques. A cervical incision is also used (Fig. 19-6). This is a complex and challenging procedure that has a steep learning curve. Early results of laparoscopic esophagectomy seem to compare favorably with open surgery, but long-term data are presently not available.

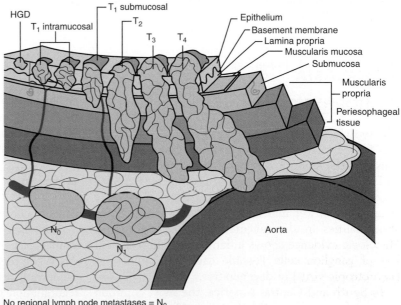

Figure 19-4 • Visual representation of TNM staging of esophageal cancer.
Reprinted with permission of The Cleveland Clinic Foundation.

No regional lymph node metastases = N_0
Regional lymph node metastases present = N_1
High grade dysplasia = HGD

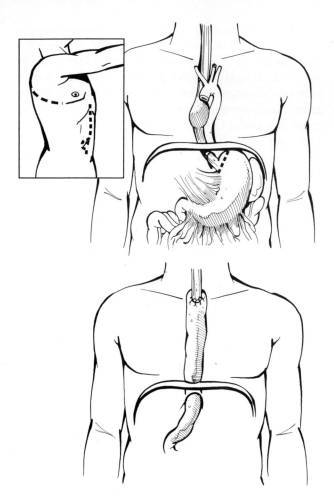

Figure 19-5 • Three-hole Mckeown modification (using additional cervical incision) of the standard Ivor Lewis abdominal and right thoracic approach.

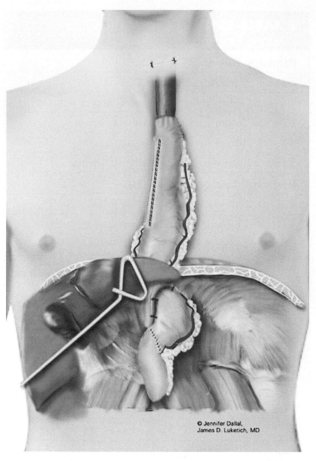

Figure 19-6 • Completed cervical anastomosis after laparoscopic transhiatal esophagectomy without thoracotomy. From Shields TW, LoCicero J III, Ponn RB, et al. *General Thoracic Surgery*. 6th ed. Philadelphia, PA: Lippincott Williams & Wilkins, 2004.

ACHALASIA

PATHOPHYSIOLOGY

The term "achalasia" is derived from the Greek, meaning "failure to relax." It is defined as absence of peristalsis in the smooth muscle of the distal esophagus and failure of the lower esophageal sphincter (LES) to relax with swallowing. The exact cause of primary achalasia is not well understood, but studies have shown abnormalities in the myenteric plexus (Auerbach). Histologic evidence shows inflammation, fibrosis, and loss of ganglion cells. Possible causes are infectious (neurotropic virus) or degenerative.

In South and Central America, the most common cause of secondary achalasia is Chagas disease (American trypanosomiasis).

EPIDEMIOLOGY

Achalasia is the most common disorder of esophageal motility but is actually rare, with an incidence of 0.5 per 100,000. Men and women are equally affected. Patients usually present between 20 and 50 years of age.

HISTORY

Patients complain of dysphagia to solids and liquids. Because ingested material is unable to pass into the stomach, a column of food or liquid rises in the esophagus. When there is a change in position, liquid spills into the mouth or into the lungs, and patients complain of regurgitation or have a history of recurrent aspiration pneumonia. Because the regurgitant does not include gastric contents, it is usually not sour tasting.

DIAGNOSTIC EVALUATION

Chest x-ray may show an air-fluid level in the esophagus. A prominent gastric bubble may be noted because of the highly competent LES. Changes from aspiration pneumonia may be present. CT scan shows a dilated, thin-walled esophagus containing food material.

Contrast esophagogram shows a dilated, smooth-walled esophagus tapering to a "bird's beak" at the LES. Dynamic video imaging or fluoroscopy reveals reduced or absent peristalsis of the distal esophagus.

Esophagoscopy should also be performed to evaluate for strictures and rule out cancer. Malignant tumors of the gastroesophageal junction can mimic the findings of achalasia, known as pseudoachalasia.

Motility and pressure studies confirm the diagnosis. The two key findings on manometry that are required to make the diagnosis are incomplete relaxation of the LES and aperistalsis of the body of the esophagus.

TREATMENT

There is no cure for achalasia, given the still unelucidated underlying process that causes esophageal neural pathology. Treatment is focused on relief of symptoms (dysphagia) caused by achalasia.

Medical treatment consists mainly of pneumatic balloon dilatation (Fig. 19-7) of the lower esophageal sphincter to reduce outflow obstruction and facilitate gravity drainage. This technique is minimally invasive, has good initial results, and can be repeated. However, it carries the risk of esophageal perforation and over the long term has inferior results when compared with surgical therapy. Another medical treatment is LES relaxation by paralysis achieved by endoscopic injections of botulinum toxin (Botox). This may be an option for frail, high-risk patients, as all patients experience symptomatic relapse.

Surgical therapy by esophageal myotomy (Heller myotomy) is the definitive treatment for achalasia.

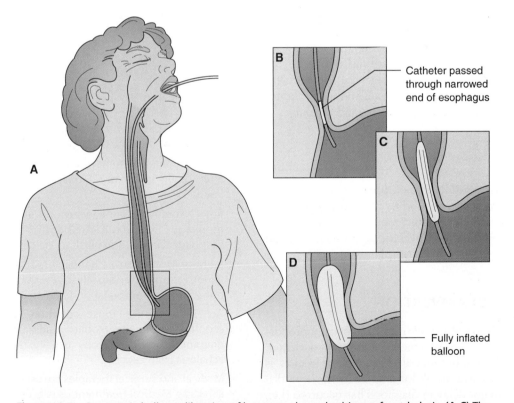

Figure 19-7 • Pneumatic balloon dilatation of lower esophageal sphincter for achalasia. **(A-C)** The dilator is passed, guided by a previously inserted guidewire. **(D)** When the balloon is in proper position, it is distended by pressure sufficient to dilate the narrowed area of the esophagus.
From Smeltzer SC, Bare BG. *Brunner & Suddarth's Textbook of Medical-Surgical Nursing*. 9th ed. Philadelphia, PA: Lippincott Williams & Wilkins, 2000.

The goal of myotomy is to reduce LES pressure to facilitate gravity drainage while also performing a partial fundoplication to ensure a degree of gastroesophageal reflux control. The procedure is performed using the laparoscopic approach, with low morbidity. Longitudinal separation of the esophageal musculature is carried from the distal esophagus onto the proximal stomach, and partial fundoplication (Dor or Toupet wrap) completes the procedure. Myotomy can also be performed through the chest by thoracoscopy or thoracotomy, but with greater morbidity. Surgical therapy provides superior long-term results over medical interventions.

ESOPHAGEAL PERFORATION

ETIOLOGY

Esophageal perforation occurs most commonly after instrumentation (iatrogenic) but also from ingested foreign bodies or penetrating trauma. Spontaneous esophageal rupture occurring after violent emesis is known as Boerhaave syndrome. The latter is named after Hermann Boerhaave, who first reported distal esophageal rupture in 1724 during the autopsy of Baron von Wassenaer, the infamous overindulging Grand Admiral of the Dutch Fleet who showed very poor judgment by engaging in self-induced, chemically assisted vomiting after feasting and drinking.

HISTORY

Recent instrumentation of the upper airway or esophagus should raise the possibility of esophageal injury. Boerhaave syndrome should be suspected in cases involving recent emesis. Epigastric abdominal pain and shoulder pain are frequent complaints.

PHYSICAL EXAMINATION

The degree of presenting symptoms is usually proportional to the time from when perforation occurred. Subcutaneous emphysema in the cervical region is often found, as well as abdominal tenderness or distention. If a major delay in diagnosis has occurred (i.e., because of lack of history in an unconscious patient), then fever, tachycardia, and hypotension resulting from sepsis is common. The presence of a hydropneumothorax can result in diminished breath sounds over the involved hemithorax.

DIAGNOSTIC EVALUATION

Chest x-ray can demonstrate pleural effusion, hydropneumothorax, and mediastinal emphysema. An esophageal contrast study with either water-soluble contrast medium or water-suspended barium sulfate can confirm the location of perforation. If diagnosis is still uncertain, then intraluminal examination by flexible endoscopy can also be used. Thoracentesis can reveal empyema.

TREATMENT

Immediate exploratory thoracotomy and repair of the perforation is indicated in almost all cases. Iatrogenic injuries can usually be closed primarily if surgical intervention is immediate. Perforations with devitalized surrounding tissue or with significant soilage and infection should be repaired with the use of a pedicled flap (i.e., intercostal muscle flap). Pleural space drainage with chest tubes continues postoperatively. Although small cervical lacerations may occasionally be managed with antibiotics and close observation alone, mortality from perforation of the thoracic esophagus is >50% if not treated within 24 hours.

KEY POINTS

- The esophagus is a muscular tube with a rich submucosal lymphatic network that lacks an outer serosal layer. Therefore, esophageal cancer is often advanced at the time of diagnosis.
- Most esophageal tumors are malignant. Survival after surgery is 20% to 30%. Overall survival remains low at 5%.
- Risk factors for esophageal cancer include Barrett esophagus from gastroesophageal reflux disease, esophageal burns, and nitrosamine ingestion.
- Surgery is the only chance for attaining cure. Various surgical approaches are used, including transthoracic, transhiatal, and minimally invasive.
- Achalasia is the most common disorder of esophageal motility. Motility studies confirm the diagnosis. Esophagoscopy usually differentiates achalasia from cancer.
- Medical and surgical therapies are used for treating achalasia. Medical treatment usually entails balloon dilation, whereas surgical esophageal myotomy provides definitive treatment and symptom relief.
- Esophageal perforation is frequently fatal if not diagnosed and treated early.

Part V

Special Topics

Chapter

20 Neurosurgery

BRAIN TUMORS

Because the brain is encased in a nonexpandable bony skull, both benign and malignant brain tumors can cause death if not appropriately diagnosed and treated. Brain tumors cause elevated intracranial pressure (ICP) by occupying space, producing cerebral edema, interfering with the normal flow of cerebrospinal fluid, or impairing venous drainage (Fig. 20-1). Patients may present with progressive neurologic deficits owing to increasing ICP, tumor invasion, or brain compression. Alternatively, they can present with headache or seizures.

PATHOLOGY

Intracranial tumors can be classified as either intracerebral or extracerebral (Table 20-1). Intracerebral tumors include glial cell tumors (astrocytomas, oligodendrogliomas, ependymomas, primitive neuroectodermal tumors), metastatic tumors (lung, breast, skin [melanoma], kidney, colon), pineal gland tumors, and papillomas of the choroid plexus. Extracerebral tumors arise from extracerebral structures and include meningiomas, acoustic neuromas, pituitary adenomas, and craniopharyngiomas.

Glial cell tumors and metastatic tumors are the most common central nervous system (CNS) tumors seen in adults. Children have a higher proportion of posterior fossa tumors.

GLIAL CELL TUMORS

Glial cells account for approximately 50% of CNS tumors in adults. Different glial cell types (astrocytes, oligodendrocytes, ependymal cells, and neuroglial precursors) give rise to various histologic types of tumors. Although the term "glioma" can be used to describe

152

the above glial tumor types, its common use refers only to astrocytic tumors.

Astrocytic tumors are graded I to IV based on histologic evidence of malignancy; grade I and II tumors are slow-growing malignancies. In children, astrocytomas located in the posterior fossa (cerebellum) usually have cystic morphologies (pilocystic astrocytoma). Grade III tumors are the more aggressive anaplastic astrocytomas. The most common as well as the most malignant astrocytoma is the grade IV glioblastoma multiforme. Glioblastoma multiforme tumors often track through the white matter, crossing the midline via the corpus callosum, resulting in the so-called butterfly glioma on computed tomography (CT). Median survival is 1 year.

Oligodendrogliomas are slow-growing calcified tumors, often seen in the frontal lobes. They are most common in adults and are often associated with seizures.

Ependymomas arise from cells that line the ventricular walls and central canal. Clinical signs and symptoms of elevated ICP are the main features of presentation. Ependymomas are mostly seen in children and usually arise in the fourth ventricle.

Classified by location, infratentorial posterior fossa tumors make up most of the lesions seen in childhood. These are most commonly cystic cerebellar astrocytomas, ependymomas, and medulloblastomas. Highly malignant medulloblastomas typically occur in the vermis in children and in the cerebellar hemispheres in young adults.

METASTATIC TUMORS

Approximately 30% of patients with systemic cancer have cerebral metastases, which usually originate in the lung, breast, skin (melanoma), kidney, and colon. Most lesions are supratentorial and located at the cortical

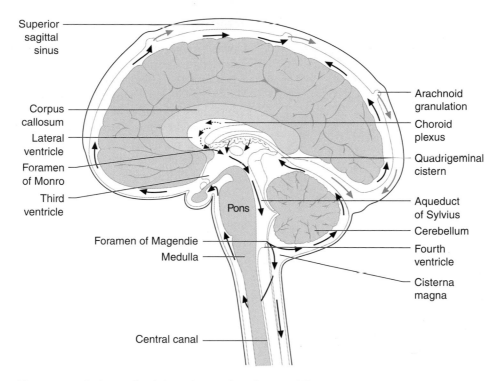

Figure 20-1 • Pathways for the circulation of cerebrospinal fluid.

white matter junction. Resection depends on the nature of the underlying malignancy, symptoms, and prognosis. Single, approachable lesions should be considered for surgical resection in the appropriate setting. Radiation usually follows surgery. Stereotactic radiosurgery is an option in patients with multiple lesions.

MENINGIOMAS

Slow-growing, meningiomas arise from the meninges lining the brain and spinal cord. Complete tumor removal is curative, and residual disease can be observed or treated with radiosurgery.

History

Patients usually present with neurologic signs and symptoms attributable to cerebral compression from the expanding tumor mass. Seizures are a common presentation. Headache, nausea, vomiting, and mental status changes are the most common generalized symptoms of elevated ICP. Classically, patients complain of diffuse headache that is worse in the morning after a night of recumbency.

Physical Examination

Bilateral papilledema may occur, especially in the later stages of disease. Personality changes may be

■ **TABLE 20-1** Intracranial Tumors
Intracerebral
Glial cell tumors—astrocytomas, anaplastic astrocytomas, glioblastoma multiforme, oligodendroglioma, ependymoma, primitive neuroectodermal tumors
Metastatic tumors—lung, breast, melanoma, kidney, colon
Pineal gland tumors
Papillomas of the choroid plexus
Extracerebral
Meningiomas
Neuromas, especially acoustic neuromas
Pituitary tumors
Craniopharyngiomas

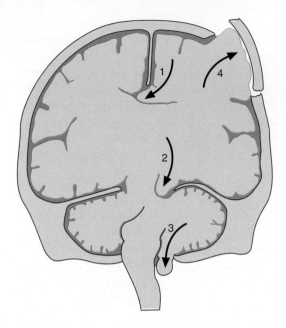

Figure 20-2 • Examples of brain herniation: (1) cingulate gyrus herniation across the falx; (2) temporal uncus herniation across the tentorium; (3) cerebellar tonsil herniation through the foramen magnum; (4) herniation of brain tissue through craniotomy defect.

noted early on and may progress to stupor and coma as ICP increases and brain herniation occurs (Fig. 20-2). Speech deficits and confusion are common with dominant hemisphere lesions. Eye deviation can be a sign of frontal lobe involvement. Ataxia is common with cerebellar tumors. Motor or sensory deficits indicate involvement around the central sulcus or deep structures, especially if combined with mental status changes.

Differential Diagnosis

The differential diagnosis for a patient presenting with central neurologic deficits and symptoms includes cerebrovascular accident, neurodegenerative diseases, abscess, vascular malformations, meningitis, encephalitis, communicating hydrocephalus, and toxic state.

Diagnostic Evaluation

CT and magnetic resonance imaging (MRI) assist in making the diagnosis and in localization of the tumor. MRI with gadolinium enhancement is useful for visualizing higher-grade gliomas, meningiomas, schwannomas, and pituitary adenomas. T2-weighted MRI is useful for low-grade gliomas.

Treatment

Correct management of primary brain tumors requires knowledge of the natural history of specific tumor types and the risks associated with surgical removal. When feasible, total tumor removal is the goal; however, subtotal resection may be necessary if vital brain function is threatened by complete tumor extirpation. If subtotal resection is performed, postoperative radiation therapy can prolong life and palliate symptoms. Chemotherapy is also used for specific tumor types.

Metastatic brain tumors are generally treated with whole-brain irradiation. Occasionally, single lesions amenable to surgery are removed first, followed by whole-brain irradiation.

Perioperative management of increased ICP caused by cerebral edema is accomplished by using corticosteroids (dexamethasone [Decadron]). If hydrocephalus is present, shunting of cerebrospinal fluid may be required.

INTRACRANIAL ANEURYSMS

Intracranial aneurysms are saccular, berry-shaped aneurysms, usually found at the arterial branch points within the circle of Willis (Fig. 20-3). Although they

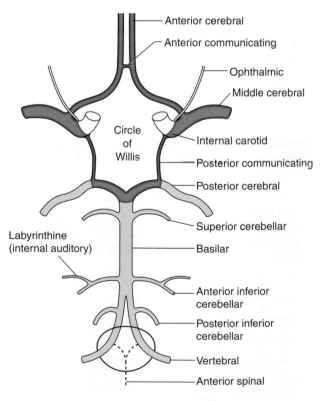

Figure 20-3 • Cerebral arterial circle of Willis.

rarely rupture, significant morbidity and mortality may result secondary to hemorrhage. Subarachnoid hemorrhage (SAH) develops when intracranial aneurysms rupture and bleed.

HISTORY

Sudden onset of a severe headache, typically described as the "worst headache of my life," usually signals the rupture of an intracranial aneurysm. ICP transiently increases with each cardiac contraction, causing a pulsating headache. Progressive neurologic deficits may develop as a result of blood clot mass effect, vasospasm with infarction, or hydrocephalus. Coma and death may occur.

A system for categorizing the severity of hemorrhage has been developed using clinical assessment based on neurologic condition. The five-point Hunt-Hess grading system ranges from grade 1, indicating good neurologic condition, to grade 5, indicating significant neurologic deficits (Table 20-2).

DIAGNOSIS

CT is useful for demonstrating SAH. If CT is negative in a patient with a highly suspicious presentation, a lumbar puncture should be performed. If SAH is present, four-vessel cerebral angiography is performed to define the aneurysm neck and relationship with surrounding vessels (Fig. 20-4).

TREATMENT

Initial medical treatment involves control of hypertension with intravenous medications. Phenytoin is administered for prophylactic treatment of seizures,

mannitol can be given to control edema, and nimodipine is used to reduce the risk of developing delayed neurologic deficits from vasospasm.

Emergency external ventricular drainage may be indicated to decrease the ICP. In rare cases with progressive neurologic deterioration, emergency craniotomy and evacuation of a blood clot are required to prevent herniation. The definitive treatment is obliteration by microsurgical clipping or endovascular coiling of the aneurysm.

EPIDURAL HEMATOMA

Epidural hematomas are usually seen in patients with head trauma who have sustained a skull fracture across the course of the middle meningeal artery, causing an arterial laceration and an expanding hematoma (Fig. 20-5). The increasing pressure of the arterial-based hematoma strips the dura mater from the inner table of the skull, producing a lens-shaped mass capable of causing brain compression and herniation.

HISTORY

The presentation of an epidural hematoma is commonly described as a head injury followed by an initial loss of consciousness, recovery (the honeymoon period), and then progressive deterioration. In reality, this sequence of events is unusual. It is more common not to have an initial period of unconsciousness or to become unconscious initially and not to regain it.

PHYSICAL EXAMINATION

Assessing the level of consciousness is the most important aspect in evaluating head injuries. The standard clinical tool for assessment is the Glasgow Coma Scale (GCS), which evaluates eye opening, verbal response, and motor response. Patients with a GCS of ≤7 have severe head injuries, those with scores of 8 to 12 have moderate injuries, and those with scores of >12 have mild injuries. Patients with severe injuries (GCS <8) require immediate endotracheal intubation for airway protection and rapid neurosurgical evaluation (Table 20-3).

DIAGNOSTIC EVALUATION

CT is crucial to establish a diagnosis and treatment plan.

■ TABLE 20-2 Hunt-Hess Classification of Subarachnoid Hemorrhage

Grade	Description
1	Mild headache and slight nuchal rigidity
2	Cranial nerve palsy, severe headache, nuchal rigidity
3	Mild focal deficit, lethargy, or confusion
4	Stupor, hemiparesis, early decerebrate rigidity
5	Deep coma, decerebrate rigidity, moribund appearance

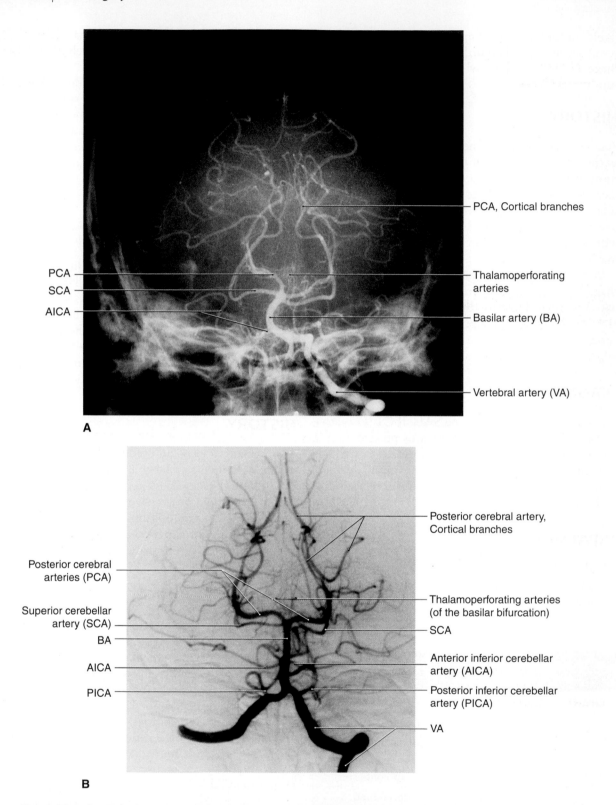

Figure 20-4 • A vertebral artery angiogram is shown in **A**; the same view, but in a different patient, is shown in **B**, using digital subtraction methods. Relevant arteries are labeled.

From Haines DE. *Neuroanatomy: An Atlas of Structures, Sections, and Systems*. 6th ed. Philadelphia, PA: Lippincott Williams & Wilkins, 2004.

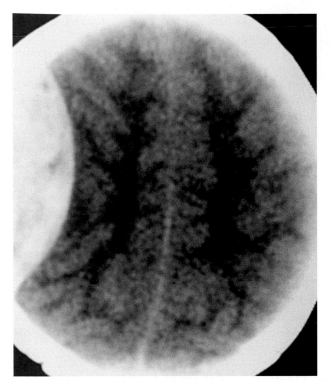

Figure 20-5 • Epidural hemorrhage: epidural hematoma. This 8-year-old boy presented after a sledding accident. He had no loss of consciousness but complained of headache and vomiting. A head computed tomography scan shows the classic biconvex hyperdensity of an epidural hematoma.

From Fleisher GR, Ludwig S, Baskin MN. *Atlas of Pediatric Emergency Medicine.* Philadelphia, PA: Lippincott Williams & Wilkins, 2004.

■ **TABLE 20-3** Calculation of Glasgow Coma Score
Best Eye Response (4 points possible)
1. No eye opening
2. Eye opening to pain
3. Eye opening to verbal command
4. Eyes open spontaneously
Best Verbal Response (5 points possible)
1. No verbal response
2. Incomprehensible sounds
3. Inappropriate words
4. Confused
5. Orientated
Best Motor Response (6 points possible)
1. No motor response
2. Extension to pain
3. Flexion to pain
4. Withdrawal from pain
5. Localizing pain
6. Obeys commands

TREATMENT

For patients presenting with a depressed skull fracture and a neurologic examination indicating a deteriorating level of consciousness, airway control and emergency cranial decompression must be performed. Burr holes are made over the area of hematoma seen on CT, a flap is quickly turned, and the clot is decompressed, with resultant decrease of the ICP. Middle meningeal artery bleeding is controlled, and the dura is fixed to the bone to prevent reaccumulation.

SUBDURAL HEMATOMA

In contrast with epidural hematomas, subdural hematomas are usually low-pressure bleeds secondary to venous hemorrhage. Both spontaneous and traumatic subdural bleeds occur. The source of hemorrhage is from ruptured bridging veins that drain blood from the brain into the superior sagittal sinus.

RISK FACTORS

Most commonly, subdural hematoma is a result of trauma. Older adult patients, those with brain atrophy, and patients treated with anticoagulants are at particularly increased risk. Less common causes include rupture of a cerebral aneurysm, arteriovenous malformation, and metastatic tumors.

HISTORY

Headache, drowsiness, and unilateral neurologic symptoms are the usual presenting symptoms. Seizure activity and papilledema are uncommon.

EVALUATION

Prompt imaging is the cornerstone of diagnosis. Head CT should be performed in patients with the appropriate history. MRI is more sensitive and may be considered. In patients without history of trauma, angiography may be useful to identify the root cause.

TREATMENT

Nonoperative management is limited to patients who are stable, have small lesions, and do not have evidence of herniation. Patients with significant neurologic deficits secondary to mass effect may need urgent burr-hole decompression or craniotomy. Other indications for surgical management include lesion size >10 mm, >5 mm of midline shift, or declining GCS. Generally, it is important to identify and ligate the bleeding vessel.

SPINAL TUMORS

Tumors are defined by anatomic location as being extradural, intradural, or intramedullary (Fig. 20-6). Extradural tumors are most commonly lesions of metastatic disease from primary cancers of the lung, breast, or prostate. Other common tumors are multiple myeloma of the spine and lymphoma. Back pain

or neurologic deficit from cord compression is the usual presenting complaint.

The most common intradural tumors are meningiomas, schwannomas, neurofibromas, and ependymomas. A nerve root tumor may transverse the intervertebral foramen, forming a bilobed lesion called a dumbbell tumor. Patients usually present with numbness progressing to weakness.

Intramedullary tumors include astrocytomas, ependymomas, and cavernous malformations. It is important to differentiate cystic tumors from syringomyelia by gadolinium-enhanced MRI, because both may present with sensory loss.

DIFFERENTIAL DIAGNOSIS

The differential diagnosis for patients presenting with signs and symptoms of spinal cord pathology are cervical spondylitic myelopathy, acute cervical disc protrusion, spinal angioma, and acute transverse myelitis.

PHYSICAL EXAMINATION

Patients with tumors of the spine typically present with complaints indicative of progressive spinal cord compression, with evidence of a sensory level.

DIAGNOSTIC EVALUATION

Plain radiographs may demonstrate bony erosion. MRI is the modality of choice, because it provides detailed anatomic definition. A CT myelogram may be performed if MRI is unavailable.

TREATMENT

The goal of spinal tumor treatment is to relieve cord compression and to maintain spinal stability. These are interrelated goals, because removing a compressing tumor usually requires surgery on the vertebral column.

The spine consists of two columns: the anterior column (vertebral bodies, discs, and ligaments) and the posterior column (facet joints, neural arch, and ligaments). Damage sustained to one of the columns may result in permanent spinal instability.

For anterior tumors that involve the vertebral body, tumor removal via the anterolateral approach is performed. The vertebral body is resected and the defect repaired with a bone graft and metal plate stabilization.

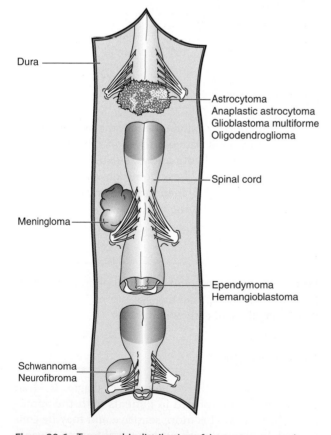

Dura

Astrocytoma
Anaplastic astrocytoma
Glioblastoma multiforme
Oligodendroglioma

Spinal cord

Meningloma

Ependymoma
Hemangioblastoma

Schwannoma
Neurofibroma

Figure 20-6 • Topographic distribution of the common neoplasms of the spinal meninges, spinal nerve roots, and spinal cord.

Posterior tumors can be removed by laminectomy that usually does not cause spinal instability. Metastatic and unresectable disease can be palliated and pain controlled with radiation therapy. Occasionally, anterior and posterior approaches are combined; therefore, appropriate spine stabilization requirements must be anticipated.

SPONDYLOSIS AND DISC HERNIATION

Degenerative changes in the spine are responsible for a large proportion of spine disease. Intervertebral discs consist of two parts: the central nucleus pulposus, which acts as a cushion between vertebrae, and the surrounding dense annulus fibrosus (Fig. 20-7). At birth, the nucleus contains 80% water, but over time the disk dehydrates, and the disc space narrows. In the cervical and lumbar spines, this narrowing causes abnormal vertebral stresses, which in turn cause osteogenesis, producing osteophytes and bony spurs. These degenerative bone growths can traumatize nerve roots. This degenerative process secondary to abnormal motion in an aging spine is called spondylosis.

Structural failure of the intervertebral disc occurs when the nucleus pulposus herniates into the spinal canal or the neural foramina through a defect in the circumferential disc annulus. Lateral disc herniation can cause nerve root compression and radicular symptoms; central disc herniation can cause myelopathy.

These two interrelated degenerative processes are responsible for most spine disease, manifested by nerve root and spinal cord compression. The most mobile segments of the spine (cervical and lumbar) are commonly affected by both processes (Fig. 20-8).

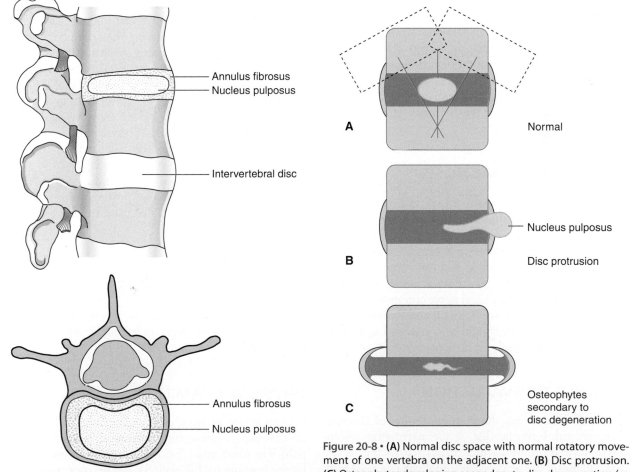

Figure 20-7 • Intervertebral disc: annulus fibrosus and centrally located nucleus pulposus.

Figure 20-8 • **(A)** Normal disc space with normal rotatory movement of one vertebra on the adjacent one. **(B)** Disc protrusion. **(C)** Osteophytes developing secondary to disc degeneration (or disc protrusion). Note the different origin of the disc protrusion and osteophytes.

CERVICAL DISC DISEASE

HISTORY

Patients with cervical spondylosis and disc disease are typically older than 50 years and can present with pain, paresthesia, or weakness. In the case of cervical spondylotic myelopathy secondary to repetitive spinal cord damage by osteophytes, patients experience progressive numbness, weakness, and paresthesia of the hands and forearms in a glove-like distribution. In contrast, patients with radiculopathy secondary to disc disease complain of pain radiating down the arm in a nerve root distribution, worsening on neck extension.

PHYSICAL EXAMINATION

Limitation of neck motion and straightening of the normal cervical lordosis are common findings. Sensory and motor deficits in a radicular pattern and careful testing for signs of diminished biceps, brachioradialis, and triceps reflexes assist with localization. Hyperreflexia and the presence of the Hoffmann (reflex contraction of thumb and index finger on tapping the nail of or flicking the middle finger) or Babinski reflex (extension of the great toe on stroking the lateral aspect of the sole of the foot) help determine the presence of myelopathy and are important signs to elicit.

DIFFERENTIAL DIAGNOSIS

All causes of cervical spinal cord or cervical nerve root compression must be considered. More common causes of cord compression are rheumatoid arthritis and ankylosing spondylitis. For nerve root compression, brachial plexus compression from a first or cervical rib and scalenus anticus syndromes (thoracic outlet syndrome) should be ruled out. Peripheral nerve entrapment (carpal tunnel syndrome, ulnar nerve palsy) and Pancoast tumor of the pulmonary apex should be considered in patients who have arm pain without neck pain.

DIAGNOSTIC EVALUATION

Cervical spine x-rays show straightening of the normal cervical lordosis, disc space narrowing, osteophyte formation, and spinal canal narrowing. If the axial diameter of the cervical spinal canal is ≤10 mm, risk is high for cervical cord compression.

CT myelography and MRI are used to evaluate the spinal cord and nerve roots and define their relationships to other vertebral structures. Areas of cord and root compression can be identified and intervention planned. MRI is the study of choice for initial evaluation of a herniated cervical disc, whereas CT is preferred when more bony detail is required.

TREATMENT

All patients should initially be managed with medical therapy, except for those with myelopathy or severe radicular weakness. Cervical traction, analgesics, and muscle relaxants are used. For acute cervical radiculopathy caused by cervical disc herniation, >95% of patients improve without surgery. However, patients with spondylosis and disc prolapse who fail to improve or who exhibit progressive worsening may require surgical treatment.

Because the pathogenesis of degenerative osteogenesis is abnormal stress and movement between vertebrae, procedures aimed at stabilizing the spine have shown significant success in obtaining symptomatic relief and promoting osteophyte reabsorption. Anterior cervical fusion produces immobilization by removal of the intervertebral disc, with bone graft replacement and internal fixation. Both cervical spondylosis and cervical disc prolapse can be treated with this procedure.

Decompression laminectomy is usually performed only on patients who have a diffusely narrow spinal canal and who are rapidly worsening as a result of spondylotic myelopathy. The posterior approach for lateral disc herniations is also used to avoid segmental fusion.

LUMBAR DISC DISEASE

Lumbar disc prolapse is a common disorder. Patients often present with pain radiating down the lower extremity.

PHYSICAL EXAMINATION

Symptoms of sciatica are caused by disc herniation compressing a nerve root, leading to severe radicular pain. The L4-5 and L5-S1 discs most commonly prolapse, leading to L5 and S1 nerve root symptoms. Paresthesia, numbness, and weakness may be present.

Straight leg raise testing can be positive for pain radiating down the affected extremity, with both ipsilateral and contralateral leg raising. Other important signs indicating disc herniation include absence of an ankle or knee reflex, weakness of foot dorsiflexion or plantar flexion, or weakness of knee extension.

DIAGNOSIS

Clinical diagnosis is confirmed by MRI that demonstrates disc protrusion at the suspected level (Fig. 20-9).

TREATMENT

Most patients improve without surgery. Elective surgery should be considered for patients with chronic, disabling, intractable pain. The standard procedure of choice is open laminectomy and discectomy of the appropriate interspace. Urgent surgery is indicated in patients with progressive neurologic deficits (e.g., foot drop) and in those with acute onset of cauda equina syndrome, which is a neurosurgical emergency and occurs as a result of a massive midline disc protrusion that compresses the cauda equina. Typical findings of cauda equina syndrome include urinary

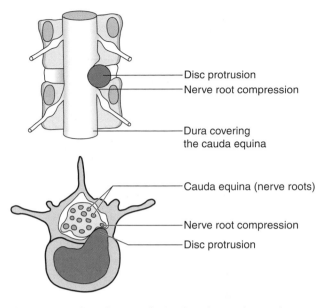

Figure 20-9 • The relations of a lumbar disc prolapse. The protruding disc causes nerve root compression.

retention or overflow incontinence, bilateral sciatica, and perineal numbness and tingling (i.e., saddle anesthesia). Bilateral laminectomy decompression with disc removal is the procedure of choice.

KEY POINTS

- Brain tumors cause elevated intracranial pressure by occupying space, producing cerebral edema, blocking cerebrospinal fluid flow, or impairing cerebral venous drainage, resulting in neurologic deficits.
- Glioblastoma multiforme tumors are the most common and most malignant astrocytic tumors. They can track across the corpus callosum and are then called butterfly gliomas.
- Most childhood tumors are located in the posterior fossa and include cystic astrocytomas, ependymomas, and medulloblastomas.
- Intracranial aneurysms are usually found at arterial branch points within the circle of Willis.
- Patients with low-grade presentations should have early aneurysm obliteration to prevent rerupture.

- Patients with high-grade presentations are stabilized with external ventricular drainage, and the aneurysm is obliterated early or in a delayed fashion, depending on brain swelling. Endovascular treatment is frequently considered for patients with higher-grade presentations.
- Epidural hematomas arise from middle meningeal artery hemorrhage after head trauma and produce a lens-shaped mass capable of causing brain herniation.
- A "honeymoon" period may precede rapid progressive deterioration.
- Emergency cranial decompression is lifesaving.
- Subdural hematomas are usually low-pressure venous bleeds arising from ruptured bridging veins that drain blood from the brain into the superior sagittal sinus.

- Older adult patients receiving anticoagulants are at increased risk.
- Neurologic deficit warrants urgent neurosurgical intervention.
- Spinal tumors are extradural, intradural, or intramedullary.
- Most extradural tumors are metastatic lesions.
- Symptoms of spinal tumors include pain, myelopathy, disc protrusion, spinal angioma, and transverse myelitis.

- Spondylosis and disc herniation can manifest with nerve root or spinal cord compression.
- Most patients with spondylosis and disc herniation improve without surgery.
- Cauda equina syndrome presents as urinary retention or overflow incontinence, bilateral sciatica, and perineal numbness secondary to lumbar disc herniation. Urgent decompressive laminectomy is indicated.

Kidneys and Bladder

ANATOMY

The kidneys are retroperitoneal structures. They are surrounded by Gerota's fascia and lie lateral to the psoas muscles and inferior to the posterior diaphragm. Blood supply is by renal arteries; usually there is a single renal artery, but there may be more than one. The renal veins drain into the inferior vena cava. The ureters course retroperitoneally, dorsal to the cecum on the right and the sigmoid colon on the left. They cross the iliac vessels at the bifurcation between internal and external and enter the true pelvis to empty into the bladder. The bladder lies below the peritoneum in the true pelvis and is covered by a fold of peritoneum. Blood supply is from the iliac arteries through the superior, middle, and inferior vesical arteries (see Color Plate 14). Sympathetic nerve supply is from L1 and L2 roots, whereas parasympathetic is from S2, S3, and S4.

URINARY TRACT INFECTION

Urinary tract infections are classified as lower if they involve only the bladder (acute cystitis), and upper if they involve the kidneys (pyelonephritis). They are considered uncomplicated if they occur in young, nonpregnant women and complicated if they occur in men, pregnant women, or older women.

ETIOLOGY

Escherichia coli is by far the most common pathogen, accounting for more than two thirds of all cases. Other Gram-negative rods, including *Proteus*, *Klebsiella*, *Staphylococcus saprophyticus*, and *Enterococcus*, are also common. In hospitalized patients, more resistant organisms, including *Pseudomonas*, may be found. In women, most infections are thought to result from fecal colonization of the vagina.

EPIDEMIOLOGY

Infections of the lower tract are more common than those of the upper tract. In young women in the United States, the incidence is approximately three in 1,000. Risk factors include diabetes, sexual intercourse, stress incontinence, and previous urinary tract infections.

HISTORY

Patients often present with frequency, dysuria, nausea, and vomiting. Flank pain is generally more associated with pyelonephritis and suprapubic pain with cystitis, but this is not reliable. Previous urinary infections and multiple or new sexual partners may help lead to the diagnosis.

PHYSICAL EXAMINATION

Patients may have fever, flank or suprapubic tenderness, or foul smelling urine. In severe cases, patients may be hypotensive.

DIAGNOSTIC EVALUATION

Pyuria is nearly ubiquitous in patients with urinary tract infections. Hematuria is also common. Culture growth of >100,000 colony-forming units/mL of urine is diagnostic, although some patients will have only 1,000 or

10,000 colony-forming units/mL. For uncomplicated cases, imaging is not necessary. Complicated cases may require cystoscopy with or without upper tract imaging.

TREATMENT

Antibiotics are the mainstay of treatment. Oral antibiotics are adequate for uncomplicated cases, but hospital admission and parenteral antibiotics should be considered for complicated cases. Fluoroquinolones are a reasonable first choice. For complicated cases, urologic evaluation should be considered.

STONE DISEASE

ETIOLOGY

The most common kidney stones are calcium phosphate and calcium oxalate (80%); struvite (15%), uric acid (5%), and cystine (1%) are other causes. Calcium stones are usually idiopathic but can be caused by hyperuricosuria and hyperparathyroidism. Struvite stones are caused by infection with urease-producing organisms, usually *Proteus*. Uric acid stones are common in patients with gout and can occur with Lesch-Nyhan syndrome or tumors. Cystine stones are hereditary.

EPIDEMIOLOGY

Approximately 20% of males and 10% of females will be affected by nephrolithiasis over their lifetime. Calcium stones and struvite stones are more common in women, uric acid stones are twice as common in men, and cystine stones occur with equal frequency in men and women.

HISTORY

Stone formation is associated with a number of dietary factors, which should be investigated. Low fluid intake is a general risk factor. Diets high in salt promote excretion and increased urinary concentration of calcium. High intake of animal protein results in increased calcium, uric acid, citrate, and acid excretion. Low-calcium diets can also be problematic, as they increase oxalate excretion.

Patients with stone disease usually present with acute onset of pain beginning in the flank and radiating down to the groin, although the pain can be anywhere along this track. The patient is often unable to find a comfortable position, and vomiting is common. Dysuria, frequency, and hematuria may be described.

DIAGNOSTIC EVALUATION

Workup includes evaluation of urinary sediment that shows hematuria, unless the affected ureter is totally obstructed. Crystals are frequently observed. It is imperative to determine the type of stone to guide therapy. Urinary sediment may be extremely useful for this purpose. Calcium oxalate stones are either dumbbell-shaped or bipyramidal and may be birefringent. Uric acid crystals are small and red-orange. Cystine stones are flat, hexagonal, and yellow. Struvite stones are rectangular prisms. Uric acid crystals and calcium oxalate crystals can be found in normal individuals and thus are less useful when found in the sediment.

Blood work should evaluate for elevated serum calcium and uric acid. Measurement of parathyroid hormone levels should be performed in patients with hypercalcemia or high urinary calcium.

Spiral computed tomography is commonly used to make the diagnosis. The stones appear bright in the thin cuts that are obtained with this technique. An abdominal radiograph will often show the stones, as calcium, struvite, and cystine stones are all radiopaque. Intravenous pyelography involves intravenous administration of an iodinated dye that is excreted in the kidneys. This allows diagnosis of stones by outlining defects in the ureter or demonstrating complete obstruction caused by stone disease. Retrograde pyelography involves injecting dye through the urethra and is useful for assessing the degree and level of obstruction. Ultrasonography of the kidneys can demonstrate the stone (Fig. 21-1) and hydronephrosis (Fig. 21-2) indicative of ureteral obstruction. The presence of fluid jets at the entrance of the ureter in the bladder precludes the diagnosis of total obstruction.

TREATMENT

In the acute setting, pain and nausea should be controlled with narcotics and antiemetics. Most stones pass spontaneously; deflazacort and nifedipine or tamsulosin may be used to facilitate stone passage. Stone size predicts spontaneous passage: asymptomatic stones <5 mm usually do not require intervention. Stones >5 mm should be considered for intervention. Less invasive options include extracorporeal shock wave lithotripsy (ESWL); percutaneous nephrolithotomy (PCNL); and endoscopic lithotripsy using ultrasonic, electrohydraulic,

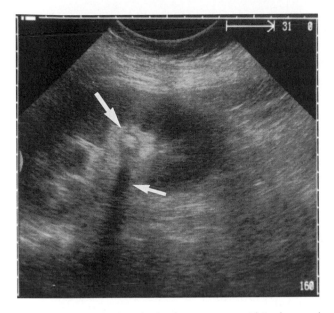

Figure 21-1 • Posterior shadowing: a stone within the renal pelvis (large arrow) casts a posterior shadow (small arrow).
From Harwood-Nuss A, Wolfson AB, Lyndon CH, et al. *The Clinical Practice of Emergency Medicine.* 3rd ed. Philadelphia, PA: Lippincott Williams & Wilkins; 2001:128.1.

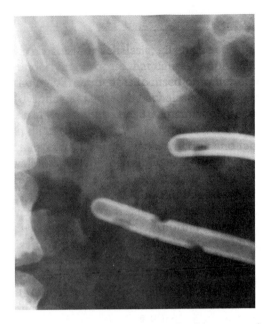

Figure 21-3 • Combined percutaneous nephrolithotomy and extracorporeal shock wave lithotripsy for staghorn calculi. A 35-year-old woman presented with a *Proteus* urinary tract infection and was found to have a large complete left staghorn calculus.
From Harwood-Nuss A, Wolfson AB, Lyndon CH, et al. *The Clinical Practice of Emergency Medicine.* 3rd ed. Philadelphia, PA: Lippincott Williams & Wilkins; 2001:63–65.

or laser energy to remove stones. ESWL is the most common approach and involves using high-energy shock waves that originate extracorporeally. Focusing the energy on the stone causes fragmentation, which facilitates passage. This technique is not ideal for struvite or staghorn calculi. PCNL involves placement of a nephrostomy tube and is more efficacious than ESWL for stones that are large, complex, or composed of cysteine. PCNL and ESWL can be combined (Fig. 21-3). Open pyelolithotomy is reserved for patients who fail multiple attempts at less invasive approaches.

To prevent recurrent stones, patients should be counseled to increase fluid intake. Dietary modifications should be recommended based on the stone type. Pharmacologic interventions include a thiazide diuretic for patients with hypercalciuria and allopurinol or potassium citrate for uric acid stones. Hypocitraturia may be treated with potassium citrate. Oxalate stones may be treated with calcium if urinary calcium is low.

RENAL CANCER

EPIDEMIOLOGY

Two percent of cancer deaths are attributable to renal cancer. Men are affected twice as often as women, and smoking may be a risk factor.

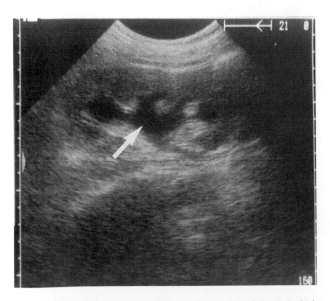

Figure 21-2 • Hydronephrosis: longitudinal view of the right kidney. There is moderate hydronephrosis, which is seen as separation of the pelvic calyces by fluid (arrow).
From Harwood-Nuss A, Wolfson AB, Lyndon CH, et al. *The Clinical Practice of Emergency Medicine.* 3rd ed. Philadelphia, PA: Lippincott Williams & Wilkins, 2001.

PATHOLOGY

Renal cell cancer is classified as clear cell (80%), papillary (15%), and chromophobe (5%; see Color Plate 15). Rare types include collecting duct carcinoma and unclassified renal cell cancer. Other tumors that may arise in the kidney include Wilms tumor and sarcoma.

HISTORY

Patients may experience hematuria and flank pain, which can be sudden in the event of hemorrhage. Fever and extrarenal pain from metastatic disease may be present. Approximately 30% of patients will present with metastatic disease.

PHYSICAL EXAMINATION

Tumors may be palpable.

DIAGNOSTIC EVALUATION

Intravenous pyelography demonstrates a defect in the renal silhouette. Computed tomography can differentiate between cystic and solid lesions.

TREATMENT

Initial treatment in most cases is radical nephrectomy with attempt to remove all tumor. For patients with metastatic disease, results with chemotherapy are disappointing. Gemcitabine and fluorouracil demonstrate limited activity against the tumor. Interleukin-2 is a drug approved by the Food and Drug Administration for renal cell cancer. Response rates are in the 15% to 20% range.

BLADDER CANCER

PATHOLOGY

Transitional cell tumors make up 90% of bladder malignancies. The remainder are squamous cell and adenocarcinoma.

EPIDEMIOLOGY

Men are more frequently affected than women by a ratio of 3:1. Smoking, beta-naphthylamine, schistosomiasis, and paraminophenol all predispose a person to the development of bladder cancer.

HISTORY

Most patients present with hematuria. Urinary tract infections are relatively common, as is bladder irritability evidenced by frequency and dysuria.

DIAGNOSTIC EVALUATION

Urinary cytology may reveal the presence of bladder cancer. Cystoscopy with biopsy confirms the diagnosis. Excretory urography may demonstrate the lesion.

TREATMENT

For local disease, transurethral resection with chemotherapy including doxorubicin, mitomycin, or thiotepa is effective. For locally advanced disease, radical cystectomy (including prostatectomy in men) is combined with radiation and gemcitabine and cisplatin.

KEY POINTS

- Kidney stones are usually composed of calcium salts.
- Symptoms of kidney stones include severe flank pain, which may radiate to the groin.
- Stones >5 mm should be considered for intervention. Most patients will respond to minimally invasive methods of stone removal.
- Renal cancer is responsible for 2% of cancer deaths, and treatment in most cases is radical nephrectomy.
- Patients with bladder cancer usually have hematuria.
- Treatment for bladder cancer may be transurethral resection for local disease; radical cystectomy is used for advanced disease.

Prostate and Male Reproductive Organs

BENIGN PROSTATIC HYPERPLASIA

Benign prostatic hyperplasia (BPH) is a common condition of the prostate gland seen in older men. BPH is clinically important because it is the most common cause of urinary outlet obstruction in men older than 50 years. Untreated, stasis occurs, which increases the risk of urinary tract infection and bladder stones. Over time, bladder decompensation can result in chronic urinary retention with overflow or renal failure secondary to high-pressure urinary retention.

PATHOGENESIS

Prostate gland growth is influenced by steroid hormones. However, the exact mechanism of prostatic hyperplasia remains unclear. Interestingly, BPH does not occur in castrated men or pseudohermaphrodites, both of whom lack dihydrotestosterone, the active metabolite of testosterone. Estrogens have also been implicated in prostatic hyperplasia, because in aging men, the levels of estrogens increase and those of androgens decrease.

The specific area of cellular hyperplasia is the transitional zone or periurethral area of the prostate. The periurethral glandular elements undergo hyperplasia, causing an increase in glandular mass that results in compression of the prostatic urethra and the onset of obstructive symptoms (Figs. 22-1 and 22-2).

EPIDEMIOLOGY

The prevalence of BPH increases with age. Autopsy studies show that at least 50% of men older than 50 years have significant enlargement of the prostate as a result of BPH. Rarely does a patient present before age 50 years, because the doubling time of the hyperplastic gland is slow. By age 90 years, roughly 90% of males have a significant degree of hyperplasia. All men with intact functional testes are at risk for development of BPH.

CLINICAL MANIFESTATIONS

History

Any older man presenting with obstructive urinary symptoms must be suspected of having BPH. Symptoms include urinary hesitancy, intermittency, decreased force of urinary stream, and a sensation of incomplete bladder emptying after voiding. Secondary symptoms are a consequence of urinary stasis. High postvoid residual volumes promote bacterial growth, leading to urinary tract infection. Stasis can also promote the formation of bladder calculi. Most seriously, high-pressure chronic retention can cause bilateral hydroureteronephrosis and subsequent renal failure.

Physical Examination

A careful rectal examination reveals an enlarged symmetric rubbery gland. The size of the gland has no relationship to symptomatology. A small gland may produce a high degree of outflow obstruction, whereas a large gland may produce no symptoms at all. The suprapubic region should be palpated to rule out a grossly distended bladder.

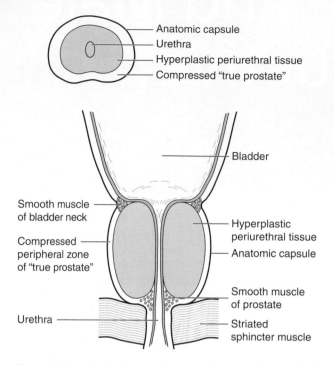

Figure 22-1 • Benign prostatic hyperplasia causing urethral compression. The enlarged periurethral glands are enclosed by the orange peel–like surgical capsule, which is composed of compressed true prostatic tissue.

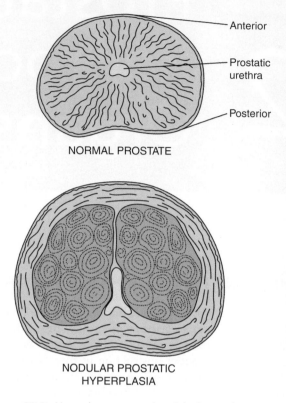

NORMAL PROSTATE

NODULAR PROSTATIC HYPERPLASIA

Figure 22-2 • Normal prostate and nodular hyperplasia. In prostatic hyperplasia, the nodules distort and compress the urethra and exert pressure on the surrounding normal prostatic tissue. Image from Rubin E, Farber JL MD. *Pathology*. 3rd ed. Philadelphia, PA: Lippincott Williams & Wilkins, 1999.

Diagnostic Evaluation

Urine should be obtained for sediment analysis and microbiologic cultures. Serum blood urea nitrogen and creatinine levels should be checked for evidence of renal insufficiency. If chronic urinary retention is suspected, a postvoid residual can be checked by straight catheterization or bladder ultrasonography. Urinary flow rate is assessed by measuring the volume of urine voided during a 5-second period. A flow rate of <50 mL in 5 seconds is evidence of bladder outlet obstruction. Ultrasonography, intravenous pyelography, or computed tomographic (CT) scan can be used for imaging the urinary tract. Information regarding size of the prostate, presence of bladder stones, the postvoid residual volume, and hydronephrosis can be obtained. Transrectal ultrasonography is used to evaluate either an irregular prostate when found on examination or an elevated prostate-specific antigen level.

Treatment

The goals of drug therapy for BPH are to relax smooth muscle in the prostate and bladder neck or to induce regression of cellular hyperplasia, thereby enhancing

urinary outflow from the bladder to the urethra. Alpha blockade of adrenergic receptors produces smooth muscle relaxation of both prostate and bladder neck. An infrequent side effect of alpha-antagonists (e.g., terazosin) is postural hypotension (2% to 8%). Prostatic hyperplasia can also be treated with 5-alpha reductase inhibitors (e.g., finasteride), which block the conversion of testosterone to dihydrotestosterone without lowering serum levels of circulation testosterone. However, the effectiveness of 5-alpha reductase inhibitors is less than half that seen with alpha-blockers.

Surgical relief of obstruction is necessary when medical therapy fails. The indications for surgery are a postvoid residual volume >100 mL, acute urinary retention, chronic urinary retention with overflow dribbling, gross hematuria on more than one occasion, and recurrent urinary tract infections. Additional indications are patient request for restoration of normal voiding pattern because of excessive nocturia or dribbling.

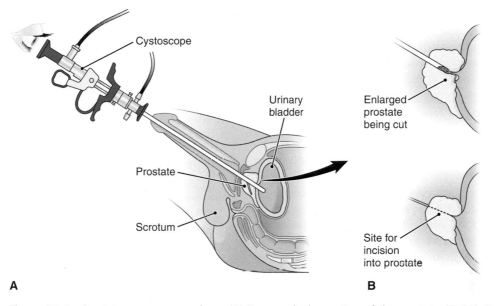

Figure 22-3 • Prostate surgery procedures. **(A)** Transurethral resection of the prostate (TURP). Portions of the prostate are removed at the bladder opening. **(B)** Transurethral incision of the prostate. One or two incisions are made in the prostate to reduce pressure on the urethra.
From Cohen BJ. *Medical Terminology*. 4th ed. Baltimore, MD: Lippincott Williams & Wilkins, 2003.

The procedure of choice is transurethral resection of the prostate (TURP). With the patient in the lithotomy position, the resectoscope is introduced via the urethra into the bladder. The occlusive prostate tissue is identified, and under direct vision, the tissue is shaved away using an electrified wire loop (Fig. 22-3).

Extravasated blood and tissue fragments are evacuated as the bladder is continuously irrigated with a nonelectrolytic isotonic solution. An indwelling catheter is left in place for 1 to 7 days. To minimize the blood loss and side effects of the standard TURP technique, alternative minimally invasive outpatient procedures have been developed and are applicable to select patients. Transurethral needle ablation and focused ultrasound—both of which are less invasive modalities than TURP—ablate prostate tissue by locally heating the tissue. Although these procedures have excellent short-term results in selected patients, long-term efficacy is not well established.

PROSTATE CANCER

Prostate cancer is the most common malignancy of the male genitourinary tract. Indolent tumor growth and a long latency period account for the majority of cases (approximately 80%) being clinically silent.

Most prostate cancers are only discovered on postmortem examination. Management and prognosis depend on stage of tumor.

PATHOGENESIS

The vast majority of prostate cancer (approximately 95%) is adenocarcinoma. Tumors arise from the glandular epithelium in the peripheral zone of the prostate. Tumor growth is hormonally influenced; testosterone exerts a stimulatory effect, whereas estrogens and antiandrogens are inhibitory. Tumors are histologically graded using the Gleason grading system, with scores from 2 (well differentiated) to 10 (poorly differentiated). Tumor grade is correlated with prognosis.

EPIDEMIOLOGY

Prostate cancer is a malignancy of older men, usually occurring after age 60 years. The disease is more common in Black men than in White men.

CLINICAL MANIFESTATIONS

History

Early prostate cancer is usually asymptomatic and is typically only detected on screening examination.

Many patients present with evidence of obstructive symptoms indicating invasion or compression (poor stream, incomplete bladder emptying, nocturia). Such patients are commonly misdiagnosed as having BPH. Metastatic disease is often manifested by bony pain or ureteric obstruction.

Physical Examination

Digital rectal examination and prostate-specific antigen level measurement are the principal methods of screening. Tumor staging is based on the degree of spread: T1 to T2 indicates localized spread within the prostate, T3 to T4 indicates local spread to seminal vesicles or pelvic wall, and M1 indicates metastatic disease. Pattern of spread is via lymphatics to iliac and periaortic nodes and via the circulation to bone, lung, and liver.

Diagnosis

As for most cancers, prostate cancer requires tissue diagnosis. Typically, a hard nodule is detected on digital rectal examination and a follow-up transrectal ultrasound is obtained for needle biopsy of the prostate. The procedure is well tolerated and performed on an outpatient basis.

Chest x-ray is performed to evaluate for lung metastases. Liver function tests may detect liver metastases. If bone metastases are suspected on the basis of presenting symptoms, a bone scan is indicated.

Treatment

Treatment for prostate cancer is based on the stage and grade of the tumor. Two common staging systems are the Gleason score and the TNM stage (Tables 22-1 and 22-2). The treatment options for localized disease (T1 to T2) include radical prostatectomy, external-beam radiotherapy, or interstitial irradiation with implants.

■ TABLE 22-2 AJCC Classification for Prostate Cancer

TNM Definitions	
Primary tumor (T)	
T0	No evidence of primary tumor
T1	Clinically inapparent tumor not palpable or visible by imaging
T2	Tumor confined within prostate
T3	Tumor extends through the prostate capsule
T4	Tumor is fixed or invades adjacent structures other than seminal vesicles: bladder neck, external sphincter, rectum, levator muscles, and/or pelvic wall
Regional Lymph Nodes (N)	
N0	No regional lymph node metastasis
N1	Metastasis in regional lymph node(s)
Distant Metastasis (M)	
M0	No distant metastasis
M1	Distant metastasis
AJCC Stage Groupings	
Stage I	
T1a, N0, M0, G1	
Stage II	
T1a, N0, M0, G2–G4	
T1b, N0, M0, any G	
T1c, N0, M0, any G	
T1, N0, M0, any G	
T2, N0, M0, any G	
Stage III	
T3, N0, M0, any G	
Stage IV	
T4, N0, M0, any G	
Any T, N1, M0, any G	
Any T, any N, M1, any G	

■ TABLE 22-1 Gleason Score

Histopathologic Grade (G)	
G1	Well-differentiated (slight anaplasia)
(Gleason 2–4)	Well-differentiated tumors with cells that are expected to grow slowly and not spread readily
G2	Moderately differentiated (moderate anaplasia)
(Gleason 5–6)	Moderately differentiated tumor cells
G3–G4	Poorly differentiated or undifferentiated (marked anaplasia)
(Gleason 7–10)	Poorly differentiated tumors with cells that are likely to grow rapidly and spread to other parts of the body (metastasize)

For local spread (T3 to T4), the treatment is external-beam radiotherapy, with the addition of hormonal therapy for more advanced cases. Treatment for metastatic disease is hormonal ablation, as most prostate cancers are androgen sensitive. Methods of androgen ablation include surgical and pharmacologic options. Bilateral surgical orchiectomy is the gold standard for ablating testosterone production. Chemical castration using luteinizing hormone-releasing hormone agonists in conjunction with antiandrogens, such as flutamide and cyproterone, produces castrate levels of testosterone. Randomized trials demonstrate that patients with hormone-refractory prostate cancer benefit from docetaxel-based chemotherapy.

TESTES

Disorders of the testes requiring surgical management include congenital abnormalities, tumors, and, in the emergent setting, testicular torsion.

CONGENITAL ABNORMALITIES

Cryptorchidism

Cryptorchidism is the failure of normal testicular descent during embryologic development. The cause of failed descent is unknown but may be due to a selective hormone deficiency, gubernaculum abnormality, or intrinsic testicular defect. Such cryptorchid testes fail in spermatogenic function, but they may retain the ability to secrete androgens. The major risk of cryptorchid testes is the increased risk of testes cancer (35 to 48 times more common than in descended testes). Inguinal hernia is also found in at least 25% of patients with cryptorchidism.

Physical Examination

The testicle remains within the abdomen and cannot be palpated on physical examination.

Treatment

Because spermatogenic failure is progressive, surgical exploration and scrotal placement of the testis should be performed before 2 years of age. If placement of the testicle into the scrotum is not possible, orchiectomy is indicated, because the incidence of cancer of abdominal testes is very high.

Incomplete Descent of the Testis

Incomplete descent of the testis implies a testicle arrested at some point in the path of normal descent

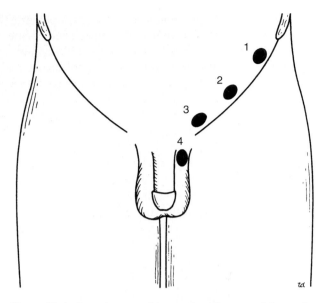

Figure 22-4 • Four degrees of incomplete descent of the testis. 1. In the abdominal cavity close to the deep inguinal ring. 2. In the inguinal canal. 3. At the superficial inguinal ring. 4. In the upper part of scrotum.
From Snell RS. *Clinical Anatomy*. 7th ed. Philadelphia, PA: Lippincott Williams & Wilkins, 2003.

but palpable on physical examination. Such testes are usually located within the inguinal canal between the deep and superficial rings (Fig. 22-4).

Incompletely descended testes are often associated with congenital indirect hernias as a result of the incomplete obliteration of the processus vaginalis.

Treatment

Because testicular function is less compromised than in a cryptorchid testicle, the usual treatment is repositioning and orchiopexy within the scrotum. If present, an indirect hernia is repaired concurrently.

Testicular Tumors

Tumors of the testicle are the most common genitourinary malignancy among young men between the ages of 20 and 35 years. Virtually all neoplasms of the testicle are malignant. Tumors are divided into either germ cell or non–germ cell tumors, depending on their cellular origin. Germ cell tumors predominate, accounting for 90% to 95% of all tumors.

Pathology

Non–germ cell tumors, which arise from Leydig and Sertoli cells, produce excess quantities of androgenizing hormones. Germ cell tumors arise from totipotential cells of the seminiferous tubules. Germ cell tumors are divided into two categories: seminomas and nonseminomatous germ cell tumors (NSGCTs). Seminomas are relatively slow growing and exhibit late invasion. They are usually discovered and surgically removed before metastasis can occur. NSGCTs exhibit greater malignant behavior and metastasize earlier. NSGCTs consist of embryonal (20%), teratoma (5%), choriocarcinoma (<1%), or mixed cell type (40%). Choriocarcinomas are fortunately rare subtypes but are highly invasive, aggressive tumors that metastasize via lymphatic and venous systems early in the disease.

Epidemiology

Seminomas are the most common malignant germ cell tumor. Embryonal carcinoma is usually seen in younger males during childhood. Non–germ cell tumors are relatively rare.

History

Tumors usually manifest as firm, painless testicular masses (Fig. 22-5). Occasionally, the mass may cause a dull ache. Hemorrhage into necrotic tumor or after minor trauma may cause the acute onset of pain. Approximately 10% of patients with testicular tumors have a history of cryptorchidism. Because of excess androgen production, non–germ cell tumors can cause

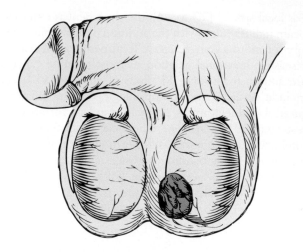

Figure 22-5 • Early testicular tumor.
From Weber J, Kelley J. *Health Assessment in Nursing.* 2nd ed. Philadelphia, PA: Lippincott Williams & Wilkins, 2003.

precocious puberty and virilism in young males and impotence and gynecomastia in adults.

Diagnostic Evaluation

Immediate evaluation should include serum for tumor markers (alpha-fetoprotein [AFP], beta-human chorionic gonadotropin [β-hCG]), serum lactate dehydrogenase, and ultrasound. Tumor markers are not always helpful because seminomas, the most

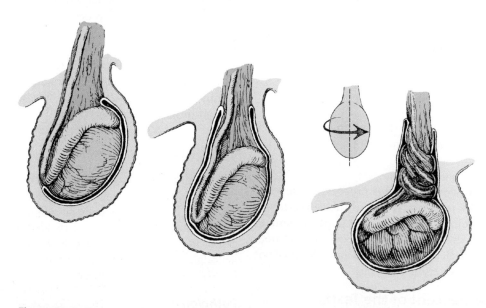

Figure 22-6 • Torsion. Left image shows normal testicular anatomy; a bell-clapper deformity in the tunica vaginalis (middle image) can permit torsion of spermatic vessels (right image).
LifeART image copyright © 2009. Lippincott Williams & Wilkins. All rights reserved.

common testicular neoplasm, are usually negative for both AFP and β-hCG. In neoplasms with tumor markers, the level of tumor burden directly relates to AFP/β-hCG levels that can be monitored during the postoperative period to evaluate the efficacy of treatment and to detect recurrence.

Treatment

Initial treatment is always radical orchiectomy. Subsequent therapy depends on tumor type, grade, and staging. Retroperitoneal lymph node dissection is standard therapy for stage I and II NSGCT.

Seminomas are usually highly radiosensitive. Adjuvant treatment with radiation and chemotherapy yields high 5-year survival rates for both localized and metastatic disease.

Torsion of the Spermatic Cord

Torsion of the spermatic cord is a urologic emergency because complete strangulation of the testicular blood supply renders the testicle surgically unsalvageable after approximately 6 hours.

Pathogenesis

Torsion results from an abnormally high attachment of the tunica vaginalis around the distal end of the spermatic cord. This abnormality allows the testis to hang within the tunica compartment, like a bell clapper within a bell—hence the name bell clapper deformity. As such, the testicle is free to twist on its own blood supply, causing pain and ischemic strangulation (Fig. 22-6).

History

Torsion is usually seen in young male patients, who present complaining of the rapid onset of severe testicle pain followed by testicle swelling.

Physical examination reveals a high-riding, swollen, tender testicle, oriented horizontally in the scrotum. Pain is worse with elevation of the testes, and the cremasteric reflex is often absent.

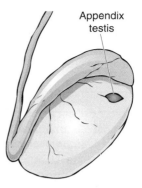

Figure 22-7 • Torsion of appendix testis or appendix epididymis (not shown) can also cause testicular pain and tenderness.

Diagnostic Evaluation

A color-flow Doppler ultrasound should be obtained to evaluate for blood flow within the testicle. Absence of flow confirms the diagnosis.

Differential Diagnosis

The differential diagnosis of an acutely swollen, tender testicle includes essentially two diagnoses: torsion of the spermatic cord and advanced epididymitis. Because one can mimic the other, it is vitally important to arrive at a timely diagnosis. Other less common diagnoses include torsion of an appendix testis or appendix epididymis (Fig. 22-7).

Treatment

Prompt surgical exploration and orchiopexy are required to save the testicle from undergoing ischemic necrosis. Because the bell clapper deformity is usually bilateral, orchiopexy of the contralateral testicle is performed concurrently. If the diagnosis is unclear, surgical exploration is required, because an uncorrected torsion will cause necrosis of the testicle.

KEY POINTS

- Benign prostatic hyperplasia causes bladder outlet obstruction and obstructive urinary symptoms. Urinary stasis leads to urinary tract infections, bladder calculi, hydroureteronephrosis, and renal failure.

- Benign prostatic hyperplasia is medically treated by alpha blockade to relax prostate and bladder neck smooth muscle and occasionally by 5-alpha reductase inhibition to block dihydrotestosterone production and cause regression of cellular hyperplasia. Surgically treatment is by transurethral resection of the prostate and other techniques.

- Prostate cancer is the most common male genitourinary tract malignancy, occurring in older men. Management depends on tumor stage. Treatment

- options include surgery, radiotherapy, and hormonal ablation.
- Cryptorchidism and incomplete testicular descent are congenital abnormalities. Abdominal testes have a high incidence of cancer.
- Testicular tumors are either germ cell tumors (seminomas [the most common] or nonseminomatous germ cell tumors [embryonal carcinoma, teratoma, choriocarcinoma, or mixed]) or non–germ cell tumors (Leydig and Sertoli cell tumors). Tumors usually manifest as firm, painless testicular masses.

- Tumor diagnosis is by ultrasound and alpha-fetoprotein and beta-human chorionic gonadotropin measurement. Orchiectomy, with or without radiation, is standard treatment for testicular tumors.
- Testicular torsion is caused by abnormally high attachment of the tunica vaginalis around the distal end of the spermatic cord. Doppler ultrasound is used for diagnosis because epididymitis can mimic torsion. Prompt surgical exploration and bilateral orchiopexy is required to reverse ischemia from strangulation.

Skin Cancer

ANATOMY

Skin is often referred to as the largest organ in the body, which, by mass, it is. The importance of the skin as a functional barrier to loss of fluids and protection from microorganisms is immediately apparent to anyone caring for patients with significant burns. The performance of these functions requires a highly specialized multi-layer construction.

The outer layer, the epidermis, comprises four layers. Moving inward, they are the keratin layer, consisting of dead skin cells, the granular layer, the squamous layer, and the basal layer. Epithelial cells originate in the basal layer and are pushed outward over time to form the upper layers. These basal cells are strongly attached to the basement membrane. Moving inward, the dermis is composed of collagen, elastin, and glycosaminoglycans. Cellular components are typically fibroblasts. Below the dermis is a layer of subcutaneous fat that is home to sweat glands, hair follicles, and sebaceous glands.

OVERVIEW AND PREVENTION

Skin cancer is the most common malignancy in the United States, with the less aggressive forms, basal cell and squamous cell, being much more prevalent than melanoma skin cancer. Approximately 1 million non-melanoma skin cancers will be diagnosed in the United States in 2007, but only 2,000 deaths will be attributable to the disease. The incidence of these types of cancers is increasing in the United States.

It is generally accepted that these cancers are due to sun exposure. Professional and public education campaigns regarding the dangers of excessive sun exposure are expected to decrease the incidence over time. Methods to reduce sun exposure include limiting daytime activity during peak sun hours, between 11 AM and 3 PM; using protective clothing, including long sleeves and hats; and using high-opacity sunscreens. Because sunburns seem to be associated with higher rates of skin cancer, these should be avoided.

Skin cancer seems to be more prevalent in people with light skin or numerous moles. Regular check-ups for both these groups are critical to make an early diagnosis and initiate treatment.

BASAL CELL CARCINOMA

Basal cell carcinoma (BCC) is the most common form of skin cancer in Caucasians. It is rare in Asians and exceedingly rare in darkly pigmented individuals. The predominant cause is long-term excess exposure to ultraviolet B (UVB) radiation. Accordingly, BCC is a disease of adults, and tumors arise from sun-exposed skin, namely the head and neck. The cellular origin of BCC has traditionally been thought to be the basal cell of the epidermis. More recently, an alternative theory posits that the originating cell type is a pluripotent epithelial cell. BCC is categorized into three types: noduloulcerative, superficial, and sclerosing.

NODULOULCERATIVE BASAL CELL CARCINOMA

Lesions have a pearly, dome-shaped, nodular appearance, with associated telangiectasia and an ulcerated center (see Color Plate 16). Telangiectasia is secondary to tumor-induced angiogenesis, and ulceration results from outgrowth of the local blood supply. Noduloulcerative lesions are the most common type of BCC.

Tumors <1 cm in diameter are rarely invasive and can be treated with cautery and curettage or cryosurgery. Tumors >1 cm are treated with surgical excision. High-risk sites of tumor growth are areas with underlying bone and cartilage (i.e., nose, ear), because the growing tumor tends to track along these structures. Such tumors have a high recurrence rate. Therefore, high-risk tumors and recurrent tumors should be treated with Moh micrographic surgery to ensure complete excision. In this procedure, the entire visible tumor is excised and the margins are carefully marked. Frozen sections are then examined to determine whether the tumor has been completely excised, and if not, to guide further resection. The wounds are not closed until the pathologist determines that all margins are negative. In this way, a maximum amount of skin and soft tissue can be saved, providing a good cosmetic result.

SUPERFICIAL BASAL CELL CARCINOMA

The second most common BCC is the superficial type. Lesions usually appear on the trunk and proximal extremities and clinically resemble thin, scaly, pink plaques with irregular margins (see Color Plate 17). These horizontally expanding tumors are often dismissed as dermatitis; subsequently, tumors may reach diameters of several centimeters by the time of diagnosis. By this late stage, ulceration and deep dermal invasion are present. Standard treatment has been wide-margin excision, with skin grafting if necessary. However, this approach may be unacceptably morbid, leaving a large skin defect. Recently, topical chemotherapy with fluorouracil, cryosurgery, and cautery/curettage has shown cure rates similar to those of traditional wide excision.

SCLEROSING BASAL CELL CARCINOMA

Sclerosing BCC is the least common type. The anatomic distribution is similar to that of the noduloulcerative type, but histologically, the lesions appear as narrow cords of tumor cells encased in a proliferation of connective tissue. Macroscopically, lesions are smooth, atrophic, and indurated and easily mimic scar tissue. This deceptive appearance is unfortunate, because sclerosing tumors are more aggressive than other basal cell tumor types. The growth pattern follows tissue planes and neurovascular bundles, resulting in deep soft tissue invasion. Moh micrographic surgery is the preferred management technique.

MELANOMA

Melanoma is the most frequent cause of death of all skin cancer types. It results from malignant transformation of the normal melanocyte, usually located in the basal layer of the epidermis. Many melanomas are curable by surgical excision.

PATHOGENESIS

Ultraviolet (UV) light is suspected to play a role in the development of all types of skin cancer, including melanoma. Although the precise etiologic role of UV light in the malignant transformation of skin cells remains unresolved, both ultraviolet A (UVA) and UVB are thought to have carcinogenic potential. UVA penetrates deep into the dermis, damaging connective tissue and intrinsic skin elasticity. Excessive UVB exposure results in sunburn.

EPIDEMIOLOGY

Melanoma accounts for 5% of all skin malignancies and 3% of all cancers. The diagnosis of melanoma carries a 50% mortality rate in the United States, and the incidence has dramatically increased during the past 10 to 15 years. Many lesions arise from preexisting moles. A mole that shows rapid growth or heterogeneous pigmentation should be evaluated and possibly biopsied to rule out melanoma. Fair-skinned individuals have a higher incidence of melanoma than the general population. The five signs of melanoma can be remembered as the ABCDE's: *a*symmetric shape, irregular *b*order, mottled *c*olor, large *d*iameter, and progressive *e*nlargement.

RISK FACTORS

Risk factors include the following: a mole that shows persistent changes in shape, size, or color; persons having more than 100 nevi; atypical nevi (5% of population); personal history or family history of melanoma; excess sun exposure (especially in childhood); fair complexion; and tendency to freckle and sunburn.

MELANOMA TYPES

Superficial spreading melanoma can occur anywhere, on both sun-exposed and nonexposed areas. The average age of diagnosis is 40 to 50 years. Lesions are commonly on the upper back and lower legs. Lesions show heterogeneous pigmentation with irregular margins. The growth phase is radial with horizontal spread (Fig. 23-1).

Lentigo maligna melanoma is usually seen in older individuals, with the average age of diagnosis being 70 years. Lesions appear on sun-exposed surfaces, particularly the malar region of the cheek and temple. Lesions exhibit horizontal spread (Fig. 23-2).

Acral lentiginous melanoma has an unusual distribution in that lesions appear on palms, soles, nail beds, or mucous membranes. The most common mucous membrane site is the vulva. Other sites include the anus, nasopharynx, sinuses, and oral cavity. The average age of diagnosis is 60 years. Spread is in a horizontal pattern.

Nodular melanoma can occur at any site and has a very early malignant potential secondary to a predominantly vertical growth phase. In contrast to the three other melanoma types exhibit which radial growth phases with horizontal spread. Nodular lesions have well-circumscribed borders and uniform black or brown coloring.

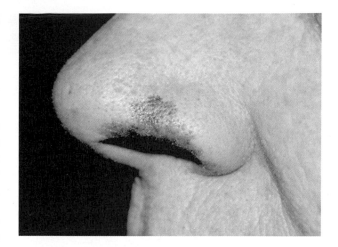

Figure 23-2 • Lentigo maligna melanoma. Biopsy of this lesion demonstrated invasion into the dermis.
From Goodheart HP. *Goodheart's Photoguide of Common Skin Disorders.* 2nd ed. Philadelphia, PA: Lippincott Williams & Wilkins, 2003.

PROGNOSIS

As with other cancers, the extent of spread is an important prognostic factor. Stage I denotes local disease <1.5 mm. Stage II denotes local disease >1.5 mm. Stage III denotes regional disease. Stage IV denotes metastatic disease. As indicated in Table 23-1, stage I disease carries a relatively good prognosis as compared with the dismal prognosis of stage IV disease.

In melanoma, tumor thickness is inversely related to survival and is the single most important prognostic indicator. Historically, there have been two systems for classifying melanomas: the Breslow thickness scale and Clark level of tumor invasion.

The Breslow scale defines primary melanomas that are <0.76 mm thick as local tumors. These tumors have >90% cure rates after simple excision. Individuals with tumors deeper than 0.76 mm have a significant risk of metastatic disease and worse survival.

Clark levels of tumor invasion provide an anatomic description of tumor invasion. The level of tumor invasion can be used for discussing prognosis and planning surgical management (Fig. 23-3).

TNM staging defines stage I tumors as T1 lesions (≤0.76 mm thick) or as T2 lesions (0.76 to 1.50 mm thick) with negative nodes and no metastases. Stage II tumors are T3 lesions (1.51 to 4.00 mm thick) or T4 lesions (>4.00 mm thick) with negative nodes and no metastases. Stage III tumors have fewer than three regional metastases (N1) and no distant metastases,

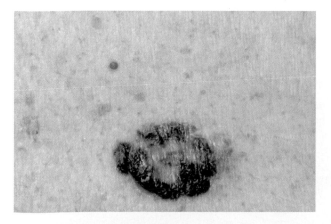

Figure 23-1 • Superficial spreading melanoma. Note the central area (whitish gray) of regression.
From Goodheart HP. *Goodheart's Photoguide of Common Skin Disorders.* 2nd ed. Philadelphia, PA: Lippincott Williams & Wilkins, 2003.

■ **TABLE 23-1** Ten-Year Survival Rates in Patients with Melanoma by Tumor Thickness and Ulceration (n = 4,568)[a]

Thickness, mm	Number of Patients with		10-Year Survival Rate		
	No ulceration, Percent	Ulceration, Percent	No ulceration	Ulceration	P value
0.01–1.00	2017 (95.5)	96 (4.5)	92.0	69.1	<0.0001
1.01–2.00	944 (78.8)	255 (21.2)	77.7	62.9	<0.0001
2.01–4.00	500 (57.4)	372 (42.6)	59.5	53.2	0.006
>4.00	146 (38.1)	238 (61.9)	54.5	35.5	0.0006

[a]Modified from Buzaid AC, Ross MI, Balch CM, et al, Critical analysis of the current American Joint Committee on Cancer staging system for cutaneous melanoma and proposal of a new staging system. J Clin Oncol 1997;15:1039.

whereas stage IV tumors have metastases in skin or subcutaneous tissue, distant lymph node metastases, or visceral metastases.

TREATMENT

Surgical excision is the treatment of choice for primary melanomas. The size of the surgical margin is based on the thickness of the primary lesion (Table 23-2).

Most tissue defects are primarily closed without skin grafting. If primary biopsy specimens are found to have tumor-negative margins, no further surgical treatment is required. Primary mucosal melanomas have poor outcomes because disease is usually extensive. Nail bed lesions require amputation at the distal interphalangeal joint for finger primaries and the interphalangeal joint for thumb primaries.

Regarding regional disease, the performance of elective regional lymph node dissection for nonpalpable nodes is not routine. The thickness of the primary melanoma is used to predict the chance of regional lymph node metastases. Thin lesions limited to the epidermis have a low likelihood of lymph node metastasis, whereas thick lesions invading the subcutaneous fat have a higher likelihood of spread. Regional lymphadenectomy is usually only performed for thick lesions with a high likelihood of nodal spread.

Because of the morbidity of formal regional lymphadenectomy and to increase the ability of detecting microscopic nodal involvement with minimal

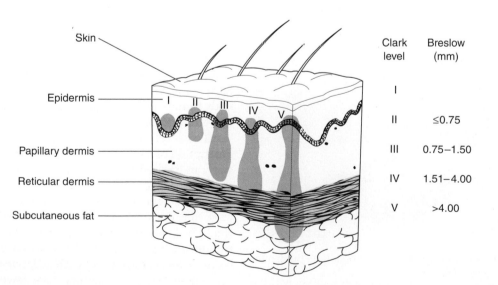

Figure 23-3 • The Clark and Breslow classifications for melanoma.

■ TABLE 23-2 Suggested Margins for Surgical Excision of Melanoma

Melanoma Thickness	Margin
In situ	5 mm
<1 mm thick	1 cm
>1 mm thick	2 cm

■ TABLE 23-3 Predisposing Factors for Developing Squamous Cell Carcinoma

Sunlight exposure
Human papilloma virus infection
Immunosuppression (transplant recipients)
Immunocompromise (HIV infection)
Chronic ulcers
Ionizing radiation (x-rays, gamma rays)
Tobacco use
Scars (burn injury)

invasiveness, the technique of sentinal lymph node biopsy was developed. Using lymphoscintigraphy, the sentinel node of the first-order lymph node basin into which the tumor initially drains is identified. In lymphoscintigraphy, technetium and a sulfur colloid are circumferentially injected around the primary lesion. The technetium drains via lymphatics to the sentinel node, which is identified using a handheld Geiger Counter. The sentinel node is excised and evaluated microscopically for evidence of metastasis. Sentinel lymph node biopsy is usually considered for lesions >1 mm in thickness.

In metastatic disease, individuals with a single identifiable metastatic lesion may benefit from surgical resection. However, resection is generally not recommended for patients with multiple metastatic lesions. Metastatic sites include skin, lung, brain, bone, liver, and the gastrointestinal tract. Treatment options include surgery, radiation, chemotherapy, and isolated limb perfusion.

SQUAMOUS CELL CARCINOMA

Squamous cell carcinoma (SCC) is the second most common form of skin cancer after BCC. Tumors arise from the skin and the oral and anogenital mucosa. Multiple predisposing factors for development of SCC have been identified (Table 23-3).

PATHOGENESIS

The predominant cause of most SCC is chronic actinic damage that induces the malignant transformation of epidermal keratinocytes. A similar effect is seen with exposure to ionizing radiation (x-rays and gamma rays). In darkly pigmented individuals, however, most lesions arise from sites of chronic inflammation, such as osteomyelitis and chronic tropical ulcerations. Tumors

also arise at mucocutaneous interfaces, secondary to tobacco use or human papilloma virus (HPV) infection. Smokers typically present with ulcerating lip and gum or tongue lesions, whereas invasive cancers of the vulva and penis are seen with HPV infection. Anogenital SCC is linked to infection with HPV types 16, 18, 31, 33, and 35. Immunosuppressed or immunocompromised individuals—namely, transplant recipients on immunosuppressive medication or those with HIV/AIDS— have an increased incidence of SCC and an elevated rate of metastasis. Rarely, tumors arise from old scars (usually sustained secondary to burn injury), which form so-called Marjolin ulcers or burn scar tumors. As a rule, actinically induced cancers infrequently metastasize, whereas tumors arising from other mechanisms have a significantly higher rate of metastasis (Table 23-3).

HISTORY

SCC appears as an indurated nodule or plaque, often with ulceration, which has slowly evolved over time. Most lesions are on sun-exposed areas, such as the face, ears, and upper extremities.

PHYSICAL EXAMINATION

Caucasians exhibit pinkish lesions, whereas darker-skinned individuals have hypo- or hyperpigmented lesions (Fig. 23-4). Regional lymphadenopathy occurs in 35% of SCCs arising in the lip and mouth. Aberrant keratinization is often seen in SCC, occasionally causing the growth of cutaneous horns. Therefore, the base of a cutaneous horn should always be examined for the presence of squamous cell cancer.

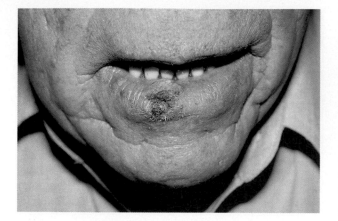

Figure 23-4 • Squamous cell carcinoma. This patient has a nodular, ulcerative lesion on his lip.
From Goodheart HP. *Goodheart's Photoguide of Common Skin Disorders.* 2nd ed. Philadelphia, PA: Lippincott Williams & Wilkins, 2003.

TREATMENT

The preferred treatment is tumor removal by surgical excision. The remaining defect is closed either primarily for smaller lesions or by skin grafting or flap reconstruction for larger lesions. Cryosurgery or cautery/curettage can also be used for small tumors.

PROGNOSIS

The overall cure rate for SCC is 90% after treatment. Tumors other than sun-induced SCC have a higher mortality rate because of the greater likelihood of metastasis.

KEY POINTS

- Basal cell carcinoma lesions appear mostly on sun-exposed areas (head and neck) and are treated by surgical excision.
- The three types of basal cell carcinoma are noduloulcerative, superficial, and sclerosing.
- The five signs of melanoma are *a*symmetric shape, irregular *b*order, mottled *c*olor, large *d*iameter, and progressive *e*nlargement.
- Prognosis for primary melanoma tumors is based on tumor thickness: Tumors <0.76 mm have >90% cure rates.
- Primary melanoma tumors require excision margins based on tumor thickness, whereas nail bed tumors require distal joint amputation.
- When indicated, sentinal lymph node biopsy confirms regional spread of melanoma.

- Sites of melanoma metastasis are lung, brain, bone, and the gastrointestinal tract.
- Squamous cell carcinoma of the oral and anogenital mucosa is associated with tobacco use and human papilloma virus infection.
- Squamous cell carcinoma has an increased incidence in immunosuppressed and immunocompromised individuals and exhibits an elevated risk of metastases.
- Squamous cell carcinoma may arise in old burn scars as Marjolin ulcers or burn scar carcinoma, or in sites of chronic inflammation, such as osteomyelitis and chronic ulcers.
- Treatment of squamous cell carcinoma consists of surgical excision.
- Overall cure rate for squamous cell carcinoma is 90%.

24 Plastic Surgery

Plastic and reconstructive surgery encompasses repair, reconstruction, and aesthetic improvement of bodily deformity resulting from congenital defects, posttraumatic tissue loss, and postablative defects, as well as overall enhancement in normal appearance. Reconstructive surgeons seek to restore form and function while simultaneously achieving aesthetic normalcy. This chapter focuses on the principles of wound healing and tissue transfer.

THE RECONSTRUCTIVE LADDER

The principles of successful wound care include healing by primary or secondary intention, vacuum-assisted closure, skin grafts, local flaps, and distant flaps. A conceptual hierarchy has been established based on a reconstructive approach. The first principle of this approach is that wounds should be managed with the simplest technique to successfully heal a wound. (Fig. 24-1). A plastic surgeon is often consulted to determine which rung (technique) of the "reconstructive ladder" is appropriate from which reconstruction can proceed. Plastic surgeons perform reconstructive surgery in almost all areas of the body. Therefore, plastic and reconstructive surgery demands thorough understanding of anatomy. Individualized patient care is critical for successful reconstructive surgery. Two nearly identical wounds can have solutions that vary greatly in their technique yet adhere to plastic surgery principles.

PRIMARY CLOSURE

This is one of the simplest and most common methods of wound closure. Surgical wounds created at the time of an operation are usually closed primarily in a linear fashion. At the termination of a procedure, typically sutures, tissue glues, or metal staples are placed to align the wound edges. Different types of suturing techniques are frequently used, depending on the dimensions and specific characteristics of a wound (see Chapter 1, Surgical Techniques, Fig 1-6).

After ensuring complete hemostasis within the wound, the skin edges (if already sharply incised) are coapted in a tension-free manner. Sutures are carefully placed to evert the skin edges as this ensures proper healing. It is important to handle skin, dermis, and subcutaneous tissues gently during closure to prevent further inflammation and scarring. Healthy patients who suffer minimal tissue injury without significant skin or subcutaneous loss heal rapidly. Wounds that result from a sharp laceration generally heal faster and with less tissue edema than avulsion and crush injuries. It is important to distinguish how a wound has occurred. Reconstructive plans should be mindful of the mechanism of injury and what tissues are missing (e.g., skin, dermis, soft tissue, cartilage, bone, and so on). Thorough wound irrigation with sterile saline solution is essential before primary closure.

DELAYED PRIMARY CLOSURE

This method of closure is often chosen when a wound is contaminated, infected, or colonized by bacteria or when skin and soft tissue are missing such that the margins of the wound cannot be closed. Infected wounds with necrotic tissue or tissues heavily colonized with bacteria require sharp debridement followed by dressing changes. Wound care may

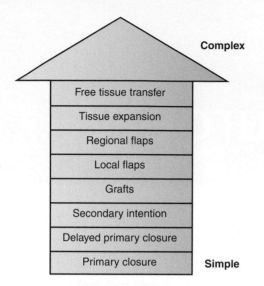

Figure 24-1 • The reconstructive ladder.

be performed for several days to weeks. Wound contraction is a normal component of the healing process. This decreases the size and depth of wounds, enabling delayed primary closure. Wound contamination must be controlled before considering delayed primary closure. Closing a wound that is not clean results in the development of an infection with further delay to definitive wound healing.

SECONDARY INTENTION

Wounds with heavy bacterial contamination or tissue devitalization requiring debridement are often left open and unsutured. The bacterial burden upon the wound is reduced by sharp debridement so that wound edges are clean and optimized for healing. The defect created by serial debridement of nonviable tissue gradually fills with beefy red fibrovascular granulation tissue, which can contract and epithelialize over time to enable complete wound closure. A major recent advance is the use of the wound vacuum to speed healing. This device consists of a sponge attached to a suction machine. The sponge is placed in the wound bed attached to suction tubing, and an airtight seal is created over the assembly. Alterations of the microenvironment allow more rapid wound healing.

GRAFTS

When tissue loss prevents primary closure and waiting for a wound to heal by secondary intention will

take months or potentially lead to wound infection, a skin graft is considered for wound closure. Skin grafting is a technique whereby skin is transferred from one area of the body to another. Most grafts are autografts (patient is both donor and recipient), although other types of grafts can be used in certain situations (isograft, allograft, or xenograft). Skin grafts lack an intrinsic blood supply. Therefore, the skin must become revascularized at the site of insertion, known as the recipient bed. Only vascularized beds are able to be covered with a skin graft. Once applied to a recipient bed, there are three phases of skin graft adherence. During the initial phase, the skin graft adheres as a result of fibrin deposition, known as plasmatic imbibition. The imbibition phase allows the skin graft to remain viable before being revascularized. This phase lasts approximately 48 hours. The second phase, called inosculation, involves anastomotic connections between the recipient bed and graft vessels. Simultaneously, capillaries from the recipient bed grow into the skin graft. Skin grafts are secured to the recipient bed with a bolster, preventing fluid accumulation and shearing between the undersurface of the graft and the wound bed. Other tissues can be used as grafts, such as cartilage, fat, nerve, bone, or tendon.

Skin is the most common tissue graft. Open wounds require barrier reconstitution to prevent bacterial invasion and fluid loss. Skin is collected as either split-thickness or full-thickness grafts.

Split-thickness skin grafts are thin sheets of skin collected from donor sites; they contain varying amounts of dermis and the overlying epidermis (Fig. 24-2). A skin graft can be meshed by creating many tiny incisions; this allows the graft to expand over a larger surface area and better conform to undulating surfaces. Meshed skin grafts also allow drainage of underlying

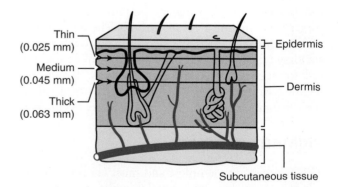

Figure 24-2 • Cross section of skin showing various thickness of split-thickness grafts.

wound exudates; however, as a disadvantage, they also leave large areas within the skin graft to heal by secondary intention. This leads to a cobblestone appearance and irregular contour. In contrast, a sheet (skin) graft often has a nicer aesthetic appearance but does not allow serum or blood to drain through it. Sheet graft survival relies solely on the recipient bed for successful adherence. Additionally, a sheet graft needs a larger donor site surface area for tissue collection. Because they are nonmeshed, sheet grafts contract considerably less than meshed grafts. The anterior thigh is a common donor site for skin graft tissue collection. Donor sites re-epithelialize from epithelial cells remaining within transected hair follicles and generally require 7 days to repopulate. Full-thickness skin grafts contain the entire dermis and epidermis. They are used to close surgical defects when durability, color match, appearance, and lack of wound contraction are required. The groin, flank, and postauricular area are common donor sites. Full-thickness donor sites require primary closure, whereas split-thickness skin grafts epithelialize (see Color Plate 18).

LOCAL FLAPS

Local flaps are blocks of tissue that maintain an intrinsic blood supply and are derived from tissue immediately adjacent to the recipient bed. A local tissue flap either advances (V-Y advancement flap, rectangular advancement flap; Fig. 24-3 and 24-5) or pivots (rotation flap

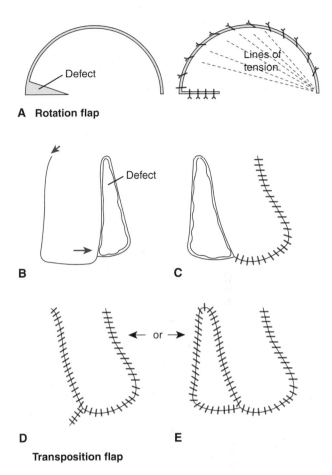

A Rotation flap

Transposition flap

Figure 24-4 • (A) Rotation flap. **(B, C, D, E)** Transposition flap. From Taylor J. *Blueprints Plastic Surgery*. Boston, MA: Blackwell Science, 2004:Fig. 5.

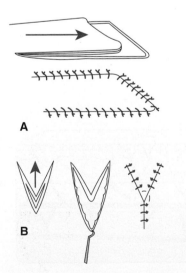

Figure 24-3 • (A) Advancement flap. **(B)** V-Y advancement flap.

or transposition flap; Fig. 24-4). It is important to distinguish and define a graft from a flap. A graft does not have its own blood supply, whereas a flap does (Fig 24-5A, B). When transferring a graft to cover a wound, it must be revascularized to survive. A flap is transferred to cover a defect with its blood supply intact.

When dealing with scar contracture that affects a patient's function and aesthetic appearance, plastic surgeons can use the Z-plasty technique to lengthen and alter the direction of the scar. A Z-plasty uses two opposing transposition flaps that switch places and gain length along the central axis of the original scar. Skin and tissue adjacent to the transposed flaps are recruited to lengthen and blend the scar with the surrounding tissues. A Z-plasty changes the direction of the central limb of scar by 90 degrees (Fig. 24-6). This technique improves the contour and aesthetic appearance of scars by camouflage. Scars become softer and less pigmented once tension is relieved via

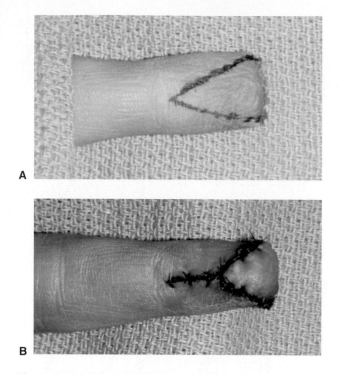

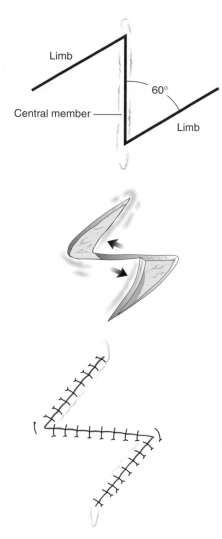

Figure 24-5 • Volar V-Y advancement flap; volar V-Y flap. **(A)** Preoperative outline of the skin incision used to create a volar skin flap in preparation for distal advancement. The tip of the V incision should be at the DIP joint flexion crease. **(B)** The flap has been advanced distally to cover the tip defect. The resultant defect has been closed, converting the V defect to a Y.
From Strickland JW, Graham TJ. *Master Techniques in Orthopaedic Surgery: The Hand.* 2nd ed. Philadelphia, PA: Lippincott Williams & Wilkins, 2005.

a Z-plasty. The actual gain in scar length depends on the angle of the flaps, the length of the central limb, and the quality of the surrounding tissues.

Figure 24-6 • Z-plasty.
Taylor J. *Blueprints Plastic Surgery.* Boston, MA: Blackwell Science, 2004; Fig. 5.

REGIONAL FLAPS

When adjacent tissue is inadequate, a flap is raised from a distant location and inset for wound closure. Flaps include adipocutaneous, fasciocutaneous, myocutaneous, osteocutaneous, or muscular flaps (Figs. 24-7 and 24-8). Flaps that are interpolated over cutaneous skin require pedicle transection once the flap becomes vascularized from the recipient tissue bed. The classic operation of this type is the Tagliacotian operation—devised by the Italian surgeon Gasparo Tagliacozzi (1546 to 1599)—in which a forearm flap is transferred to the nose (Italian rhinoplasty). Other examples are groin flaps to the hand and cross leg flaps. Prolonged awkward positioning is often required postoperatively until the pedicle is eventually transected.

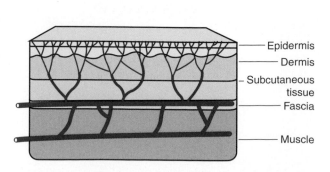

Figure 24-7 • Cross section of soft tissues used for flaps.

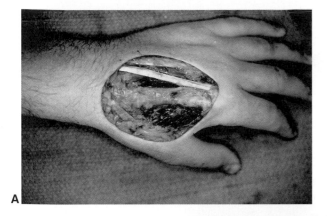
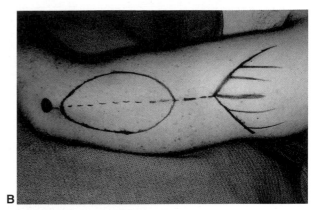
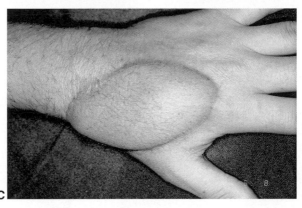

Figure 24-8 • Lateral arm flap. **(A)** Debridement of ulcer and surrounding induration creating exposure of a metacarpal and extensor tendon. **(B)** Flap borders outlined slightly larger than the size of the defect. **(C)** Flap in place 6 months after operation, before final defatting procedure.
From Strickland JW, Graham TJ. *Master Techniques in Orthopaedic Surgery: The Hand.* 2nd ed. Philadelphia, PA: Lippincott Williams & Wilkins, 2005.

A common pedicled musculocutaneous flap used for breast reconstruction is the transverse rectus abdominis myocutaneous flap. The contralateral rectus abdominis muscle is mobilized, with the superior epigastric artery left intact to supply the large attached skin paddle. The bulky paddle and muscle pedicle are tunneled superiorly and inserted into the breast defect, while the abdominal donor site is closed (abdominoplasty; Fig. 24-9).

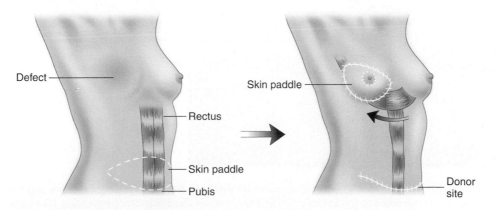

Figure 24-9 • Transverse rectus abdominis myocutaneous flap.
From Taylor J. *Blueprints Plastic Surgery.* Boston, MA: Blackwell Science, 2004;Fig. 7.

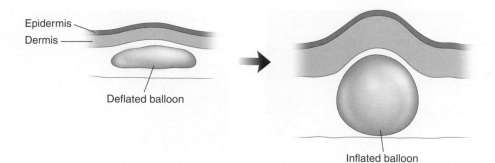

Epidermis

Dermis

Deflated balloon

Inflated balloon

Figure 24-10 • Tissue expansion with silicone balloons.
From Taylor J. *Blueprints Plastic Surgery*. Boston, MA: Blackwell Science, 2004;Fig. 8.

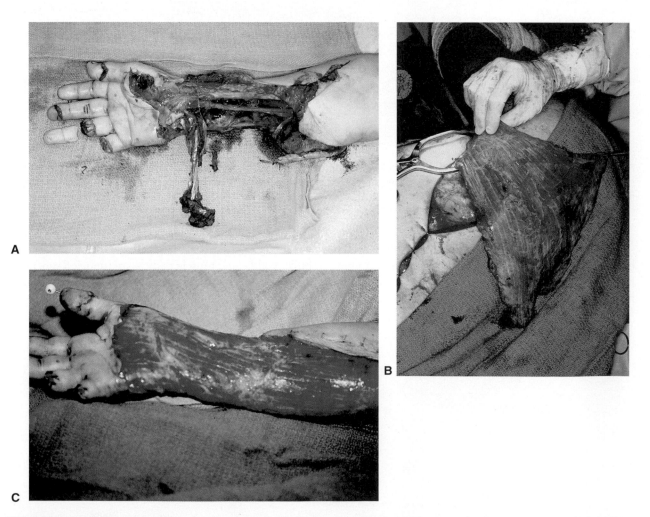

Figure 24-11 • Latissimus dorsi flap. **(A)** A 42-year-old woman with extensive trauma to the right forearm and hand after a riding lawnmower injury **(B)** Muscle elevated to tendon insertion and final pedicle identification commencing. **(C)** Muscle flap applied to the upper limb, vascular hookup performed, and muscle trimming and insertion completed.
From Strickland JW, Graham TJ. *Master Techniques in Orthopaedic Surgery: The Hand*. 2nd ed. Philadelphia, PA: Lippincott Williams & Wilkins, 2005.

TISSUE EXPANSION

Tissue expanders are placed beneath the dermis in a subcutaneous pocket. Their purpose is generally to recruit skin. This is achieved via gradual expander inflation over weeks to months to expand the skin superficial to the expander. The creation of additional skin surface area can be used for breast reconstruction, scalp reconstruction, or any defect requiring local tissue transfer (Fig. 24-10). Benefits of tissue expansion include good skin color match, as well as preservation of hair and sensation. Tissue expansion can be complicated by pain, infection, and contour deformity of surrounding structures.

FREE TISSUE TRANSFER

Free tissue transfer is used to reconstruct defects lacking local and regional pedicle flap options. Advances in microsurgery have enabled distant tissue transfer to become a reliable and predictable reconstructive option. Tissue (i.e., skin, subcutaneous fat, and muscle) can be transferred to a distant site based on its feeding nutrient artery. The free flap is collected from a distant donor site to cover a complex wound often with exposed vessels, bone, or other critical structures. The arterial blood supply and vena comitantes of a free flap are coapted to a target artery and vein within or adjacent to the defect using microvascular techniques (Figs 24-11A, B, and C).

KEY POINTS

- Goals of plastic surgery are to restore form and maximize function.
- Complex wounds require thoughtful individualized solutions.
- Methods of wound closure are based on the principles of the reconstructive ladder.
- Grafts do not have a blood supply; they become vascularized from a recipient bed.
- A flap has its own blood supply, generally rotated or advanced into complex wounds.
- Free tissue transfer involves collection of a distant flap with its arterial and venous vessels.

Orthopedic Surgery

OSTEOARTHRITIS

BACKGROUND

Osteoarthritis (OA) is the single most common disease of the joints; as such, it is one of the most important causes of morbidity in the United States. Loss of articular cartilage in the synovial joint is the primary pathologic lesion. This loss can be due to repetitive load-bearing stress or intrinsic properties of either the cartilage or bone or in the body's ability to repair these structures. Joints commonly involved include the first carpometacarpal joint, hip, knee, and spine. Risk factors include age, obesity, and female sex. Secondary OA can occur after major trauma to the joint; repetitive stress; prior inflammatory joint disease; metabolic disease, including ochronosis, hemochromatosis, and Wilson disease; and endocrine disease, including acromegaly, diabetes, and hyperparathyroidism.

HISTORY AND PHYSICAL EXAMINATION

Patients are usually older than 55 years. Typical complaints include a deep ache in the affected joint that is exacerbated by activity. Stiffness is common, especially after inactivity, but usually resolves with use. There are no systemic symptoms. Although OA is not considered an inflammatory arthritis, inflammation does play a significant role in the development of associated pain and swelling.

Physical examination reveals limitation of motion secondary to pain. Localized tenderness and soft tissue swelling may be present. Motion of the joint may produce bony crepitus. As the disease progresses, there may be gross deformities of the joint, with loss of motion.

Hip OA may be experienced as groin pain. On examination, internal rotation is often the first motion to become painful and restricted.

Knee OA may result in stiff knees that are more painful with prolonged sitting, walking, and climbing stairs.

First carpometacarpal OA often results in stiffness and pain in the joint. On examination, the "grind test," in which the joint is compressed, is positive.

DIAGNOSTIC EVALUATION

Radiographic examination reveals narrowing of joint spaces (Figs. 25-1 and 25-2). Subchondral cysts, bone sclerosis, and osteophytes may be present. In primary OA, laboratory values are normal. Specific lab tests may be useful to diagnose causes of secondary OA. Synovial fluid usually reveals a mononuclear leukocytosis; this test may be useful to exclude other diagnoses, including a septic joint.

It is important to note that radiographic findings of osteoarthritis are not always correlated with symptoms. A patient with significant OA on x-ray may be symptom-free. The reciprocal is also true: a patient with minimal x-ray findings of OA may have significant symptoms. The patient with OA must be treated, not the film.

TREATMENT

Therapy for osteoarthritis should be based on the severity of the symptoms. In general, exercises to stretch and strengthen the muscles surrounding the

Nutritional supplements such as glucosamine and chondroitin sulfate have received much attention for the prevention and treatment of osteoarthritis. Their usage remains controversial. However, because of their low side-effect profile (in contrast with nonsteroidal anti-inflammatory drugs), their use has become more widespread. Superficial joints, such as those of the fingers and toes, may benefit from topical analgesics.

Intra-articular corticosteroids can be extremely effective for pain. The number of corticosteroid injections that can be performed per joint remains controversial. Some physicians advocate a total of three corticosteroid injections in the life of a joint, whereas others argue that three injections per year are safe.

Hyaluronic acid injections may also be of benefit. These injections are approved by the U.S. Food and Drug Administration for knee OA, and they are being used with increasing frequency, off-label, for hip OA. Some studies are also investigating their use for ankle, shoulder, and elbow OA.

Surgical treatment should be reserved for patients with debilitating pain or compromised quality of life after nonsurgical options are exhausted. In patients with mild disease, particularly younger patients who want to remain more active, osteotomy may produce significant pain relief. In the knee, an osteotomy is not an option if the patient is unable to flex the knee past 90 degrees or if he or she has more than 15 to 20 degrees of valgus deformity.

Total joint arthroplasty for hip and knee OA has excellent results in patients with more advanced disease. In the hip, a polymethylmethacrylate cemented or cementless prosthesis may be used. A cemented prosthesis has the advantage of allowing the patient full weight bearing and quicker healing immediately after the procedure. Cementless prostheses have the potential advantage of ultimately achieving longer life and durability once they have matured. The disadvantage is that the patient may have greater postoperative pain and must remain toe-touch weight bearing (putting less than 10% of body weight on the affected limb) for at least 6 to 8 weeks. In general, a cemented prosthesis is recommended for an older, less active patient, and a cementless prosthesis is recommended for a younger, more active patient. A hemiarthroplasty in the hip is another option. In contrast to a total joint arthroplasty, which involves replacing the femoral head and the acetabulum, a hemiarthroplasty involves only replacing the femoral head.

The most common surgical approach for a total hip replacement is posterior. After a posterior approach,

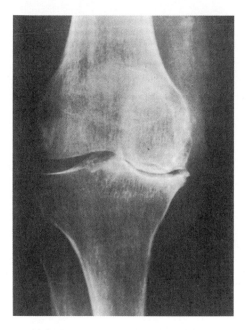

Figure 25-1 • X-ray appearance of osteoarthritis of the knee.
Reproduced with permission from Duckworth T. *Lecture Notes on Orthopaedics and Fractures.* 3rd ed. Cambridge, MA: Blackwell Science, 1995.

joint are critical. Joints face an enormous amount of daily stress. Descending stairs, for example, results in the knee bearing five to six times the body weight load. Weak or tight muscles result in excessive forces being placed through the joint itself, rather than being relieved by the muscles.

No pharmacologic interventions can reverse the lesions of osteoarthritis, but nonsteroidal anti-inflammatory agents, as well as analgesics (e.g., acetaminophen), can provide symptomatic relief for pain.

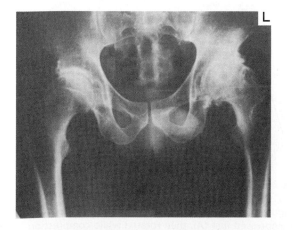

Figure 25-2 • X-ray appearance of osteoarthritic hip.
Reproduced with permission from Duckworth T. *Lecture Notes on Orthopaedics and Fractures.* 3rd ed. Cambridge, MA: Blackwell Science, 1995.

hip precautions include (1) no hip flexion beyond 90 degrees, (2) no hip adduction past neutral, and (3) no hip internal rotation beyond neutral.

In the knee, cemented, cementless, and hybrid prostheses are available. However, cement fixation is by far the most common. After a cemented total knee replacement, patients should expect to gradually return to their activities in 1 to 3 months.

When considering any major surgery, it is vital to consider anticoagulation after the procedure. This is particularly true with total knee and hip replacements. After a total knee replacement, as many as 64% of patients may develop a clot if not anticoagulated. Only 6% to 24% may develop a clot if properly anticoagulated. In the hip, >50% of patients who do not receive adequate anticoagulation may develop a clot. Anticoagulation options include warfarin (keeping the international normalized ratio between 2 and 3), aspirin 325 mg orally twice per day, subcutaneous heparin 5,000 U twice per day, low molecular heparin, and possibly an inferior vena cava filter for patients who are not candidates for anticoagulation.

JOINT PAIN

It is important to distinguish between acute and chronic causes of pain. Critical questions include history of trauma, swelling, decreased range of motion, and problems with weight bearing. Positions or circumstances that alleviate or exacerbate the pain may yield clues to the diagnosis.

On physical examination, a careful assessment for swelling, joint effusion, range of motion, deformity, tenderness, and instability should be made.

KNEE PAIN: COMMON DIAGNOSES

Meniscal Injury

Meniscal injuries are more common in men but can occur in women. Injury to the medial meniscus is more common than injury to the lateral meniscus. Pain is the most common symptom. Patients also may complain of knee locking or clicking. Effusions may be present, and weight bearing may be difficult. Examination usually reveals joint line tenderness. A McMurray test is often positive. In this test (Fig. 25-3), the patient is in the supine position. The examiner flexes the knee while palpating the joint line. Using the ankle as a fulcrum, the leg is externally rotated and a valgus stress is applied as the knee is extended.

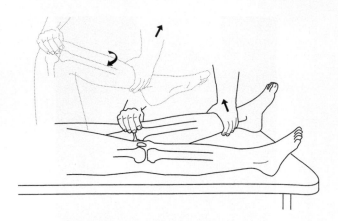

Figure 25-3 • The McMurray test is performed with the leg externally rotated and applying a valgus stress to test the medial meniscus.
Reproduced with permission from Gross JM, Fetto J, Rosen E. *Musculoskeletal Examination.* 2nd ed. Malden, MA: Blackwell, 2002.

A palpable or audible click, or recreation of symptoms in the knee, is considered a positive test result. The grinding and distraction test of Apley is also useful (Fig. 25-4). In this test, the patient lies prone with the knee flexed to 90 degrees. Using the ankle as a fulcrum, again, the examiner first internally and externally rotates the leg while compressing the tibia into the table. The examiner then internally and externally rotates the leg while distracting the tibia. If pain is produced while grinding but not while distracting, the meniscus is implicated as the cause of

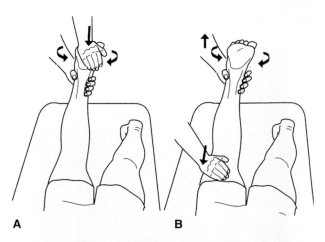

A   **B**

Figure 25-4 • The grinding/distraction test of Apley. The tibia is compressed first **(A)**, then rotated while compression force is maintained **(B)**. Distraction with rotation tests the collateral ligaments, whereas compression with rotation tests the menisci.
Reproduced with permission from Gross JM, Fetto J, Rosen E. *Musculoskeletal Examination.* 2nd ed. Malden, MA: Blackwell, 2002.

pain. If pain is produced during both distraction (when the meniscus is unloaded) and grinding, the ligaments are more likely involved.

Magnetic resonance imaging (MRI) is accurate and sensitive for meniscal injury. Not all meniscus lesions require surgery. Conservative therapy is indicated, particularly if the tear is ≤10 mm or partial thickness or if a radial tear is ≤3 mm. However, even larger tears may respond to conservative therapy. If locking is present and significant, surgical intervention should be considered sooner. Surgical options include arthroscopic meniscectomy and meniscus repair. For tears in the vascular region (in the peripheral part of the meniscus), arthroscopic meniscus repair with fixation using the outside-in, inside-out, or all-inside method is recommended.

Cruciate Ligament Injury

The cruciate ligaments stabilize the knee to translational motion. Acute pain in the setting of trauma and subsequent swelling should alert the examiner to this possibility. Typically, a twist or hyperextension trauma causes these lesions. The pain may improve after the initial injury, but chronic pain may develop. The anterior cruciate ligament (ACL) is most commonly torn. Between 30% and 50% of people will report hearing a popping sound at the time of tearing their ACL. The most sensitive diagnostic maneuver for ACL is the Lachman test (Fig. 25-5). In this test, the knee is flexed 20 to 30 degrees and the examiner

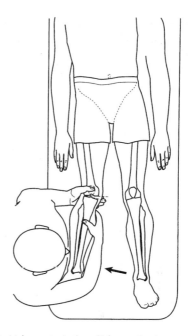

Figure 25-6 • Valgus strain (medial gapping).
Reproduced with permission from Gross JM, Fetto J, Rosen E. *Musculoskeletal Examination.* 2nd ed. Malden, MA: Blackwell, 2002.

applies an anteroposterior glide. A few degrees of anteroposterior glide may be normal. It is important to always compare side-to-side findings. A loose end point or excessive glide is a positive finding for an ACL tear.

The medial collateral ligament is evaluated by applying a valgus stress and comparing glide side-to-side (Fig. 25-6). The posterior cruciate ligament and lateral collateral ligament are likewise evaluated by stressing those ligaments.

Treatment is typically conservative, focusing on strengthening the surrounding muscles and gradually returning to activity. Depending on the severity of injury, the ACL may be repaired by arthroscopic allograft or autograft. The allograft, taken from a cadaver, has the advantage of not requiring tissue collection of the graft from the patient. Allografts are irradiated to greatly reduce the chance of infection. Autografts are performed by either taking a segment of the patient's hamstrings or patella tendon. The disadvantage of these procedures is primarily the occurrence of increased postoperative wound pain. Both surgical approaches have similar long-term outcomes.

Medial collateral ligament and posterior cruciate ligament injuries are generally treated conservatively unless the ligament is severely torn.

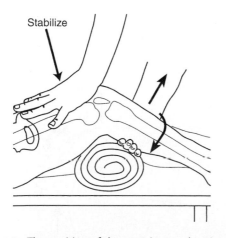

Stabilize

Figure 25-5 • The position of the examiner and patient for the Lachman test. It is important that the patient be relaxed for this test.
Reproduced with permission from Gross JM, Fetto J, Rosen E. *Musculoskeletal Examination.* 2nd ed. Malden, MA: Blackwell, 2002.

Patellofemoral Syndrome

Patellofemoral syndrome is common in young adults. The pain is generally anterior. A positive "theatre sign" is characteristic. When positive, the patient has trouble sitting for a long period of time (such as at a theatre) and must extend the knee (placing his or her foot into the aisle) to relieve the discomfort. Pain is also exacerbated by running and ascending/descending stairs. Tenderness is usually present under the patella. The Q-angle, which is the angle formed by a line drawn from the anterior superior iliac spine to the mid patella and transected by a line drawn from the mid patella to the tibial tubercle with the knee in full extension, is usually increased (>17 degrees in women and >14 degrees in men; Fig. 25-7).

The problem is primarily caused by patellar misalignment and abnormal tracking. Classically, the patella tracks excessively laterally. Treatment focuses on strengthening the quadriceps, particularly the vastus medialis oblique, and stretching the iliotibial band. Patellar taping or bracing may also be somewhat helpful. Surgical correction is rarely indicated but may be used when conservative care is not sufficient and an identifiable anatomic abnormality is present, such as isolated lateral patellar tilt that may be arthroscopically released.

SHOULDER PAIN: COMMON DIAGNOSES

A variety of structures within the shoulder can be injured or inflamed, but most problems respond to conservative therapy.

Impingement Syndrome

Impingement syndrome includes rotator cuff tendonitis and subacromial bursitis. These two conditions often coexist and are treated in much the same way. To diagnose impingement syndrome, Neer and Hawkins' tests are useful. In the Neer test, the examiner stabilizes the patient's scapula with one hand and internally rotates and flexes the shoulder with the other. As the shoulder is elevated, the greater tuberosity of the humerus abuts the coracoacromial arch, placing pressure on the rotator cuff tendon. Result for this test is considered positive when symptoms are reproduced. The same maneuver but with the shoulder in external rotation often produces less or no pain. In the Hawkins' test, the patient's shoulder is abducted to 90 degrees in the plane of the scapula and the elbow is flexed to 60 to 90 degrees. The shoulder is then placed firmly into internal rotation (Fig. 25-8). When this reproduces pain, the test result is considered positive for impingement syndrome.

The best test for impingement syndrome is to inject 3 to 5 mL of 1% lidocaine into the subacromial space and repeat the Neer and Hawkins' tests. With the lidocaine injected, these maneuvers should be significantly less painful. If so, the patient likely has impingement syndrome.

Impingement syndrome responds well to physical therapy that focuses on scapular stabilization and rotator cuff strengthening exercises. A subacromial corticosteroid injection can also be very effective and help speed recovery.

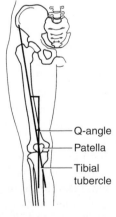
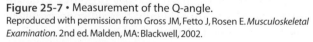

Figure 25-7 • Measurement of the Q-angle.
Reproduced with permission from Gross JM, Fetto J, Rosen E. *Musculoskeletal Examination.* 2nd ed. Malden, MA: Blackwell, 2002.

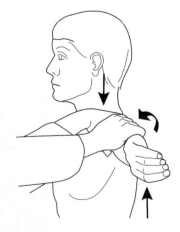

Figure 25-8 • The supraspinatus impingement test (Hawkins' test) being performed.
Reproduced with permission from Gross JM, Fetto J, Rosen E. *Musculoskeletal Examination.* 2nd ed. Malden, MA: Blackwell, 2002.

Biceps Tendonitis

The biceps tendon crosses the shoulder joint and may become inflamed where it traverses the bicipital groove. This is best identified by tenderness to palpation and a positive Speed test result. In the Speed test, the patient's shoulder is flexed to 90 degrees with the elbow extended. The patient then resists the examiner who applies an inferior force to the patient's arm. Reproduction of pain is consistent with bicipital tendonitis.

Glenohumeral Labral Tear

A labral tear may be identified on physical examination by the O'Brien test. In this test, the patient's shoulder is flexed, adducted, and externally rotated. An inferior force is applied by the examiner. The arm is then placed in internal rotation and an inferior force is again applied (and resisted by the patient). If symptoms are reproduced when the shoulder is internally rotated (thumb facing down) but not in external rotation (thumb facing up), the test is considered positive for a labral tear. An MRI is the best way to evaluate for a labral tear. Not all labral tears require surgery. Conservative care includes physical therapy and, in some cases, an intra-articular corticosteroid injection.

Rotator Cuff Tear

The rotator cuff is a collection of the tendons of the supraspinatus, infraspinatus, subscapularis, and teres minor. The most common tendon to tear is the

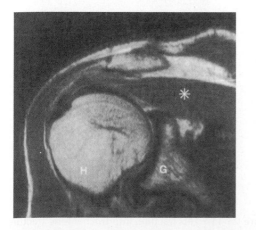

Figure 25-9 • Magnetic resonance imaging of normal rotator cuff (*) and surrounding structures. H, humerus, G, glenoid.
Reproduced with permission from Gross JM, Fetto J, Rosen E. *Musculoskeletal Examination.* 2nd ed. Malden, MA: Blackwell, 2002.

supraspinatus. On examination, a supraspinatus tear will result in weak abduction, particularly from 0 to 30 degrees. MRI is sensitive and specific for rotator cuff injuries (Fig. 25-9). Surgery is an option if conservative measures fail.

BACK PAIN

Back pain is an epidemic in the United States, causing chronic disability in 1% of the population, with a cost of approximately $50 billion annually. Back pain can be divided into acute pain from a muscle strain or spasm and subacute or chronic pain that is more likely a result of intervertebral disc irritation, zygapophysial (facet) joint pain, or sacroiliac joint pain. A radiculitis can also result if a nerve root is irritated. A radiculitis characteristically involves pain radiating into the lower extremity.

FACET JOINT PAIN

The facet joints in the spine are synovial joints (similar to the knee joint). These joints can become arthritic, just like the knee. These joints are a common source of lower back pain. Pain is usually exacerbated by trunk extension and oblique extension. Treatment options include physical therapy, facet joint injections, and radiofrequency neurotomy to essentially sever the medial branches of the dorsal rami that innervate the involved joints.

DISCOGENIC PAIN

The disc is the most common cause of chronic lower back pain in the younger population and is also a common cause of pain in older populations. A herniated disc is not synonymous with discogenic back pain. When discs cause pain, it is because the annulus of the disc has torn internally and the nucleus pulposus (which is full of inflammatory proteins) is irritating the pain receptors in the outer third of the annulus. A painful disc may appear normal on MRI. Reciprocally, a herniated disc may not be the source of back pain. A herniated disc is more commonly associated with nerve root impingement or irritation, which would result in a radiculitis, causing electric, radiating pain into the lower extremity.

Discogenic pain is typically worse with trunk flexion. Prolonged sitting may make the pain worse. Though somewhat controversial, definitive diagnosis is accomplished using provocative discography in which dye is injected under x-ray guidance into the disc. When this reproduces the patient's pain at low injection pressures, the disc is considered positive. Postdiscography computed tomography will often reveal the extent of the torn annulus (when present).

Treatment includes physical therapy that focuses on extension-based lumbar stabilization and stretching and strengthening the surrounding muscles. Fusion is reserved for patients for whom more conservative measures have failed.

NEOPLASM

Metastatic cancer must always be included in the differential diagnosis of back pain. Cancer pain in the back tends to be worse at night, and may wake the patient up from sleep. X-rays, bone scan, and MRI all may be used as part of the workup, depending on the index of suspicion. Though much less common, primary bone tumors in the spine can also occur.

INFECTION

Osteomyelitis of the spine most commonly occurs in debilitated patients or intravenous drug abusers and is usually associated with some type of systemic infection. Patients will usually have tenderness at the site and with movement. Pain is typically constant, and signs of systemic infection are present. The sedimentation rate is often elevated. Plain films may be negative initially, MRI is usually diagnostic, and a tagged white cell scan may light up the affected area.

HIP FRACTURE

Hip fracture is the most common fracture causing hospital admission. Approximately 300,000 hip fractures occur each year in the United States. The generally advanced age of patients with this problem leads to a staggering 50% 1-year mortality rate after injury. Hip fractures are twice as common in women. Three general types of fracture occur: fractures of the femoral neck, intertrochanteric fractures, and subtrochanteric fractures (Fig. 25-10). The first two are by far the most common and usually occur in older adults as a result of a relatively low-impact type of injury.

The typical history involves an older adult patient who falls and has subsequent hip, groin, or knee pain. Weight bearing is often difficult. On examination,

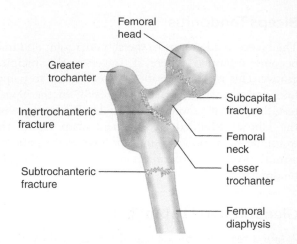

Figure 25-10 • Diagram of common points of femoral fracture. Reproduced with permission from Uzelac A, Davis RW. *Blueprints Radiology*. 2nd ed. Philadelphia, PA: Lippincott Williams & Wilkins, 2006.

patients with femoral neck fractures may have a shortened and externally rotated extremity. Hip motion may be painful. Diagnosis is usually confirmed with plain radiograph films (Fig. 25-11). MRI should be obtained if x-rays appear normal but clinical evidence is suggestive

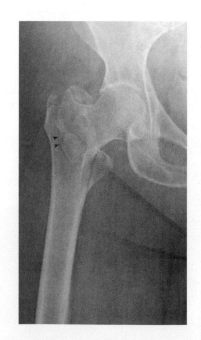

Figure 25-11 • Hip fracture. Intertrochanteric fracture in the right hip of an 83-year-old woman who fell after getting out of bed.
Courtesy of Cedars-Sinai Medical Center, Los Angeles, CA.

■ **TABLE 25-1**	Garden Classification and Treatment	
Garden Type	**Findings**	**Treatment**
I	Femoral head valgus impaction	Open reduction and internal fixation
II	Complete, nondisplaced fracture	Open reduction and internal fixation
III	Varus displacement of femoral head	Open or closed fixation versus total hip replacement
IV	Complete loss of fragment continuity	Open or closed fixation versus total hip replacement

of possible fracture (x-rays may miss up to 67% of acute hip fractures, according to one study).

Treatment is based on comorbidities and degree of fracture (Tables 25-1 and 25-2). If the acetabulum is involved in the fracture, total hip replacement must be considered.

Both stable and unstable intertrochanteric fractures are typically treated with open reduction and internal fixation using the sliding screw hip implant. Fracture healing time after surgery is approximately 12 weeks.

It is critical to properly anticoagulate patients after a hip fracture. Failure to do so may lead to a lower-extremity deep venous thrombosis and/or fatal pulmonary embolism in 40% to 83% of patients. These numbers are greatly reduced (to 4% to 38%) in patients who receive appropriate anticoagulation. High-risk patients, or patients who are not candidates for anticoagulation, may require an inferior vena cava filter.

SEPTIC JOINT CONSIDERATIONS

A septic joint requires appropriate, prompt attention. Clinical signs and symptoms of a septic joint include fevers, chills, and a hot, red, swollen joint. A low index of suspicion should be used for septic joint,

because failure to diagnose and treat this condition quickly may result in destruction of the joint. If suspected, the joint should be aspirated and the fluid sent for analysis. Blood tests should also be performed. If clinical suspicion is high, treatment should be started before lab results have been obtained. Treatment includes intravenous and/or oral antibiotic treatment.

Laboratory studies should include a complete blood cell count with differential and erythrocyte sedimentation rate. If positive, complete blood cell count may show increased white blood cell count ($>12,000$/mL) with a left shift. Erythrocyte sedimentation rate is typically elevated (>40 mm/h). Other laboratory tests may include a Lyme test and blood cultures.

If suspected, a urethral or cervical culture may be obtained to evaluate for *Neisseria gonorrhoeae*. The fluid aspirate should be sent for Gram stain, culture, cell count, and crystal analysis. Table 25-3 presents results analysis.

Corticosteroid injection should NOT be administered if sepsis is suspected.

If infection is confirmed, drainage in combination with continued intravenous antibiotics is the treatment of choice. Drainage may be attempted by percutaneous aspiration; however, surgical drainage is often required if percutaneous aspiration is not adequate.

■ **TABLE 25-2**	Jensen Classification of Intertrochanteric Fractures	
Type	**Findings**	**Stability**
I	Nondisplaced two-fragment fracture	Stable
II	Displaced two-fragment fracture	Stable
III	Three-fragment fracture without posterolateral support	Unstable
IV	Three-fragment fracture without medial support	Unstable
V	Four-fragment fracture without posterolateral and medial support	Unstable

■ TABLE 25-3 Synovial Fluid Classification

Quality	Reference Range	Noninflammatory	Inflammatory	Septic	Crystal
Volume	<3.5 mL	>3.5 mL	>3.5 mL	>3.5 mL	<3.5 mL
Viscosity	High	High	Low	Variable	Low
Color	Clear	Straw-yellow	Yellow	Variable	Yellow-milky
Clarity	Transparent	Transparent	Translucent	Opaque	Opaque
WBC	<200/mL	200–2,000/mL	2,000–75,000/mL	Often >100,000/mL	500–200,000/mL
PMN	<25%	<25%	>50%	>75%	<90
Culture result	Negative	Negative	Negative	Often positive[a]	Negative
Mucin clot	Firm	Firm to friable	Friable	Friable	Friable
Glucose	~Blood	~Blood	Decreased	Very decreased	Decreased
Crystals	Negative	Negative	Negative	Negative	Present

[a]Synovial fluid culture results are positive in 85% to 95% of nongonococcal arthritis cases and approximately 25% of gonococcal arthritis cases.
WBC, white blood cell count; PMN, polymorphonuclear neutrophils.
Modified from Schumacher HR. Pathologic findings in rheumatoid arthritis. *Arthritis: An Illustrated Guide to Pathology, Diagnosis and Management.* Philadelphia, PA: JB Lippincott, 1988. Available at: http://www.emedicine.com/orthoped/topic437.htm.

 KEY POINTS

- Orthopedic injuries are a tremendous cause of economic loss, morbidity, and mortality in the United States.

- Osteoarthritis is caused by loss of articular cartilage and is best managed conservatively, unless symptoms are debilitating.

- X-ray findings of osteoarthritis do not necessarily correlate with symptoms. The patient must be treated, not the film.

- Causes of knee pain include meniscal injury, cruciate ligament injury, and patellofemoral syndrome. Magnetic resonance imaging is the study of choice to delineate the anatomy and to help guide treatment.

- In the United States, back pain is an epidemic, with an economic cost of $50 billion per year. The most common causes of back pain include discogenic and facet arthropathy.

- Discogenic lower back pain is not necessarily caused by a herniated disc, but rather by internal derangement of the disc, which may appear normal on magnetic resonance imaging.

- Conservative therapy for back pain is usually best, unless there are neurologic symptoms or intractable pain.

- Hip fracture is a common lesion in older adults and carries high mortality at 1 year.

- It is important to keep a high index of suspicion for a septic joint. Failure to recognize and promptly treat this pathology may lead to rapid destruction of the joint.

Organ Transplantation

OVERVIEW

Organ transplantation is one of the great achievements of 20th-century medicine. Fueled by technological advances in immunology and surgical technique, transplantation of the liver, kidney, small bowel, heart, and lung is possible with good outcomes. Using various protocols, it is possible to perform transplantation when patient and donor do not have compatible blood types, and even if the recipient is sensitized to the donor. Researchers at various centers are also experimenting with hand, face, and uterus transplantation. The decision to perform transplantation must take into account the risk of the surgery as well as long-term immunosuppression.

BASIC SCIENCE

The key to successful organ transplantation, after the technical aspects have been performed successfully, is the ability to prevent the recipient immunologic response from destroying the graft. In most cases, the donor and recipient blood type will be matched, and control of the host's response to the donor's major histocompatibility (MHC) antigens determines the success or failure of organ transplantation. MHC antigens are coded by a single chromosomal complex. In humans, the MHC is named the HLA antigen (human leukocyte antigen), which is located on the short arm of chromosome 6. HLA antigens are classified according to their structure and function. Class I antigens are present on virtually all nucleated cells in the human body and act as targets for cytotoxic T cells. Class II antigens are located on B cells, monocytes, macrophages, activated T cells, and other antigen-presenting cells. The rejection

reaction of a transplant recipient directed against mismatched donor HLA antigens is a complex event that involves the actions of cytotoxic T cells, activated helper T cells, B lymphocytes, activated macrophages, and antibodies. The reaction is primarily cellular in nature and is T cell–dependent. Class I antigens stimulate cytotoxic T cells, directly causing donor tissue destruction. Class II antigens activate helper T cells, which, along with activated cytotoxic T cells, elaborate interleukin-1 (IL-1) and IL-2. IL-1 and IL-2, in turn, further activate macrophages and antibody-releasing B cells.

Although most rejections are cell-mediated, humoral rejections are also possible. The exact pathogenesis of humoral rejection is not well understood. When it occurs early after transplantation, it is generally due to preformed antibodies against class I antigens in the recipient. These antibodies are commonly acquired via blood transfusions, pregnancy, or prior transplantations. If this occurs in the period immediately after the transplantation procedure, it is termed "hyperacute rejection." To avoid this, cross-matching of the recipient's serum against the donor's lymphocytes is performed to confirm the absence of preexisting antibodies against donor tissue antigens. Types of rejection are listed in Table 26-1.

Immunosuppressive regimens use a combination of agents among a number of classes. In the past, most patients were treated with three drug regimens, but more and more transplantations are being performed with corticosteroids only in the immediate postoperative period. Generally, patients will receive an antibody as an induction agent for a few days at the time of the transplantation. In general, antibodies bind white blood cells and trigger a destructive immune reaction. The most common agent is rabbit anti-thymocyte

TABLE 26-1 Classification Criteria for Allograft Rejection Responses			
Type	**Time Course**	**Target**	**Response**
Hyperacute	Minutes to hours	Vessels	Humoral
Acute	Early after transplantation	Parenchyma/vessels	Cellular/humoral
Chronic	Late after transplantation	Parenchyma/vessels	Cellular/humoral

globulin (Thymoglobulin), which profoundly depletes T cells. Also common are basiliximab and daclizumab, both of which are humanized antibodies to the IL-2 receptor on T cells.

Currently, the foundation of maintenance immunosuppression is a calcineurin inhibitor (either tacrolimus or cyclosporine). This agent binds to immunophilins and inhibits calcineurin activity, which is necessary for the transcription of genes that activate T cells, including IL-2, IL-3, IL-4, and interferon. Unfortunately, nephrotoxicity of these medicines is associated with high rates of renal failure. The major alternative is rapamycin, which does not seem to have nephrotoxicity but can impair wound healing, increase lipid levels, and cause pulmonary toxicity and edema. Most regimens include an antimetabolite, such as mycophenolate mofetil. Mycophenolate mofetil is rapidly converted to the morpholino ethyl ester of mycophenolic acid, which inhibits inosine monophosphate dehydrogenases, blocking proliferation of T and B lymphocytes and inhibiting antibody formation and the generation of cytotoxic T cells. Mycophenolic acid also down regulates the expression of adhesion molecules on lymphocytes. Other drugs in this category include azathioprine, a purine synthesis inhibitor.

Use of corticosteroids, once the mainstay of immunosuppression, is decreasing rapidly. Given the significant long-term complications associated with corticosteroids (e.g., diabetes, heart disease, edema, avascular necrosis of the hip, and easy bruisablity), alternatives have been actively sought. Current data suggest that if an induction agent is included at transplantation, then maintenance corticosteroids are not required. Corticosteroids alter the transcription and translation of several genes responsible for cytokine synthesis; they inhibit T-cell activation by blocking IL-1, IL-2, IL-6, and interferon synthesis; and they have local anti-inflammatory effects.

It is unusual to lose a graft from acute rejection. Antibody therapy that profoundly depletes T cells halts most rejections. The most potent agents are antithymocyte globulin and OKT3, an antibody to CD3 which binds to and depletes T cells.

DONORS

Organs can be used from living people or cadavers. Live donors for kidney transplants are routine, and the majority of kidneys come from this source. The risk of death to the donor is approximately three in 10,000, and complication rates are in the range of 2% to 3%. Live donors can be used for liver transplantation, but donor risk is greater, with a mortality rate of approximately 0.2%, in addition to a biliary complication rate that is much higher. Adult-to-child transplantation procedures usually use the left lateral segment of the liver, which is safer than using the right lobe, as is common in adult-to-adult live-donor liver transplantation.

Other than the kidney and liver, organs are generally not obtained from living people. There are two types of cadaver donors: heart beating or after cardiac death. Heart beating donors are pronounced brain-dead well before the time of donation. In this case, the cadaver is taken to the operating room with full life support, which is withdrawn after the aorta is cannulated. Cold perfusion is instituted immediately after the aorta is clamped, so the organs are preserved immediately. In donation after cardiac death, the decision has been made independent of the transplantation procedure that the patient's condition is terminal and life support will be withdrawn. After this occurs and the heart has stopped by natural causes for 5 minutes, the patient is pronounced dead and the organs are removed. This waiting period when the heart has stopped renders the organs relatively ischemic, and outcomes using livers from these patients may not be as good as from heart-beating donors.

LIVER TRANSPLANTATION

EPIDEMIOLOGY

There are approximately 17,000 patients on the waiting list for liver transplants in the United States, and 2,000 people on the waiting list die each year.

TABLE 26-2 Categories of Liver Disease Leading to Transplantation

Categories of Disease	Examples
Noncholestatic cirrhosis	Hepatitis B
	Hepatitis C
	Alcoholic cirrhosis
	Autoimmune hepatitis
	Nonalcoholic steatohepatitis
Cholestatic cirrhosis	Primary biliary cirrhosis
	Primary sclerosing cholangitis
	Caroli disease
Metabolic	Wilson disease
	Alpha-1 antitrypsin deficiency
	Tyrosinemia
	Ornithine carbamoyl-transferase deficiency
Cancer	Hepatoblastoma
	Hepatoma
Congenital	Biliary atresia
Acute fulminant liver failure	Tylenol overdose
	Halothane hepatitis
	Cryptogenic cirrhosis
	Viral hepatitis
Miscellaneous	Budd-Chiari syndrome
	Polycystic liver disease

INDICATIONS

Liver transplantation is indicated for life-threatening or debilitating liver failure or early-stage hepatocellular cancer that is not resectable because of tumor location or underlying liver disease. Disease states leading to end-stage liver disease are listed in Table 26-2.

LIVER ALLOCATION

Assignment of livers to patients depends on the Model for End-Stage Liver Disease (MELD), a formula that uses the patient's creatinine, international normalized ratio (INR) of prothrombin time, and bilirubin.

$$MELD = 10(0.957\ln[\text{creatinine mg/dL}] + 0.378\ln[\text{bilirubin mg/dL}] + 1.12\ln[\text{INR}])$$

Values <1.0 are set to 1.0; maximum creatinine level that may be used is 4.0 mg/dL, which is also the score for dialysis patients. "Ln" is the natural logarithm.

This equation produces a number that directly correlates with mortality; livers are offered to the patients with highest mortality. Waiting time is no longer a factor in liver allocation, unless patients have identical MELD scores. This system has been prospectively analyzed and has resulted in fewer deaths on the waiting list. Extra points are offered for certain early-stage tumors in recognition of excellent outcomes with liver transplantation.

PROGNOSIS

Outcome after transplantation depends on a number of factors, including donor quality, recipient health, and indication for operation. Overall, patient survival after liver transplantation is 93% at 3 months, 88% at 1 year, 80% at 3 years, and 74% at 5 years. Graft survival rates are 88% at 3 months, 81% at 1 year, and 66% at 5 years. Fulminant hepatic failure carries poor prognosis after transplantation.

After successful liver transplantation, many patients return to a normal life, including work.

THE OPERATION: LIVER TRANSPLANTATION

Before beginning, it is imperative that adequate blood, platelets, and fresh frozen plasma are available. After the organ is verified to be the correct ABO type, the entire abdomen is prepped, as is the groin in case bypass will be necessary. Intravenous antibiotics are administered, and central monitoring is established. A wide bilateral subcostal incision with midline extension is made. Goals are dissecting the suprahepatic cava, isolating the portal vein in the porta hepatis, and freeing the liver from the diaphragm above the bare area of the liver. The liver can be removed with or without the inferior vena cava. Most commonly, the liver is removed with the retrohepatic cava (straight orthotopic). The new liver is sewn to the supra and infrahepatic portions of the cava. In this case, because the cava is clamped, veno-venous bypass can be useful to preserve venous return to the heart (Fig. 26-1). This also decreases bowel edema. It is also possible to leave the cava intact in the recipient. In this case, the hepatic veins are

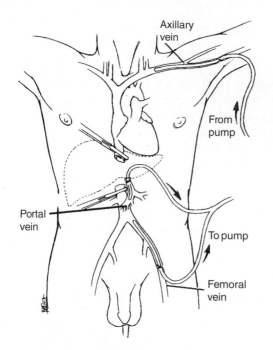

Figure 26-1 • An example of veno-venous bypass during orthotopic liver transplantation. The cannula drains the inferior vena cava, and the centrifugal pump returns blood to the axillary vein. This circuit helps returns blood to the heart during the anhepatic phase of the operation when the inferior vena cava is occluded.
From Blackbourne LH. *Advanced Surgical Recall.* 2nd ed. Baltimore, MD: Lippincott Williams & Wilkins, 2004.

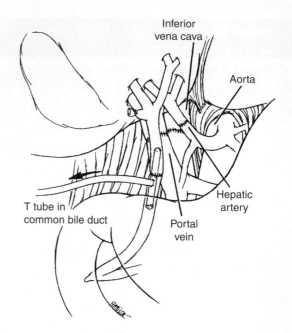

Figure 26-2 • Diagram of orthotopic liver transplantation demonstrating the hepatic artery, portal vein, bile duct, and infrahepatic caval anastomosis. Not shown is the suprahepatic caval anastomosis.
From Blackbourne LH. *Advanced Surgical Recall.* 2nd ed. Baltimore, MD: Lippincott Williams & Wilkins, 2004.

clamped, the liver is cut from the hepatic veins, and the new liver is sewn so it "hangs down" from the hepatic veins (piggyback technique). In both techniques, the portal vein is then reconstructed, followed by the hepatic artery, and finally the bile duct (Fig. 26-2). Drains are placed, and the abdomen is closed.

Complications

Technical complications after liver transplantation include caval stenosis, which can cause lower extremity edema, or outflow problems for the liver, which causes swelling of the graft and dysfunction. A particularly dangerous complication is hepatic arterial stenosis or thrombosis, which often leads to graft loss when acute and intrahepatic abscesses when chronic. Portal vein stenosis or thrombosis can cause portal hypertension and varices, as well as graft dysfunction or graft loss. Bile duct complications include stenosis and leak and may be managed with operative repair, hepaticojejunostomy, or stents.

All patients with hepatitis C will experience recurrence in the graft. This can be a cause of graft loss

both early and late. Rejection typically presents with increasing liver function tests.

KIDNEY TRANSPLANTATION

EPIDEMIOLOGY

There are currently >60,000 people in the United States waiting for a kidney transplant, among a group of more than 300,000 patients on dialysis.

INDICATIONS

Kidney transplantation is indicated for end-stage renal disease in patients otherwise healthy enough to tolerate the surgery and subsequent immunosuppression. Common causes are given in Table 26-3.

KIDNEY ALLOCATION

Kidney allocation is based on a formula that incorporates the kidney's degree of match, the waiting time, whether a person has been a kidney donor, the recipient's age, and the recipient's degree of sensitization (Table 26-4).

■ **TABLE 26-3** Disease States Leading to End-Stage Renal Disease
Glomerulonephritis
Chronic pyelonephritis
Hereditary conditions—polycystic kidney disease; nephritis, including Alport syndrome; tuberous sclerosis
Metabolic conditions—diabetes mellitus, hyperoxaluria, cystinosis, Fabry disease, amyloid, gout, porphyria
Obstructive uropathy
Toxic insults
Multisystem disease (lupus, vasculitis, scleroderma)
Hemolytic-uremic syndrome
Tumors
Congenital—hypoplasia, horseshoe
Irreversible ATN
Trauma
Recurrences That Cause Graft Loss
FSGS: 30%
Mesangiocapillary type I glomerulonephritis: 20%
Hemolytic-uremic syndrome: 50%
Oxalosis: 90%
Recurrences That Do Not Result in Graft Loss (generally)
Membranous glomerulonephritis
IgA nephropathy
ATN, acute tubular necrosis; FSGS, focal segmental glomerulosclerosis; IgA, immunoglobulin A.

■ **TABLE 26-4** Kidney Allocation	
Criteria	**No. of Points**
Each year on the waiting list	1
Very high preformed antibodies	4
<10 years old	4
11–17 years old	3
Previous organ donor	4
No mismatch	7
One mismatch	5
Two mismatches	2

PROGNOSIS

The half-life of a cadaver kidney, censoring for patient death, is >10 years, whereas for a live donor kidney, half-life is close to 30 years. Transplantation is superior to dialysis for quality of life and survival, even in older people.

THE OPERATION: KIDNEY TRANSPLANTATION

Before beginning, it is imperative to verify that the proper kidney has been received and is ABO compatible and cross-match negative. Placement of the kidney on the right side is usually easier, as the right iliac vein is more accessible than the left for anastomosis. Incising from the pubis to two fingerbreadths medial to the anterior-superior iliac spine allows exposure of the anterior rectus sheath and the external oblique. Incision through the muscular and fascial layers permits entry into the retroperitoneal space. Care is taken to preserve the spermatic cord in males. Dissection of the retroperitoneal space allows the renal vessels to be anastomosed to the external iliac artery and vein. Anastomosis of the ureter directly to the bladder re-establishes drainage.

Complications

Technical complications after renal transplantation include venous and arterial thrombosis, which generally result in graft loss. Ureteral complications include stricture and leak. Early problems should be fixed with re-operation, either via direct repair or ureteroureterostomy with the recipient's native ureter. For chronic problems, dilation and stenting can be attempted. Rejection typically presents with decreased urine output, increasing creatinine, or edema.

PANCREAS TRANSPLANTATION

Pancreas transplantation is generally reserved for patients with severe type I diabetes who also need a kidney transplant. In this setting, there is no additional risk of immunosuppression. In patients with hypoglycemic unawareness, who can lose consciousness from low blood sugars, and other patients with severe complications, pancreas transplantation alone is indicated. Transplantation will generally arrest the development, but not reverse, diabetic complications. One- and 3-year graft survival of the pancreas in kidney plus pancreas recipients is 85% and 71%, respectively. One- and 3-year graft survival of the pancreas with pancreas transplantation alone is 73%, and 53%, respectively.

The pancreas is prepared with the donor duodenum intact to allow control of exocrine secretions. A bifurcated arterial graft is placed to connect the splenic artery and superior mesenteric artery of the pancreas so that the entire gland receives blood. The gland is drained via its portal vein. The graft is placed either in the right iliac fossa or in the middle of the abdomen. Right iliac placement requires inflow from the right common iliac artery and drainage via the right common iliac vein, although the aorta and vena cava can both be used. The pancreas can also be placed in the middle of the abdomen and have venous drainage through the superior mesenteric vein (portal drainage). The duodenum may be anastomosed to the bowel or bladder to control exocrine secretions.

Major complications include arterial or venous thrombosis, leak of the duodenal anastomosis, and pancreatitis. Bladder drainage can lead to hematuria from bladder irritation and metabolic acidosis owing to loss of bicarbonate secretions.

SMALL BOWEL TRANSPLANTATION

Small bowel transplantation is indicated for short bowel syndrome or intestinal failure, commonly resulting from surgical resection. It is commonly performed in combination with liver transplantation. One- and 3-year graft survival is 78% and 40%, respectively.

HEART TRANSPLANTATION

Heart transplantation is indicated for patients with end-stage heart failure whose symptoms cannot be controlled with medications. The most common causes are coronary artery disease (45%) and congestive heart failure (40%). Valvular disease, congenital, and other causes account for fewer than 10% of all transplant recipients. One- and 3-year graft survival is 88% and 79%, respectively. Allograft vasculopathy is a major cause of late graft loss.

LUNG TRANSPLANTATION

Lung transplantation is indicated for symptomatic end-stage lung disease. Chronic obstructive pulmonary disease/emphysema accounts for >50% of transplants, and idiopathic pulmonary fibrosis another 26%. Less common causes include alpha-1 antitrypsin deficiency, cystic fibrosis, sarcoidosis, and re-transplantation. One- and 3-year graft survival is 83% and 64%, respectively. Because the lung is in direct contact with the

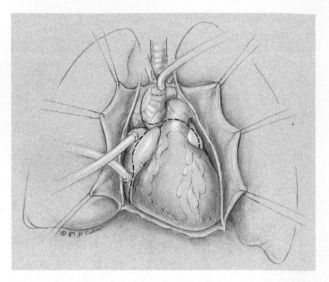

Figure 26-3 • Heart/lung transplantation, step 1. Anterior view of recipient heart and lungs before removal. Resection lines are shown dashed.

environment, infection is a major problem, and there is a constant struggle between overimmunosuppression and rejection. Bronchiolitis obliterans syndrome is a poorly understood entity that is a major source of morbidity and mortality in these patients.

Heart and lung transplantation are often performed together, and the operation is depicted in Figures 26-3, 26-4, 26-5, and 26-6.

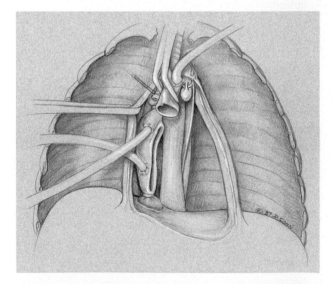

Figure 26-4 • Heart/lung transplantation, step 2. Anterior view of recipient mediastinum after heart and lungs have been removed. Shunts are in place. Aorta is clamped.

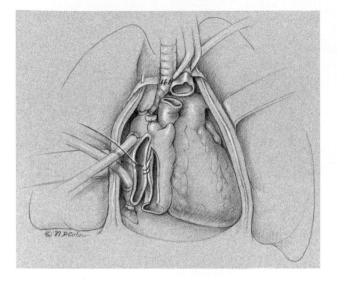

Figure 26-5 • Heart/lung transplantation, step 3. Anterior view of recipient mediastinum after presentation of donor heart and lungs. Suturing has begun along inferior vena cava and right atrium. Shunts are in place. Aorta is clamped.

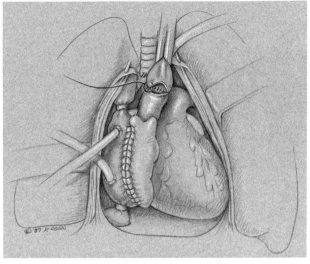

Figure 26-6 • Heart/lung transplantation, step 4. Anterior view of recipient mediastinum during last stages of transplantation. Recipient aorta is being sutured to donor aorta.

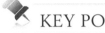

KEY POINTS

- Control of the host response to donor major histocompatibility antigens is necessary for successful organ transplantation.

- Most current immunosuppressive regimens have moved away from long-term use of corticosteroids.

- Cadaver donors can be divided into heart-beating and non–heart-beating donors.

- Liver transplantation is indicated for end-stage liver disease or unresectable early-stage hepatocellular cancer and can be performed with removal or preservation of the recipient vena cava.

- Kidney transplantation is superior to dialysis for long-term patient survival and quality of life.

- Pancreas transplantation is indicated for patients with type I diabetes receiving a kidney, but transplantation will generally not reverse diabetic complications.

- Small bowel transplantation is indicated for patients with small bowel syndrome or irreversible bowel failure.

- Heart transplantation is a successful therapy for end-stage heart disease.

- Allograft vasculopathy is a major source of morbidity in heart transplantation.

- Bronchiolitis obliterans syndrome is an important cause of morbidity after lung transplant.

27 Trauma

Trauma is the leading cause of death in the first four decades of life and the third leading cause of death overall, trailing only cancer and coronary artery disease. Approximately 60 million injuries occur annually in the United States. Although approximately 150,000 traumatic deaths occur annually, the rate of disability from trauma is three times greater than mortality. Therefore, issues relating to trauma care are of importance to all medical and surgical specialists, from the trauma surgeon to the rehabilitation specialist.

Death due to trauma has been shown to occur in a trimodal distribution, during three identifiable time periods. The first peak of death occurs within seconds to minutes of injury. Lethal injury to the body's vital anatomic structures leads to rapid death, unless immediate advanced intervention is performed. The second peak of death occurs within minutes to several hours after the injury. Death during this second period is usually due to progressive neurologic, cardiovascular, or pulmonary compromise. It is during this intermediate period that patients have the greatest chance of salvage and toward which organized trauma care is focused. Rapid resuscitation, coupled with the identification and treatment of potentially lethal injuries, is the goal. The final third peak of death occurs several days to weeks after initial injury, usually secondary to sepsis and multiorgan system failure.

This chapter discusses trauma management during the aforementioned second period. Specifically, the steps of the initial assessment performed when the trauma patient arrives at the hospital emergency room, the primary survey of the patient (ABCs), resuscitation, the secondary survey (head to toe), and the institution of definitive care are examined.

PRIMARY SURVEY

The focus of the primary survey is to identify immediately life-threatening conditions and to prevent death. Without a patent airway, adequate gas exchange, or sufficient intravascular volume, any patient will die. Therefore, a simple mnemonic—ABCDE—is used to direct the primary survey:

Airway with cervical spine control
Breathing and ventilation
Circulation and hemorrhage control
Disability and neurologic assessment
Exposure to enable examination

The principle here is that injuries are fixed as they are discovered, and this algorithm is to remind the physician not to get distracted by obvious injuries. For example, a common exam question goes something like this: "A patient is admitted to the emergency department after a crush injury to the left upper extremity such that three fingers have been severed and one is attached only by a thin piece of skin. What is your first intervention?" It is important to demonstrate awareness that the airway should be assessed first. This should take approximately 15 to 30 seconds if there are no abnormalities.

(A) AIRWAY

The airway is immediately inspected to ensure patency and that any causes of airway obstruction are identified (foreign body, facial fracture, tracheal/laryngeal disruption, cervical spine injury). Cervical spine control must be maintained at all times—patients with multitrauma must be assumed to have cervical spine injury until cleared radiographically. The chin thrust and jaw lift are methods of initially establishing airway patency while simultaneously protecting the cervical spine. Conscious patients should be asked to open their mouths, which should be inspected, and then to talk. This establishes at least a partially open conduit from the lungs to the outside world.

Airway control in the conscious patient can be achieved with an easily inserted nasopharyngeal trumpet; an oropharyngeal airway is used in the unconscious patient. Definitive control of the airway and enhanced ability to ventilate and oxygenate the patient are achieved with endotracheal intubation. Tube placement may be via the nasal or oral route. Nasotracheal intubation is a useful technique for patients with cervical spine injuries; however, it is contraindicated when midface or basilar skull fractures are suspected. When the trachea cannot be intubated, as might occur with severe swelling or multiple fractures, a surgical airway is indicated and should not be delayed. Jet insufflation of the airway after needle cricothyroidotomy can adequately oxygenate patients for 30 to 45 minutes. Surgical cricothyroidotomy with the insertion of a tracheostomy or endotracheal tube allows prolonged ventilation and oxygenation. This is best achieved via a longitudinal incision that avoids the anterior jugular veins, which can bleed significantly. The cricoid cartilage is palpated, and a transverse incision is made, into which a tracheostomy tube can be placed.

(B) BREATHING

Once airway patency is established, the patient's ability to breathe must be assessed. Normal function of the lungs, chest wall, and diaphragm is necessary for ventilation and gas exchange to occur. Four entities should be of particular concern: open pneumothorax, tension pneumothorax, hemothorax, and flail chest. Each can lead to rapid death resulting from respiratory compromise. A mnemonic to remember this is to repeat "open, tension, hemo, flail" a number of times. It has a regular cadence, and with enough repetition, it will come quickly back to you when performing the breathing survey.

Open pneumothorax occurs when the integrity of the chest wall is compromised so that diaphragmatic motion and decreased intrathoracic pressure cause air to enter the chest through the hole in the chest instead of through the mouth. In this case, the lung will not expand. Treatment requires closure of the chest wall defect and placement of a chest tube. Intubation will

also solve this problem because the positive pressure will expand the lungs.

Tension pneumothorax occurs when an injury to the lung parenchyma allows air to escape into the pleural space. Often this will result in a simple pneumothorax, but if a valve effect occurs in which the air cannot escape out of the plural space back into the lung, pressure in the pleural space will continue to increase. This will render half of the lung useless for gas exchange, and cause tremendous pressure (tension) on the mediastinum, pushing all structures away from the side of the tension pneumothorax. This will impair venous return to the heart and will be fatal if not recognized and treated (Fig. 27-1). The clinical picture of hypotension, tachycardia, tracheal deviation, neck vein distention, and diminished unilateral breath sounds suggests the diagnosis of tension pneumothorax. Immediate decompression by inserting a needle catheter into the second intercostal space in the midclavicular line is indicated, followed by definitive treatment with chest tube insertion into the fifth intercostal space at the anterior axillary line just lateral to the nipple.

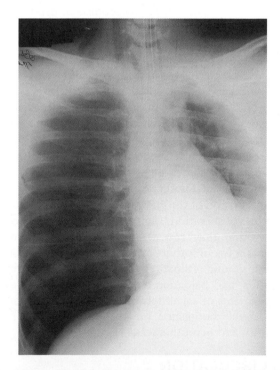

Figure 27-1 • Chest x-ray reveals a right-sided tension pneumothorax. The right lung is collapsed and the increased pressure in the right chest displaces the heart and other mediastinal structures to the left.
From Fleisher GR, Ludwig S, Baskin MN. *Atlas of Pediatric Emergency Medicine*. Philadelphia, PA: Lippincott Williams & Wilkins, 2004.

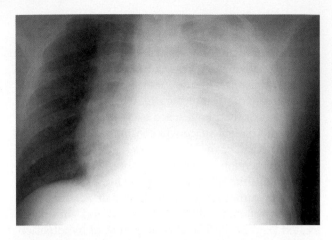

Figure 27-2 • Chest film reveals a left-sided hemothorax. The left lung is compressed by the blood, and the mediastinum is shifted to the right.

From Harwood-Nuss A, Wolfson AB, Lyndon CH, et al. *The Clinical Practice of Emergency Medicine.* 3rd ed. Philadelphia, PA: Lippincott Williams & Wilkins, 2001.

Hemothorax occurs as a result of a ruptured blood vessel in the pleural space, which fills up with blood and compromises gas exchange (Fig. 27-2). This can cause life-threatening pulmonary compromise or hypotension. Treatment involves tube thoracostomy and operation if bleeding continues.

Flail chest occurs when multiple rib fractures prevent normal expansion of the lungs. In this case, there may be paradoxical collapse of a portion of the chest on inspiration (Fig. 27-3). This can be life-threatening if severe and is intensely painful. Often there is severe underlying lung contusion, which impairs gas exchange. Treatment of pain with rib blocks may improve ventilation. Intubation will allow lung expansion for the same reason for open pneumothorax.

Examination of the chest during the primary survey includes observation, palpation, and auscultation. Observation may reveal asymmetries in expansion, suggesting pneumothorax or hemothorax, or an open, sucking wound. Palpation of the trachea may reveal deviation, and palpation of the chest wall may reveal flail segments or asymmetrical excursion. Auscultation may reveal diminished breath sounds as occurs in pneumo- and hemothoraces.

(C) CIRCULATION

Hypotension in the trauma patient is caused by blood loss until proven otherwise. There are only five places to put enough blood to make someone hypotensive, so these areas require specific attention: chest, abdomen,

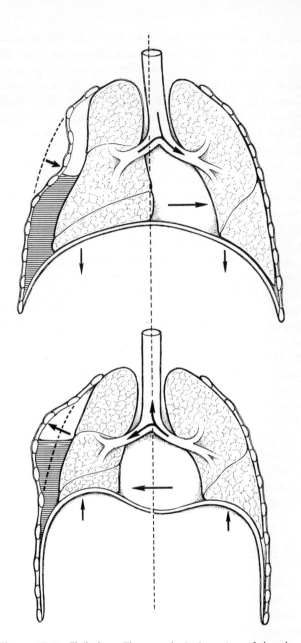

Figure 27-3 • Flail chest. The paradoxical motion of the chest cavity is shown. (top) As the patient inhales (diaphragm moves down), the flail segment collapses, because the compromised chest wall can no longer resist the decreased intrathoracic pressure. In contrast, on expiration (bottom), exhalation causes a bowing out of the flail segment. In these ways, flail chest results in dramatic impairments in lung function.

Illustration by Neil O. Hardy, Westpoint, CT.

retroperitoneum, thighs, and outside world. External hemorrhage can usually be identified and controlled by direct manual pressure. Tourniquets should be avoided, because they cause distal ischemia. Internal hemorrhage is more difficult to identify. Therefore, hypotension without signs of external hemorrhage must be assumed to be due to intra-abdominal or intrathoracic injury or from fractures of the pelvis or long bones. The hypovolemic hypotensive patient usually exhibits a diminished level of consciousness as cerebral blood flow is reduced, the pulse is rapid and thready, and the skin is pale and clammy.

(D) DISABILITY

Traumatic injuries may cause damage to the central and peripheral nervous systems. Spinal cord injuries are most commonly seen in the cervical and lumbar regions. The thoracic spine is less prone to injury because of the rigidity of the bony thorax. Complete spinal cord injury affects all neurologic function below a specific level of the cord. Incomplete spinal cord injury exhibits sacral sparing and may involve the central portion of the cord, as in central cord syndrome; a single side of the cord, as in Brown-Séquard syndrome; or the anterior portion of the cord, as in anterior cord syndrome. A rapid assessment of disability and neurologic function is vital so that drug therapy and physical maneuvers can be initiated to prevent further neurologic injury.

(E) EXPOSURE

Exposure of the trauma patient is important for the entire body to be examined and injuries diagnosed. Complete exposure entails removing all clothing from the patient so a thorough examination can be performed, allowing for identification of entry and exit wounds, extremity deformities, contusions, or lacerations; sometimes this is considered part of the secondary survey. The patient should be rolled onto one side with the neck and back supported in a rigid position to determine whether there are additional injuries. If there is suggestion of spinal injury and no obvious hemorrhage is coming from the back, this maneuver can be postponed. After the examination, attention should be paid to maintaining the patient's core body temperature.

EMERGENCY DEPARTMENT THORACOTOMY

In the severely injured, hypotensive patient, the question sometimes arises whether to perform thoracotomy in the emergency department as a life-saving maneuver. In the blunt trauma patient, this intervention is rarely successful and should be avoided, unless the vital signs are lost just before or during the resuscitation and all other measures have failed to improve the situation. In victims of penetrating trauma, this maneuver can be successful, especially if cardiac tamponade is found. This can temporize until the patient can be taken to the operating room for definitive repair.

VOLUME RESUSCITATION

Hemorrhage leading to hypovolemic shock is the most common cause of postinjury death in the trauma patient. Rapid fluid resuscitation and hemorrhage control are the keys to restoring adequate circulating blood volume. The fluid status of patients can be quickly evaluated by assessing their hemodynamics (hypotension and tachycardia), their level of consciousness (adequacy of cerebral perfusion), the color of their skin (pale skin indicates significant exsanguination), and the presence and character of the pulse (absent central pulses indicate profound hypovolemic shock). All sources of external hemorrhage must be identified and treated by applying direct pressure. Indiscriminate hemostat usage should be avoided, because it may crush and damage surrounding neurovascular structures. Sources of internal hemorrhage are usually hidden and are suspected by unstable hemodynamics. Internal bleeding may occur in the thorax as a result of cardiovascular or pulmonary injury, in the abdomen from splenic or liver lacerations, or into the soft tissues surrounding femur or pelvic fractures.

Fluid resuscitation of the hypovolemic, hypotensive patient requires establishing adequate intravenous access. Two large-bore catheters (14 gauge) should be placed in upper extremity veins and rapid infusion of a balanced salt solution (Lactated Ringer's or normal saline) initiated. If the pattern of injury allows, central access via the femoral vein approach using larger-diameter catheters maximizes the rate of fluid administration. If percutaneous access is unsuccessful, a cut-down of the greater saphenous vein at the anteromedial ankle is required. After intravenous access is established, bolus infusion of crystalloid solution should be replaced with O-negative or type-specific blood, once it becomes available.

TRAUMA RADIOGRAPHS

For patients with blunt trauma (automobile crashes, falls), three standard radiographic studies are required to assess the neck, chest, and pelvis: cross-table lateral cervical spine, anteroposterior chest, and anteroposterior pelvis. Obtaining these three x-rays early in the resuscitation process allows potentially neurologically disabling cervical spine injuries, life-threatening chest wall and cardiopulmonary injuries, and pelvic injuries to be identified and immediately treated. For patients with penetrating trauma (gunshot, stabbing, impaling), an anteroposterior chest film and other films pertaining to the site of injury should be obtained.

SECONDARY SURVEY

The secondary survey begins after the airway, breathing, and circulation have been assessed and resuscitation has been initiated. This secondary survey is a head-to-toe evaluation of the body, during which additional areas of injury are identified. A meticulous examination during this phase of the trauma evaluation minimizes the chance of missing an important finding.

The final phase of acute trauma care is instituting definitive treatment. This may entail simple wound care in the emergency room for minor injuries or, if the injuries warrant, transportation to the operating room for surgical treatment.

THORACIC TRAUMA

Because of the great importance of the structures in the chest, thoracic trauma is second only to head trauma as a cause of death in injured patients. After the interventions described in the primary survey, many injures will remain that will require expeditious repair.

Open pneumothorax will generally require chest wall repair. The timing of this depends on whether the defect can be controlled, how large it is, and the severity of the patient's other injuries.

Tension pneumothorax, after emergent decompression, will require chest tube placement.

Hemothorax, after initial chest tube placement, requires careful monitoring to decide whether the patient needs emergent thoracotomy. If the initial blood removed from the chest is >1,500 mL, or if ongoing blood loss is >200 mL/hr, the patient should be explored in the operating room for hemorrhage control. Even if the patient does not require emergent thoracotomy, many centers will aggressively clean the pleural space of blood with thoracoscopy at some point in the future when the patient is stable.

Flail chest is often a sign of significant pulmonary contusion, which will cause a ventilation perfusion mismatch. These patients can be very difficult to oxygenate. Treatment consists of diuresis, pain control, and if necessary, prolonged intubation with positive end-expiratory pressure. The flail chest itself can be stabilized operatively, but this is rarely necessary.

Cardiac tamponade is a life-threatening condition in which blood escapes into the pericardium. Because the pericardium does not expand well, the blood compresses the heart and dramatically decreases venous return and cardiac output. The diagnosis is made from the Beck's triad of hypotension, distant heart sounds, and elevated central venous pressure. Pericardiocentesis can remove blood from the space and temporarily restore normal hemodynamics. These patients should generally be taken to the operating room to diagnose and repair cardiac injuries or other sources of the bleeding.

Severe impact on the sternum can cause blunt cardiac injury or cardiac contusion. This lesion can decrease cardiac output and predispose patients to arrhythmias. Although there is no specific therapy, these patients should be monitored and supported if the cardiac output is inadequate to perfuse the body.

Thoracic aortic injury from blunt trauma usually involves disruption of the aorta just distal to the take-off of the left subclavian artery where the aorta is tethered by the ligamentum arteriosum. This lesion requires tremendous energy to produce and is most commonly due to falls or high-speed frontal impacts. This lesion should be suspected in the appropriate clinical circumstances. Chest radiograph may reveal a wide mediastinum, loss of aortic knob contour, nasogastric tube deviation to the right, first or second rib fracture, or pleural cap, which is an accumulation of blood above the pleura. Aortography, contrast computed tomography (CT), or transesophageal echocardiogram can be used in diagnosis.

Diaphragmatic rupture may occur from penetrating or blunt trauma. Tremendous force is required to cause this injury. Diagnosis is made with chest x-ray, demonstrating a nasogastric tube or bowel in the chest, or with CT scan or contrast study. On the right side, the liver prevents most cases, so that the left diaphragm is most commonly affected. Operative exploration is indicated for repair and evaluation of other injuries.

Esophageal injury is diagnosed on contrast swallow or endoscopy. In general, operative repair with wide drainage is necessary to prevent mediastinitis, which can be fatal.

Tracheal injury can present on physical examination with crepitus, difficulty speaking, respiratory distress, or hemoptysis. Bronchoscopy is necessary to define the lesion. Treatment is expectant or operative depending on the nature and severity of the injury.

ABDOMINAL TRAUMA

Complete examination of the abdomen is extremely difficult in the emergency department because of the noise and number of people. Although classic teaching is to listen, observe, palpate, and auscultate bowel sounds, findings can be unreliable because of altered states of consciousness of the patient, ambient noise, and multiple procedures occurring at the same time. The abdominal examination is best thought of in the context of all of the patient's injuries, and it may be necessary to act definitively in spite of physical examination findings. For example a hypotensive patient with no other injuries with a significant mechanism and no abdominal tenderness may still have a hemoperitoneum. A soft abdomen does not preclude a hollow viscous injury.

In addition to examination of the abdomen, rectal examination is performed to look for blood, indicative of a rectal or colonic injury, and tone, lack of which may suggest a spinal cord injury. In the male, a high-riding or nonpalpable prostate may suggest a urethral injury, and a suprapubic tube should be placed instead of a Foley catheter. Blood at the urinary meatus or a scrotal hematoma in the male also suggests a urethral injury, and again, a Foley should be avoided. Pressure should be placed on the anterior-superior iliac spine to test for fractures.

Patients who are stable with a suspected abdominal injury should undergo abdominal CT scan. Other options include focused assessment by sonography in trauma (FAST) ultrasound examination or diagnostic peritoneal lavage. Diagnostic peritoneal lavage is performed through a small infraumbilical incision. A supraumbilical incision is preferred if there is significant pelvic trauma because of the possibility of a hematoma in the preperitoneal space below the umbilicus. A catheter is placed in the abdomen, it is aspirated, and 1 L of Lactated Ringer's solution is instilled. The test result is considered positive if the initial aspiration returns blood or bowel contents, the aspirate after the liter contains >100,000 red blood cells or 500 white blood cells/mL, if bacteria or bowel contents are returned, or if the fluid has a high amylase.

Injuries to the liver and spleen are generally treated conservatively unless there is ongoing hemorrhage, making the patient unstable. Hollow viscous injuries are fixed immediately by resection and either diversion or primary anastomosis, depending on the situation. Pancreatic injuries can be treated by simple drainage or resection of a portion of the gland with or without pancreaticojejunostomy. In general, "damage control" is used to describe the initial operation in the multi-injured patient. Life-threatening injures are treated, and definitive treatment is delayed in favor of resuscitation in the intensive care unit as necessary. This is to prevent ongoing hypothermia and worsening coagulopathy, which can be fatal.

OPHTHALMIC TRAUMA

More than 1 million cases of ophthalmic trauma after penetrating or blunt injury are reported annually in the United States. Prompt and appropriate care of many ophthalmic injuries may prevent much visual disability.

CHEMICAL BURNS

Chemical burns to the eye represent an ophthalmologic emergency. If treatment is not begun immediately, irreversible damage may occur. Alkaline substances (e.g., household cleaners, fertilizers, and pesticides) cause the most severe damage, but acids may cause significant ocular morbidity as well.

Treatment

A detailed history is not required before beginning copious irrigation with any available water source for at least 15 to 20 minutes. After initial irrigation, visual acuity and pH should be measured. If the pH has not returned to the normal value of 7.5, irrigation should be continued. Prompt ophthalmologic referral should be obtained in all cases of acid or alkali burns and for patients with decreased visual acuity, severe conjunctival swelling, or corneal clouding. All other patients should see an ophthalmologist within 24 hours.

SUPERFICIAL FOREIGN BODIES

Foreign bodies that have an impact on the surface of the cornea or conjunctiva represent approximately 25% of all ocular injuries.

History

An accurate history often provides the diagnosis and should be used to judge the risk of intraocular foreign body (see below). Symptoms range from mild ocular irritation to severe pain. If symptoms began gradually rather than suddenly, other causes, such as infectious keratitis, should be considered.

Diagnostic Evaluation

Careful inspection of the cornea and conjunctiva using bright light and magnification often reveals the foreign body.

Treatment

One should always measure visual acuity before making any attempt at removing the foreign body. Superficial foreign bodies can usually be removed using topical anesthesia and a cotton swab. After the foreign body is removed, Wood's lamp examination with fluorescein should be performed to ascertain the size of any residual corneal epithelial defect. Eversion of the upper eyelid should be carried out to look for residual foreign material under the lids. Ophthalmologic referral is indicated when a foreign body cannot be safely removed or for any patient with a large corneal epithelial defect.

BLUNT OR PENETRATING INJURY

Blunt or penetrating trauma to the eye represents a leading cause of vision loss in young people. Blunt trauma most often causes ocular contusion or damage to the surrounding orbit. Penetrating trauma causes corneal or scleral laceration (a ruptured globe) and represents an ophthalmologic emergency requiring early intervention and repair. The possibility of a retained intraocular foreign body should always be considered (see below). A high degree of suspicion must be maintained in all cases of head and facial injuries.

History

History should include the mechanism of injury, the force of impact, the likelihood of a retained foreign body, and any associated ocular or visual complaints.

Diagnostic Evaluation

Eyelid integrity, ocular motility, and pupillary reaction should be tested. Use a penlight to detect conjunctival swelling or hemorrhage, corneal or scleral laceration, or hyphema (blood behind the cornea obscuring details of the underlying iris or pupil). Pain and decreased vision with a history of trauma should always lead to suspicion of perforation of the globe. Severe subconjunctival hemorrhage, a shallow anterior chamber or space between the cornea and iris, hyphema, and limitation of extraocular motility are often, but not invariably, present. Radiologic studies, including CT of the head and orbits, should be obtained in cases of suspected blowout fracture or to rule out a retained intraocular foreign body (see below).

Treatment

If the eye is lacerated or the pupil or iris is not visible, a shield should be placed over the eye, and the patient should be referred immediately to an ophthalmologist. Eyelid lacerations that involve the lid margin or lacrimal apparatus require meticulous repair to avoid severe functional and cosmetic morbidity. If the eyelid margin and inner one sixth of the eyelid are not damaged, the wound can be closed with fine sutures. If the eyelid margin is lacerated, accurate realignment of the lid margin must be ensured before wound closure. Disruption of the inner one sixth of the eyelid requires intubation of the lacrimal drainage system, with stent placement before surgical repair, and should be carried out by an ophthalmologist or other appropriately trained physician. Ophthalmologic referral after trauma is determined by ocular symptoms and findings, as set forth in Table 27-1.

INTRAOCULAR FOREIGN BODIES

A high-speed missile may penetrate the cornea or sclera while causing minimal symptoms or physical findings. Foreign-body composition is important, because certain metals, such as iron, steel, and copper, produce a severe inflammatory reaction if left in the eye, whereas other materials, such as glass, lead, and stone, are relatively inert and may not require surgical removal. Retained vegetable matter is especially dangerous and may cause a severe purulent endophthalmitis. A retained foreign body should be suspected in all cases of perforating injuries of the eye or whenever the history suggests high-risk activities, such as drilling, sawing, or hammering.

History

One should inquire about high-risk activities, a sensation of sudden impact on the eyelids or eye, and any complaint of pain or decreased vision.

Physical Examination

Visual acuity should always be recorded before any manipulation of the eye or eyelids. Inspection may reveal an entry wound, although this may be quite subtle and easily overlooked. Specifically, one should look for a hyphema, pupillary distortion, or any alteration of the red reflex on funduscopic examination.

■ **TABLE 27-1** Management of Ophthalmic Trauma

Treat on Site and Refer Immediately
Acid or alkali burn
Unremovable corneal or conjunctival foreign body
Refer Immediately
Severe pain
Subnormal visual acuity
Irregular pupil
Deformed globe
Corneal or scleral laceration
Corneal clouding
Severe lid swelling
Severe conjunctival chemosis
Proptosis
Hyphema
Absent red reflex
Suspected intraocular foreign body (history of being struck by high-speed missile)
Eyelid laceration that is deep, large, avulsed, exposes fat, or extends through lid margin or lacrimal drainage apparatus
Refer Within 24 Hours
Pain
Photophobia
Diplopia
Foreign-body sensation but no visible foreign body or corneal abrasion
Large corneal abrasion
Moderate eyelid or conjunctival chemosis but normal visual acuity
Suspected contusion of globe
Suspected orbital wall fracture
Refer Within 48 Hours
Mild contusion injury to orbital soft tissues

Diagnostic Evaluation

Accurate localization may require soft tissue radiographs, orbital ultrasound, or CT. Magnetic resonance imaging is contraindicated in all cases of suspected intraocular foreign body.

Treatment

If the history strongly suggests the possibility of a retained foreign body, urgent ophthalmologic referral is indicated, even in the absence of physical findings. Prompt surgical removal of intraocular debris is usually indicated to avoid the toxic effect of metallic foreign bodies on intraocular tissue and secondary intraocular infection from retained organic material.

BURNS

Burns are characterized by their thickness and the extent of the body surface area they cover. First-degree burns are limited to the dermis, do not blister, and are red and painful. Because the dermis is intact, they heal without scarring. Second-degree burns extend partially into the dermis and form blisters which are red and painful. The extent of dermal involvement determines the extent of scar formed. Third-degree burns occur when the entire dermis is destroyed. These areas of burn are insensate, because the nerve endings have also been destroyed. They generally require skin grafting for healing.

Patients presenting with burns must be evaluated for inhalation injury if the burn was caused by a fire. Carbon monoxide inhalation, heat causing edema of the oropharynx and larynx, and damage caused by inhalation of hot embers can also be fatal. Patients with significant injury of this type should be intubated early to maximize respiratory support and prevent airway compromise.

Severely burned patients will lose tremendous amounts of fluid, and resuscitation forms a major portion of the care of these patients. Percentage of body burn can be estimated by the rule of nines: the head has 9% of body-surface area, the dorsal and ventral torso each 18%, each arm 9%, and each leg 18%. On this basis, the Parkland formula determines the amount of fluid given and should be initiated for patients with >10% to 15% of total body-surface affected. This is calculated as the body weight in kilograms × percent of total body surface with second- or third-degree burns × 4 mL. Half of this total should be given as Lactated Ringer's solution in the first 8 hours after injury, and the rest over the next 16 hours. Urine output and blood pressure should be carefully monitored and infusions adjusted accordingly.

As treatment begins, eschars in the torso may constrict breathing, or eschars in the extremities may compromise circulation. In this case, escharotomy should be performed to relieve the compression (Fig. 27-4). In skin grafting is performed. For large burns, this procedure is limited by hypothermia and blood loss, and is often done in sequential fashion. Local care with topical antibiotics and frequent dressing changes is critical.

Burn patients often have tremendous nutritional requirements, with calorie and protein requirements approaching twice normal. Enteral feeding should be initiated as quickly as possible.

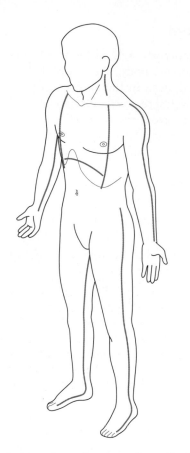

Figure 27-4 • Incisions for escharotomy. From Blackbourne LH. *Advanced Surgical Recall*. 2nd ed. Baltimore, MD: Lippincott Williams & Wilkins, 2004

this procedure, full-thickness incisions are made in the skin to release the constriction.

Sepsis is an ongoing problem for burn patients. The burn itself sterilizes the skin, but bacterial repopulation occurs quickly. Great improvements in burn care have come from early excision and grafting, which decrease the risk of infection. In this procedure, thin slices of skin are removed with a dermatome until viable tissue is encountered, as determined by bleeding. At this point,

KEY POINTS

- Trauma is the leading cause of death in the first four decades of life.
- Trauma is the third leading cause of death overall, after cancer and heart disease.
- Traumatic death occurs in a trimodal distribution.
- Trauma care involves the primary survey, resuscitation, secondary survey, and definitive care.
- The primary survey identifies immediately life-threatening injuries involving the airway, breathing, and circulation.
- Resuscitation involves airway control and ventilation and fluid infusion after intravenous access is obtained.
- The secondary survey is a head-to-toe examination to identify additional areas of injury.
- Standard radiographs required for trauma include lateral cervical spine, anteroposterior chest, and anteroposterior pelvis.
- "Open, tension, hemo, flail" is a pneumonic for life-threatening thoracic injuries diagnosed during the primary survey.
- Total surface burn area determines fluid requirements for burn patients, which are calculated using the Parkland formula.
- Chemical burns to the eye are a true ophthalmologic emergency.

Appendix: Sample Operative Reports

After each operation, a complete and concise description, outlining the indications for surgery, the operative findings, and the conduct of the operation, should be composed. This report is vital for communication among health care providers, and it documents the intervention for future reference. When dictating a report, follow a defined format, introduce only relevant information to the narrative, and maintain an orderly flow from incision to closure. The following operative reports are examples of routine general surgery procedures: open hernia repair and laparoscopic cholecystectomy.

INGUINAL HERNIA

PREOPERATIVE DIAGNOSIS: Right inguinal hernia

POSTOPERATIVE DIAGNOSIS: Right indirect inguinal hernia

PROCEDURE PERFORMED: Open-mesh repair of right indirect inguinal hernia

SURGEON: James Morris, MD

ANESTHESIA: Local and intravenous sedation

INDICATIONS FOR OPERATION: Mr. Robert Hall is a 75-year-old male who presented complaining of a symptomatic right inguinal hernia of 6 months' duration. On physical examination, a nontender reducible right inguinal hernia was noted. Operative and nonoperative management options, as well as the risks and potential complications of each approach, were discussed with the patient. After all questions were answered, he requested open-mesh hernia repair. A request-for-surgery form was signed and witnessed preoperatively.

INTRAOPERATIVE FINDINGS: Moderate indirect inguinal hernia sac, ligated and resected. Polypropylene mesh plug inserted into deep ring with mesh overlay.

DESCRIPTION OF PROCEDURE: The patient was positioned supine on the operating table, and preoperative antibiotics and intravenous sedation were administered. The right inguinal region was prepped and draped sterilely. Combined lidocaine 1% and bupivacaine 0.25% was injected subdermally, and an oblique skin incision was made above the inguinal ligament. The superficial epigastric vessels were divided between clamps and tied. Scarpa's fascia was divided and the external oblique fascia identified. A subfascial local anesthetic infiltration was performed, and the external oblique fascia was opened in the line of its fibers down through the external ring. The iliohypogastric nerve was identified and preserved. The ilioinguinal nerve was dissected away from the cord structures and retracted caudad. Both nerves were preserved and uninjured during the entire procedure. The cord was encircled at the pubic tubercle with a Penrose drain and the floor inspected. There was no evidence of direct herniation; however, the floor was somewhat attenuated. The cord was interrogated, and a moderate-sized indirect hernia sac was identified and dissected free from the surrounding structures. The vas deferens and testicular vessels were preserved and uninjured. Once the proximal sac was fully mobilized into the deep inguinal ring, the distal sac was suture ligated with a 3-0 absorbable stitch and the redundant sac excised and passed off the table as a specimen. A large-sized polypropylene plug was placed into the indirect defect and sutured superiorly for fixation. Given the previously noted attenuated floor, a polypropylene patch was sutured for reinforcement to the conjoined tendon, pubic tubercle, and shelving edge of the inguinal ligament with interrupted 3-0 absorbable suture. The ilioinguinal nerve was returned to its anatomic position alongside the cord structures, and the lateral legs of the patch were positioned around the cord as it exited the deep ring, the legs being secured with a single stitch. The iliohypogastric nerve was then returned to its anatomic position, and the external oblique fascia was closed with a running 3-0 absorbable suture, taking care to avoid entrapment of the ilioinguinal nerve. The Scarpa fascia and then the subdermal layer were reapproximated with interrupted 3-0 absorbable sutures. Skin was further closed with a running 4-0 absorbable subcuticular stitch. Paper reinforcing strips were applied across the incision, followed by a sterile dressing. The patient was then transferred to the recovery room awake and in stable condition. Total intravenous fluids were 300 mL of crystalloid, and blood loss was nil. The only specimen was the hernia sac.

LAPAROSCOPIC CHOLECYSTECTOMY

PREOPERATIVE DIAGNOSIS: Symptomatic cholelithiasis

POSTOPERATIVE DIAGNOSIS: Same

OPERATION PERFORMED: Laparoscopic cholecystectomy

SURGEON: Seth Karp, MD

ASSISTANT: James Morris, MD

ANESTHESIA: Local, general endotracheal

INDICATIONS FOR OPERATION: Ms. Gloria Brillantes is a 45-year-old female with a 2-year history of episodic postprandial right upper quadrant abdominal pain radiating to the right flank, with associated nausea and occasional emesis. Ultrasonography reveals multiple gallstones with normal gallbladder wall thickness and normal common bile duct caliber. Liver function tests were normal. After surgical consultation and review of her clinical situation, I discussed with the patient the operative and nonoperative management options, including the risks and potential complications of each approach. After all questions were answered, she requested laparoscopic cholecystectomy. A request-for-surgery form was signed and witnessed preoperatively.

INTRAOPERATIVE FINDINGS: Normal-appearing, thin-walled gallbladder without adhesions containing multiple small 5-mm cholesterol gallstones. Liver, stomach, and small and large intestines were grossly normal.

DESCRIPTION OF PROCEDURE: The patient was positioned supine on the operating room table, and preoperative antibiotics and general endotracheal anesthesia were administered. The abdomen was prepped and draped sterilely. The Veress needle was inserted uneventfully through a tiny subumbilical incision, after skin infiltration with combined lidocaine 1% and bupivacaine 0.25%. The abdomen was insufflated with carbon dioxide to 15 mm Hg pressure. A 5-mm port was then placed subumbilically and the 5-mm 30-degree endoscope inserted. The abdomen was inspected and appeared grossly normal. Under additional local anesthesia, a 10-mm port was placed in the epigastric region, and two more 5-mm ports were placed further laterally on the right. The table was placed in reverse Trendelenburg position, with mild rotation to the patient's left side. The gallbladder fundus was retracted cephalad, and the infundibulum was retracted toward the right lower quadrant. Using careful blunt dissection, normal biliary anatomy was encountered. The cystic duct and the artery were easily identified and divided between surgical clips. The gallbladder was then dissected out of the fossa using electrocautery, removed from the abdomen via the epigastric port, and passed off the table as a specimen. The operative field was then inspected and found to be hemostatic and without bile leak. Intact clips were again seen securing the duct and artery stumps. All trocars were then removed under vision, and no port site bleeding was noted. The 10-mm epigastric fascial defect was closed with a figure-of-eight 0 absorbable suture, and all skin incisions were closed with buried simple 4-0 absorbable sutures. Paper reinforcing strips were applied to the incisions, followed by sterile dressings. The patient was uneventfully extubated and transferred to the recovery room in stable condition. Administered intravenous fluids were 500 mL of crystalloid, and blood loss was negligible. Specimens included the gallbladder and contained stones.

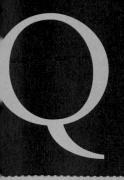

Questions

1. A 71-year-old man with sudden onset of severe abdominal and back pain is brought to the emergency department for evaluation. He has a history of hypertension. He weighs 300 lb. He has a 45-pack-a-year history of smoking. Physical examination reveals a pulsatile abdominal mass. Both lower extremities reveal pallor with diminished pedal pulses. What is the most likely cause of this patient's condition?
   a. Atherosclerosis
   b. Marfan syndrome
   c. Meningococcal infection
   d. Syphilis
   e. Trauma

2. A 78-year-old man is brought to the emergency department with a 12-hour history of abdominal pain, diarrhea, and vomiting. He has a history of atrial fibrillation and was previously treated for congestive heart failure with digoxin. Physical examination reveals a distended abdomen with significant guarding. Rectal examination reveals guaiac positive stool in the vault. White blood cell count is 24,000/mL. Abdominal x-ray reveals edema of the bowel wall. What is the most appropriate treatment for this patient?
   a. Angiographic embolization
   b. Antibiotic therapy with ampicillin and gentamicin
   c. Antibiotic therapy with gentamicin
   d. Heparinization followed by oral warfarin
   e. Surgical exploration

3. A 20-year-old male tennis player crashes into a fence trying to chase a ball he thought he could catch up to during an important match. His right knee sustains the brunt of injury. Physical examination reveals edema and decreased range of motion of the knee in flexion and extension. Magnetic resonance imaging (MRI) is performed and reveals dislocation of the joint. No pulse is palpable behind the knee joint. What is the most likely explanation for this finding?

   a. Anterior tibial artery rupture
   b. Peroneal artery hematoma
   c. Popliteal artery spasm
   d. Posterior tibial artery hematoma
   e. Superficial femoral artery spasm

4. A 25-year-old woman found a lump in her right breast on self-examination. She has no family history of breast cancer. The lump is freely mobile and well circumscribed. What is the best option to evaluate a breast mass in a young female?
   a. Biopsy
   b. Mammography
   c. Testing for breast cancer (*BRCA*) gene
   d. Ultrasound
   e. Watchful waiting

5. A 19-year-old woman began breast-feeding for the first time. At first, it was difficult for her infant to feed. Now, her breasts are red, warm, and sore. She has continued to breast-feed, despite the pain; however, she has recently begun to use a breast pump instead of breast-feeding. She is begun on a course of oral antibiotics. What condition is this patient at risk of developing?
   a. Breast abscess
   b. Fibrocystic disease
   c. Inflammatory breast cancer
   d. Prolactinoma
   e. Tuberculosis

6. A 31-year-old premenopausal woman with a left breast mass undergoes a left modified radical mastectomy. Pathology reveals infiltrating ductal carcinoma measuring 3 cm in size with negative lymph nodes. Estrogen receptor status is negative. What is the most appropriate adjuvant therapy for this patient?
   a. Chemotherapy (multiagent)
   b. External-beam radiotherapy

c. High-energy focused ultrasound therapy
d. Tamoxifen
e. Watchful waiting

7. A 31-year-old woman complains of a 6-month history of bloody diarrhea, abdominal pain, and intermittent fevers. She has a history of irritable bowel syndrome but has had a worsening of her symptoms during the above time period. Her past medical history is unremarkable. Physical examination reveals abdominal distension. Bowel sounds are present in all quadrants. Rectal examination reveals multiple anal fissures. What is the most appropriate diagnostic testing for this patient?
a. Anoscopy
b. Colonoscopy
c. Flexible sigmoidoscopy
d. Rigid sigmoidoscopy
e. No further diagnostic testing is required for this patient.

8. A 71-year-old woman presents to her primary care physician complaining of rectal bleeding. She had some mild left-sided abdominal cramps that subsided within a few minutes. She has never had a prior episode of rectal bleeding. Physical examination reveals mild left lower quadrant abdominal pain without evidence of guarding or rebound tenderness. Rectal examination reveals no fresh blood in the rectal vault. Colonoscopy reveals several outpouchings of the sigmoid colon wall without evidence of bleeding or perforation. The remainder of the colonoscopy is within normal limits. White blood cell count is normal. What is the most appropriate treatment for this patient?
a. Antibiotic therapy with ampicillin and gentamicin
b. Left hemicolectomy
c. Right hemicolectomy
d. Subtotal colectomy
e. Watchful waiting

9. An 85-year-old man is brought to the emergency department because of acute abdominal pain and progressive abdominal distention. He is a resident of a local nursing home. He has not been eating because of progressive nausea. Abdominal radiographs reveal a massively sigmoid colon. What is the initial treatment for this patient?
a. Gastrografin enema
b. High-fiber diet
c. Lactulose
d. Rectal tube decompression
e. Surgical resection

10. A 41-year-old woman complains of constant headaches for the past 6 months. She has also complained of female infertility and has been unable to have children,

despite having unprotected sexual intercourse with her husband during the past 15 years. Physical examination reveals deficits in the extraocular movements bilaterally. Breast examination reveals bilateral female gynecomastia. Which of the following laboratory tests would be most useful in diagnosing this patient?
a. Ferritin
b. Hemoglobin
c. Hematocrit
d. Iron
e. Prolactin

11. A 41-year-old woman with Crohn's disease has undergone multiple surgical procedures. She has recently undergone an ileostomy but still has evidence of some distal jejunal disease. Her current medications include prednisone and aminosalicylic acid. Which of the following effects of prolonged therapy with glucocorticoids are possible for this patient?
a. Antibody production
b. Collagen formation
c. Fibroblast dysfunction
d. Inflammatory cell migration
e. Impaired Wound healing

12. A 49-year-old obese man presents to his primary care physician for a follow-up examination. He has a history of uncontrolled diabetes mellitus and bipolar disorder. His current medications include lithium and milk of magnesium. Physical examination of the heart, lungs, and abdomen are within normal limits. Laboratory studies reveal serum calcium of 14 mg/dL. What is the most likely explanation for these findings?
a. Dietary indiscretion
b. Medication overdose
c. Milk-alkali syndrome
d. Parathyroid adenoma
e. Parathyroid hyperplasia

13. A 41-year-old man has chronic gastroesophageal reflux. He is currently managed with an H_2-blocker. Physical examination of the heart, lungs, and abdomen are within normal limits. Which of the following factors would be least protective of the esophagus in terms of the continued exposure induced by this condition?
a. Arcuate ligament
b. Gastric emptying ability
c. Gravitational effect
d. Salivary gland secretory products
e. Secondary peristaltic waves

14. A 40-year-old woman complains of chest pain and dysphagia to solids. She presents to a specialist for evaluation. Esophageal manometric studies are performed

and reveal high-amplitude contractions and eventual normal relaxation of the lower esophageal sphincter. Barium swallow is normal. What is the most likely diagnosis?

a. Cricopharyngeal muscle spasm
b. Diffuse esophageal spasm
c. Scleroderma
d. Tuberculosis
e. Psychogenic swallowing disorder

15. A 5-year-old boy is brought to the emergency department after ingesting liquid drain cleaner. The boy was left unattended while his baby-sitter was on the telephone. The boy is hoarse and has obvious stridor. What is the most appropriate initial treatment for this patient?

a. Antibiotics
b. Corticosteroids
c. Induction of vomiting with ipecac
d. Placement of nasogastric tube and lavage
e. Tracheostomy

16. A 76-year-old man with a history of vague right upper quadrant pain, a 25-lb weight loss, and anorexia presents to his primary care physician for evaluation. Physical examination reveals scleral icterus. Abdominal examination reveals a right upper quadrant mass. Kidney, ureter, and bladder (KUB) reveals a circular calcification in the right upper quadrant. Exploratory laparotomy reveals a neoplastic process involving the gallbladder and liver. What is the most likely pathology causing this condition?

a. Adenocarcinoma
b. Sarcoma
c. Squamous cell carcinoma
d. Transitional cell carcinoma
e. Tuberculosis granuloma

17. A 38-year-old woman presents to her primary care physician for evaluation of intermittent vague right upper quadrant pain. She has a history of hypothyroidism and hypertension. Her current medications include synthetic thyroid hormone replacement and a calcium channel blocker. Physical examination reveals mild right upper quadrant pain to deep palpation. Ultrasound reveals a 3-cm gallstone. What is the most likely type of stone to be present in this patient?

a. Black gallstone
b. Brown gallstone
c. Calcium oxalate gallstone
d. Type I cholesterol stone
e. Type II cholesterol stone

18. A 46-year-old woman presents to the emergency department complaining of right upper quadrant pain

and a fever to 102°F. Physical examination reveals scleral icterus and significant right upper quadrant pain to palpation. Peritoneal signs are absent. Bowel sounds are present. Which of the following should be included in the initial treatment of this patient?

a. Antibiotics
b. Choledochojejunostomy
c. Decompression with T-tube
d. Endoscopic sphincterotomy
e. Percutaneous transhepatic drainage

19. A 17-year-old boy is brought to the emergency department after suffering from chest pain and dyspnea during a pickup basketball game. Physical examination reveals a systolic crescendo-decrescendo murmur, heard best at the second right intercostal space. The murmur radiates to the right carotid artery. Chest x-ray reveals a normal heart size. Which of the following findings would be expected to be seen on an electrocardiogram in this patient?

a. Inversion of T waves in leads V1–V4
b. Left ventricular hypertrophy
c. Right bundle branch block
d. Right ventricular hypertrophy
e. Right atrial hypertrophy

20. A 72-year-old man collapses while walking in a shopping mall. He is pulseless and apneic. There is no history of trauma. Cardiopulmonary resuscitation is started until a rescue squad arrives. Advanced cardiac life support protocol is initiated. He is pronounced dead 40 minutes later. Autopsy reveals myocardial necrosis with rupture of the left ventricle. Which of the following is the most likely risk factor that contributed to his death?

a. Family history of diabetes mellitus
b. Hypotension
c. Obesity
d. Sedentary lifestyle
e. Trauma

21. A 57-year-old man is brought to the emergency department complaining of dyspnea and chest pain. He also admits to a 20-lb weight loss. He complains of fevers, chills, and night sweats. Physical examination reveals supraclavicular adenopathy. Chest examination reveals distant heart sounds. Laboratory studies reveal a white blood cell count of 170,000/mL. Chest x-ray and echocardiography reveal a pericardial effusion. What is the most likely explanation of these findings?

a. Atrial myxoma
b. Atrial fibrillation
c. Lymphoma
d. Metastatic colorectal carcinoma
e. Pericarditis

22. A newborn male has an opening of the abdominal wall at the umbilicus. He has no other prior medical or surgical history. Birth history was unremarkable. During the remainder of the physical examination and diagnostic testing, which of the following findings are most likely?
 a. Cleft lip
 b. Cleft palate
 c. Diaphragmatic hernia
 d. Pericardium
 e. Urinary bladder in retroperitoneum

23. A 44-year-old male construction worker undergoes a right inguinal hernia repair. The surgical procedure is uneventful. He has no prior medical or surgical history. He returns for follow-up on postoperative day 3 for a wound check. The wound is clean, dry, and intact. What is the optimal convalescent period required before returning to work for this patient?
 a. 1 week
 b. 4 weeks
 c. 6 to 8 weeks
 d. 12 weeks
 e. Unknown

24. A 40-year-old woman undergoes repair of a right femoral hernia. During the procedure, the femoral canal is dissected. The anatomic boundaries of the femoral canal include which of the following?
 a. Cooper ligament
 b. Inguinal ligament
 c. Ischial spine
 d. Lacunar ligament
 e. Nerve (femoral)

25. A 53-year-old man undergoes a radical prostatectomy for presumed organ-confined prostate cancer. The most important factor in maintaining continence after radical prostatectomy is preservation of the:
 a. Bladder neck
 b. External urethral sphincter
 c. Levator ani muscle complex
 d. Nervi erigentes
 e. Puboprostatic ligaments

26. A 27-year-old man has bulky retroperitoneal adenopathy after radical orchiectomy for a mixed germ cell tumor. His chest x-ray is normal. Serum beta-human chorionic gonadotropin (β-hCG) and alpha-fetoprotein (AFP) are markedly elevated. Liver enzymes are slightly elevated, and the patient relates a history of ethanol excess. He receives three cycles of chemotherapy. Restaging reveals a 3-cm retroperitoneal mass, a normal chest x-ray, and normal serum β-hCG. However, the serum AFP is 20 IU/mL (normal = 0 to 9 IU/mL). What is the next step in the management of this patient?
 a. Computed tomography (CT)—guided needle biopsy
 b. External-beam radiotherapy
 c. Retroperitoneal lymph node dissection
 d. Salvage chemotherapy
 e. Serial markers and CT scans

27. A 63-year-old man is disease-free two years after bacillus Calmette-Guerin therapy for carcinoma in situ and a grade 2, stage T1 bladder cancer. In addition to physical examination, cystoscopy, and urinary cytology, evaluation at this time should include:
 a. Intravenous pyelogram
 b. Prostatic urethral biopsy
 c. Random biopsies of the bladder
 d. Selective upper tract cytology
 e. Urinary voided cytology, repeated three times

28. A 78-year-old man presents to the emergency department for evaluation of progressive right upper quadrant pain, nausea, vomiting, and a 30-lb weight loss in the past 3 months. He has a prior medical history of cholelithiasis, diabetes mellitus, hypertension, and dementia. Physical examination reveals scleral icterus bilaterally. Abdominal examination reveals right upper quadrant tenderness and a palpable mass. Peritoneal signs are absent. CT scan reveals pancreatic, duodenal, and choledochal lymph nodes. There is an asymmetric thickening of the gallbladder. What is the most likely pathologic finding at exploratory laparotomy and biopsy?
 a. Adenocarcinoma
 b. Fibroma
 c. Lipoma
 d. Myxoma
 e. Myoma

29. An 8-year-old boy undergoes a right upper quadrant ultrasound for persistent right upper quadrant discomfort. He has no prior medical or surgical history. He has no known allergies and takes no medications. His mother has a history of gallstones. Ultrasound findings include a fusiform dilation of the common bile duct. What is the most likely explanation for these findings?
 a. Type I choledochal cyst
 b. Type II choledochal cyst
 c. Type III choledochal cyst
 d. Type IV choledochal cyst
 e. Type V choledochal cyst

30. An 18-year-old man is stabbed in his abdomen multiple times by an assailant during an altercation involving sale of illicit drugs. He is brought to the emergency department for evaluation. He has four stab wounds of the abdomen—three are in the right upper quadrant, and one is in the left lower quadrant. Physical examination of the abdomen reveals guarding and rebound tenderness. The patient is brought to surgery for an exploratory laparotomy. A penetrating injury to the gallbladder is found. Which of the following associated viscera are likely to be injured?

a. Aorta
b. Colon
c. Kidney
d. Liver
e. Urinary bladder

31. A 62-year-old woman presents to her primary care physician with a cough. She also complains of hemoptysis. Social history reveals a 55-pack-a-year history of smoking. She is a recovering alcoholic. Physical examination reveals bilateral wheezes. Cardiac, pulmonary, and abdominal examinations are unremarkable. Laboratory values reveal serum calcium of 13 mg/dL. Serum protein electrophoresis shows no abnormal spikes. What is the most likely diagnosis?

a. Goodpasture's syndrome
b. Myeloma
c. Renal adenoma
d. Small-cell carcinoma of the lung
e. Squamous cell carcinoma of the lung

32. A 10-year-old boy is brought to his primary care physician for evaluation of persistent hoarseness. He has just begun to participate with his school chorus and notes that his hoarseness worsens with singing. Physical examination of the heart, lungs, and abdomen are unremarkable. Fiber-optic flexible laryngeal examination reveals multiple lesions on his true vocal cords. What is the most likely diagnosis?

a. Gastroesophageal reflux
b. Granulomatous inflammation of the pharynx
c. Laryngeal papilloma
d. Singer's nodule
e. Thyroid carcinoma

33. A 75-year-old man presents to his primary care physician because of hoarseness. He has a 60-pack-a-year history of smoking. He also complains of a 25-lb weight loss over the past 4 months. Direct laryngoscopy reveals a sessile mass on the high right vocal cord. He also has a palpable lymph node along the right anterior cervical lymph node chain. If dysplasia is found on biopsy of the laryngeal lesion, what is the most likely diagnosis?

a. Adenoma
b. Laryngeal polyp
c. Laryngitis

d. Mucoepidermoid cystic disease
e. Squamous cell carcinoma

34. A 21-year-old male college student presents to the outpatient clinic for a routine examination at the beginning of the fall semester. He has a history of irritable bowel syndrome. Physical examination of the heart, lungs, and abdomen are unremarkable. Genitourinary examination reveals that the testes are descended bilaterally. A left grade 1 varicocele is present. There are no testicular masses. The penis is uncircumcised, and the foreskin is unable to be retracted behind the glans. What is the most likely diagnosis?

a. Balanitis
b. Hypospadias
c. Epispadias
d. Paraphimosis
e. Phimosis

35. A 71-year-old white male presents to his primary care physician complaining of a 1-month history of nocturia, polyuria, and difficulty starting and stopping his urinary stream. His American Urological Association Symptom Score is 17/35. Physical examination of the prostate reveals an enlarged gland without masses. His testes are descended bilaterally. He has a small right hydrocele that transilluminates. His prostate-specific antigen (PSA) level is 6 ng/mL, and urinalysis is negative. The patient is begun on dutasteride 0.5 mg daily. What is a likely result of taking this medication?

a. Ejaculatory dysfunction
b. Maximal change in urinary flow rate
c. Prostate size decreases by 25%
d. Serum PSA increases by 50%
e. Symptom score remains unchanged

36. A 34-year-old white male has a painless enlargement of his right testis in the past 4 months. He is brought to his primary care physician by his girlfriend, who urges him to seek evaluation. He has recently become depressed because of this problem. He had a cryptorchid right testis as an infant, which was surgically corrected. A scrotal ultrasound confirms the presence of a 3 cm hypoechoic right testicular mass. What is the most likely diagnosis?

a. Choriocarcinoma
b. Embryonal (mixed germ cell) carcinoma
c. Endodermal (yolk sac) tumor
d. Seminoma
e. Teratoma

37. A 51-year-old man is found to have an intracranial mass and will undergo resection. The surgical procedure is performed via a transoccipital approach. In this

approach, the patient develops a cerebrospinal fluid (CSF) leak. Which of the following statements is true regarding CSF?
a. Arachnoid villi act as two-way valves.
b. Arachnoid villi open at a pressure of 5 mm Hg.
c. CSF is absorbed through the spinal roots.
d. CSF enters through the foramen of Magendie.
e. Total CSF volume is 150 L.

38. A 19-year-old college student is driving under the influence of alcohol, despite recommendations from friends not to drive. She is struck by another driver. The force of impact causes her to strike the temporal area of her skull against the window. She develops a mild headache but does not lose consciousness. Several hours later, she develops a severe headache with nausea and vomiting. Which is the most likely diagnosis?
a. Bacterial infection
b. Berry aneurysm
c. Epidural hematoma
d. Subarachnoid hematoma
e. Subdural hemorrhage

39. A 59-year-old man presents to his primary care physician complaining of progressive right-sided hearing loss and gait unsteadiness. He states that when he uses the phone, he must use his left ear to listen instead of his right ear. He has a past medical history of hypertension. His current medications include a calcium channel blocker. Physical examination reveals loss of the right corneal reflex and facial weakness. Cardiac, pulmonary, and abdominal examinations are within normal limits. What is the most appropriate next best step in the diagnosis of this patient?
a. Audiometric testing
b. Brainstem-evoked potential testing
c. CT scan of the head without contrast
d. MRI of the head
e. Nystagmography

40. A 47-year-old man with a history of end-stage pulmonary disease of his right lung is scheduled for lung transplantation. Preoperative cardiac function is good. He has no history of congenital defects. Which of the following is the most appropriate surgical incision for this patient to have?
a. Chevron abdominal
b. Lateral thoracotomy
c. Midline abdominal
d. Transverse anterior thoracotomy
e. Pfannenstiel

41. A 47-year-old man with multiple medical problems and end-stage pulmonary parenchymal disease undergoes

lung transplantation. He has a prior medical history of obstructive lung disease. He has an uncle with cystic fibrosis. His father has restrictive lung disease, and his brother has pulmonary hypertension. Which of the following portends the best survival after lung transplantation for this patient?
a. Bronchogenic carcinoma
b. Cystic fibrosis
c. Obstructive lung disease
d. Pulmonary hypertension
e. Restrictive lung disease

42. A 4-year-old boy is on the waiting list for a liver transplant. He has end-stage hepatic disease and is currently hospitalized for esophageal variceal hemorrhage. What is the most likely cause of liver failure in this patient?
a. Biliary atresia
b. Hepatitis A
c. Primary biliary cirrhosis
d. Primary sclerosing cholangitis
e. Tuberculosis

43. A 23-year-old woman who complains of greasy and odorous stools, generalized weakness, and hair loss presents to her primary care physician for evaluation. Physical examination of the heart, lungs, and abdomen are unremarkable. She has no guarding or rebound tenderness. Bowel sounds are present in all quadrants. Female pelvic examination was deferred at the patient's request. What is the most likely explanation of these findings?
a. Gastric ulcer with bleeding
b. Glucose malabsorption
c. Menstruation
d. Pancreatic insufficiency
e. Pituitary tumor

44. A 27-year-old woman is 12 hours status after cadaveric pancreas transplantation and currently in the surgical intensive care unit. She has a medical history of insulin-dependent diabetes since age 5. Her vital signs are normal. Chest is clear to auscultation, and cardiac examination reveals a regular rate with a regular rhythm. Wound dressing is clean, dry, and intact. Which of the following is the best method of monitoring the transplanted pancreas?
a. Serum amylase level
b. Serum glucose level
c. Serum insulin level
d. Ultrasonography of the pancreatic vessels
e. Urinary amylase level

45. A 44-year-old man with recurrent pancreatitis is brought to the emergency department with another bout of pancreatitis. Which of the following is the most reassuring factors regarding the severity of his condition?

a. Age
b. Blood glucose level of 300 mg/dL
c. Lactate dehydrogenase level of 400 IU/L
d. Serum calcium of 6 mg/dL
e. Serum hematocrit level of 29%

46. A 41-year-old man with a long history of renal stones and hypercalcemia is found to have an adenoma of the right superior parathyroid gland. He is going to undergo surgical excision of this lesion. What is the best surgical landmark for this lesion?
a. Bifurcation of the carotid arteries
b. Carotid sinus
c. Junction of the inferior thyroid artery and recurrent laryngeal nerve
d. Junction of the upper and middle third of the thyroid gland
e. Recurrent laryngeal nerve

47. Which of the following techniques is best used to define an enlarged parathyroid gland?
a. CT scan of the neck
b. Dual tracer imaging
c. MRI of the neck
d. Thyrocervical angiography
e. Ultrasonography

48. A 44-year-old man with end-stage renal disease successfully undergoes renal transplantation. He has a prior medical history of hyperparathyroidism. Six months after renal transplantation, his serum calcium is still 13 mg/dL. Which of the following laboratory findings are possible in this patient?
a. Elevated serum phosphate
b. Elevated serum lactic acid dehydrogenase
c. Elevated urine calcium
d. Elevated urine creatinine
e. Elevated urine protein

49. A 46-year-old man presents to his primary care physician for evaluation of a skin lesion. He complains of hypopigmentation of the skin of his lower back. He has a prior medical history of eczema and basal cell carcinoma. He is a farmer who spends a great deal of time outdoors. What cells are responsible for this condition?
a. Adipocytes
b. Keratin-producing cells
c. Langerhans cells
d. Melanocytes
e. Merkel cells

50. A 69-year-old male presents to his dermatologist with a lesion present on his nose. He is a gardener who spends a great deal of his time outdoors. He has a prior medical

history of allergic rhinitis, hypertension, and diabetes mellitus. His current medications include a beta-blocker and an oral hypoglycemic. Physical examination of his nose reveals a raised, shiny, papular lesion with small blood vessels. What is the most likely diagnosis?
a. Basal cell carcinoma
b. Histiocytosis X
c. Melanoma
d. Seborrheic keratosis
e. Squamous cell carcinoma

51. A 29-year-old Black woman presents to her primary care physician because of a growth on her left ear, which occurred after she had her ear pierced for the first time a week ago. She noticed that her ear seemed to develop a growth on it quite rapidly. She had never had her ear pierced before. What is the most likely explanation for these findings?
a. Basal cell carcinoma
b. Blue nevus
c. Juvenile melanoma
d. Keloid
e. Molluscum contagiosum

52. A 52-year-old Asian American female has melanotic pigmentation of the buccal mucosa, lips, and digits. Colonoscopy reveals hamartomas throughout the gastrointestinal tract. The polyps were removed because of her increased risk of cancer. What other cancer is associated with this condition?
a. Cervical cancer
b. Kidney cancer
c. Liver cancer
d. Ovarian cancer
e. Pancreatic cancer

53. A 45-year-old female complains of chronic diarrhea and sweating. Colonoscopy is performed, and a biopsy of a lesion in her ileum is performed. The pathology report shows that the tumor is composed of neuroendocrine cells. What is a medical treatment for this condition?
a. Corticosteroids, intravenous
b Corticosteroids, topical
c. Furosemide
d. Octreotide
e. Tetracycline

54. An 18-year-old male is brought to the emergency department with sudden excruciating abdominal pain localized to the right lower quadrant, nausea and vomiting, mild fever, and slight tachycardia. He has a prior medical history of recurrent otitis media. Physical examination reveals marked right lower rebound tenderness and guarding. Serum white blood cell count is 18,000/mL.

KUB x-ray reveals bowel gas in the small and large bowel. What is the most likely diagnosis?

a. Appendicitis
b. Crohn's disease
c. Diverticulitis
d. Pancreatitis
e. Ulcerative colitis

55. A 39-year-old woman presents to the emergency department complaining of severe abdominal pain. She has a history of peptic ulcer disease. Physical examination reveals guarding and rebound tenderness. She is taken to the operating room for exploratory laparotomy. During the procedure, the surgeon who opens the gastrosplenic ligament to reach the lesser sac accidentally cuts an artery. Which of the following vessels is the most likely one injured?

a. Gastroduodenal artery
b. Left gastric artery
c. Left gastroepiploic artery
d. Right gastric artery
e. Splenic artery

56. A 2-year-old female is brought to the emergency department because of several episodes of rectal bleeding. A technetium-99m perfusion scan reveals a 3-cm ileal outpouching located 50 cm from the ileocecal valve. Which of the following types of ectopic tissue does this structure most likely contain?

a. Duodenal
b. Esophageal
c. Gastric
d. Hepatic
e. Jejunal

57. A 39-year-old woman complains of epigastric pain with eating over the past 3 or 4 months. She admits to a history of chronic back problems. She notes weight gain of 20 lb in the past 4 months. She denies the use of non-steroidal anti-inflammatory agents. She denies nausea and vomiting. Physical examination of the heart, lungs, and abdomen are within normal limits. What is the most likely pathogen associated with this condition?

a. Enterohemorrhagic *Escherichia coli*
b. *Escherichia coli*
c. *Helicobacter pylori*
d. *Shigella sonnei*
e. *Streptococcus pyogenes*

58. A 59-year-old man was injured in a car accident. An abdominal CT scan reveals a ruptured spleen. His blood pressure is 90/40 mm Hg, and his pulse is 140 beats per minute. The patient is taken for laparotomy. Splenectomy is performed. Which of the following laboratory abnormalities is likely after this procedure?

a. Anemia
b. Basophilia
c. Eosinophilia
d. Thrombocytopenia
e. Thrombocytosis

59. A 19-year-old man was kicked in the abdomen during a fight in a bar. He went to his primary care physician, who ordered a CT scan, which revealed a subcapsular splenic hematoma. The man was told to restrict physical activity. Two weeks later, he presents to the emergency department because of severe abdominal pain. He undergoes a splenectomy. Postoperatively, a peripheral smear is ordered. Which type of cell can be found in this patient?

a. Basophilic stippling
b. Blister cells
c. Howell-Jolly bodies
d. Nucleated red blood cells
e. Spherocytes

60. A 15-year-old African American male underwent a splenectomy after sustaining a knife injury during a fight. He presents to his primary care physician for a sports physical. His mother read on the Web that he is at increased risk for infection. He should receive which of the following vaccines to prevent serious infections?

a. Rubella
b. Measles
c. Tetanus
d. Vaccines against common encapsulated organisms
e. Varicella

61. A 53-year-old woman presents to her primary care physician with a 12-month history of neck pain. She complains of a 15-lb weight gain and generalized malaise. She has a past medical history of hypertension and diabetes mellitus. Her current medications include an oral hypoglycemic. Physical examination reveals tenderness along the course of the thyroid gland without evidence of a discrete mass. What is the most likely diagnosis?

a. Acute thyroiditis
b. Hashimoto thyroiditis
c. Papillary thyroid carcinoma
d. Riedel thyroiditis
e. Subacute thyroiditis

62. A 47-year-old woman with a history of a left thyroid mass undergoes left thyroid lobectomy. Pathology reveals a 1.3-cm papillary carcinoma with no evidence of extracapsular extension. What is the most appropriate next step in the treatment of this patient?

a. External-beam radiotherapy
b. Multiagent chemotherapy

c. Subtotal thyroidectomy
d. Total thyroidectomy
e. Watchful waiting with periodic follow-up

63. A 34-year-old man with a thyroid nodule is undergoing a neck exploration. During the procedure, it is possible that he will undergo thyroidectomy. Which of the following statements about the superior laryngeal nerve and the innervation of the thyroid gland is correct?
    a. Injury to the nerve causes bowing of the vocal cords during phonation.
    b. Nerve injury may be unnoticeable in singers.
    c. The nerve is rarely at risk during thyroid surgical procedures.
    d. The superior laryngeal nerve is chiefly a motor nerve.
    e. The superior laryngeal nerve is chiefly a sensory nerve.

64. A 19-year-old man leaps from the third floor of his dormitory in an apparent suicide attempt. He is brought to the emergency department unconscious. He has visible head and lower extremity injuries. He has a pulse of 110 beats per minute but is apneic. What is the best airway management for this patient?
    a. Nasotracheal intubation
    b. Oral intubation
    c. Oral intubation with head-chin lift
    d. Tracheostomy
    e. Intubation is not necessary for this patient.

65. A 21-year-old woman is stabbed in the chest by her boyfriend. She is brought to the emergency department for evaluation. Her blood pressure is 130/80 mmHg, and her pulse is 90 beats per minute. Physical examination reveals a single stab wound to the left fifth intercostal space in the midclavicular line. Neck examination is normal. Trachea is midline, and the jugular veins are not distended. She does have decreased breath sounds in the left lung fields. Which of the following diagnoses can be ruled out on the basis of the above information?
    a. Large left hemothorax
    b. Open pneumothorax
    c. Pericardial tamponade
    d. Rupture of the left main stem bronchus
    e. Tension pneumothorax

66. A 41-year-old man suffers a traumatic amputation of three of his fingers in a meat slicer. He has no prior medical or surgical history. Which of the following modalities should be used to transport the amputated fingers with the patient?
    a. Place in clean plastic bag and pack with dry ice.
    b. Place in clean plastic bag filled with room temperature water.
    c. Place in clean plastic bag in a chest filled with crushed ice and water.

d. Place in clean plastic bag filled with hot water.
e. Wrap the amputated fingers in sterile dry gauze.

67. A 19-year-old woman presents to the emergency department after sustaining an injury to her right eye while placing her contact lens. She has significant right eye pain. She has a prior medical history of seasonal allergies. Physical examination reveals a simple abrasion. Fluorescein testing is performed and reveals no evidence of a stained epithelial defect. This rules out the possibility of which of the following?
    a. Bacterial infection
    b. Iritis
    c. Trauma
    d. Viral infection
    e. Ulcer

68. A 29-year-old man who works in a factory sustained a foreign body injury to his right eye when a piece of metal shot off a conveyer belt. He is brought to the emergency department for evaluation. Physical examination of the right eye reveals a metallic foreign body on the eye with an epithelial rust ring. What is the most useful instrument to remove this foreign body?
    a. Cyanoacrylate glue
    b. Eye burr
    c. Eye spud
    d. Fine needle tip
    e. Sterile water and alcohol

69. A 37-year-old chemistry teacher sustains a chemical splash of acid to his right eye while attempting to perform a demonstration to his high school science class. He is in significant pain. While in the classroom and waiting for an ambulance to transport him to the hospital, which of the following interventions should be performed?
    a. Eyedrop instillation with normal saline
    b. Eye patch placement
    c. Flush eye with 1 to 2 L of normal saline
    d. Placement of eye under direct sunlight
    e. Watchful waiting until ambulance arrives

70. A 37-year-old construction worker sustained a crush injury to his right thigh after a crane fell on his leg at the work site. He is brought to the emergency department for evaluation. He has significant right leg pain and pain with passive stretch. The leg is tense to palpation. What is the most likely intracompartmental pressure measurement of this patient's right leg?
    a. 5 mm Hg
    b. 10 mm Hg
    c. 15 mm Hg
    d. 25 mm Hg
    e. 35 mm Hg

71. A 41-year-old woman who cleans houses for a living presents to her primary care physician complaining of tenderness in her right knee. The pain is constant and has been present for 3 weeks. She is in a monogamous relationship. Physical examination reveals that her knee is slightly swollen and tender. Cardiac, pulmonary, and abdominal examinations are within normal limits. A synovial aspiration is performed. The evaluation reveals no evidence of crystals or bacteria. What is the most likely diagnosis?
   a. Bursitis
   b. Infectious arthritis
   c. Rheumatoid arthritis
   d. Septic thrombophlebitis
   e. Trauma-induced infectious arthritis

72. A 12-year-old boy who is the star pitcher of his little league team complains of right shoulder pain. This is his pitching arm. He has no prior medical or surgical history. Physical examination reveals weakness of the rotator cuff tendon. What is the most appropriate treatment for this patient?
   a. Injection of corticosteroids
   b. Intravenous corticosteroids
   c. Rest, elevation, and anti-inflammatory agents
   d. Sling placement
   e. Surgical repair

73. A 65-year-old man with a history of coronary artery disease is undergoing an aortobifemoral bypass. Which of the following intraoperative management maneuvers will decrease his risk of intraoperative myocardial infarction?
   a. Beta blockade
   b. Calcium channel blockade
   c. Administration of normal saline instead of Lactated Ringer's solution
   d. Use of propofol
   e. Use of morphine

74. A 35-year-old healthy man is diagnosed with an inguinal hernia. He has no history of abnormal bleeding. Which of the following tests is absolutely required prior to taking him to the operating room?
   a. Hematocrit
   b. Platelet count
   c. Potassium
   d. White blood cell count
   e. None of the above

75. A 50-year-old man has diarrhea after an uncomplicated bowel resection. The fluid choice that most closely resembles his output is
   a. Normal saline
   b. Half normal saline with 20 mEq of potassium
   c. D5W with 3 amp bicarbonate

   d. Lactated Ringer's solution
   e. D5NS

76. A 27-year-old man is brought to the emergency department after slashing his hand with a knife while attempting to slice a bagel. He has a prior medical history of recurrent sinus infections. His prior surgical history is notable for repair of a nasal fracture. Physical examination reveals a 4-cm clean laceration along the palmar aspect of his hand. The principles most relevant for this case would be:
   a. Gentle handling of tissue and closure without tension
   b. Skin grafting when necessary to cover area
   c. Debridement of devitalized tissue
   d. Use of vacuum sponge to promote healing
   e. Flap reconstruction with vascularized tissue

77. A 68-year-old man is brought to the emergency department complaining of abdominal and leg pain for 2 weeks. He has a history of hypertension and hypercholesterolemia; he weighs 290 lb. Physical examination reveals a pulsatile midline abdominal mass. The lower extremities have unequal pulses. Which of the following is the best next step in the evaluation of this patient?
   a. Aortogram
   b. CT scan of the abdomen and pelvis
   c. Ultrasound, kidneys and bladder
   d. Ultrasound, liver and spleen
   e. Venacavogram

78. A 28-year-old woman presents to her physician for evaluation of a lump in her right breast found on self-examination. She has a family history of breast cancer in that her mother died in her early 40s from this condition. The mother had a modified radical mastectomy followed by chemotherapy. Physical examination reveals a breast lump that is freely mobile and well circumscribed. There is no dimpling, asymmetry, or retractions. The lesion measures 2 cm. What is the next step in the management of this patient?
   a. Biopsy of the lesion with sonographic guidance
   b. Mammography followed by stereotactic CT scan
   c. Testing for *BRCA* gene
   d. Ultrasound of the breast and consideration for breast biopsy
   e. Watchful waiting and follow-up examination by primary care physician in 1 year

79. A 28-year-old man with a history of recurrent abdominal pain and bloody diarrhea presents to his physician complaining of significant rectal pain with bowel movements. He has lost 15 pounds in the last 3 months. Physical examination reveals right and left lower quadrant pain to palpation. Laboratory values reveal a hematocrit of 28% and an elevated erythrocyte sedimentation rate. Colonoscopy performed in this patient would likely reveal:

a. Colonic mass lesion
b. Diverticulosis
c. Internal hemorrhoids
d. Normal bowel
e. Thickened friable colonic and rectal mucosa

80. A 55-year-old male presents to his physician complaining of polyuria, polydipsia, polyphagia, and a red, scaly rash on his face within the past 2 weeks. He voids 18 times/day with a good force of stream. Fasting blood glucose was 325 mg/dL. He has lost 20 pounds in the past 2 months and has never had elevated blood glucose levels in the past. Physical examination of the heart, lungs, and abdomen are normal. What is the most likely explanation for these findings?

a. Diabetes mellitus type I
b. Diabetes mellitus type II
c. Glucagonoma
d. Insulinoma
e. Verner-Morrison Disease

81. A 72-year-old man with an 80 pack-year history of smoking presents to his physician complaining of weakness and malaise. He has recently developed dysphagia to solid foods. He has lost 15 pounds in the last 3 months. Physical examination reveals right supraclavicular lymphadenopathy. Cardiac and pulmonary examinations are unremarkable. He has no guarding or rebound tenderness. Which of the following studies will provide the most definitive diagnosis?

a. Barium esophagogram
b. CT scan of the abdomen and pelvis
c. Esophagogastroscopy with biopsy
d. MRI of the abdomen
e. Ultrasound of the right upper quadrant

82. A 42-year-old African American female undergoes a laparoscopic cholecystectomy for chronic right upper quadrant pain. CT scan demonstrated gallstones and pericholecystic fluid. The surgical procedure was uncomplicated. Pathologic analysis of the gallstones revealed calcium bilirubinate stones. What is the most likely explanation of these findings?

a. High serum cholesterol levels
b. High serum lipid levels
c. High-fat diet
d. Sickle cell anemia
e. Tumor

83. A 36-year-old female complains of jaundice and peripheral swelling. An echocardiogram is ordered and the patient is determined to have right-sided heart failure with hepatic congestion and peripheral edema. No murmur is detected. What is the most appropriate explanation for these findings?

a. Aortic stenosis
b. Atrial septal defect
c. Patent ductus arteriosus
d. Tetralogy of Fallot
e. Ventricular septal defect

84. A newborn male born at term to a 27-year-old intravenous drug-abusing female is found to have a small umbilical hernia. His vital signs are stable. His cardiac and pulmonary examinations are noncontributory. Which of the following is the most likely explanation for this finding?

a. Patent foramen ovale
b. Patent omphalomesenteric duct
c. Patent umbilical ring
d. Patent urachus
e. Patent vitelline duct

85. A 28-year-old man presents to the emergency department complaining of left flank pain, nausea, and vomiting. Physical examination of the heart and lungs are normal. There is left costovertebral (CVA) tenderness. Urinalysis reveals microhematuria (5 red blood cells/high-power field). CT scan reveals a left-sided 4-mm renal stone, whereas KUB reveals a normal bowel gas pattern and no evidence of calcifications. What is the most likely explanation of these findings?

a. Calcium oxalate stone
b. Calcium phosphate monohydrate stone
c. Calcium phosphate dehydrate stone
d. Small struvite stone
e. Uric acid stone

86. A 47-year-old woman with gallstone pancreatitis is hospitalized. She has a history of hypertension and hypercholesterolemia. Early cholecystectomy is indicated to prevent which of the following complications?

a. Cholangitis
b. Recurrent pancreatitis
c. Gastric ulcer
d. Gallstone ileus
e. Gallbladder perforation

87. A 56-year-old man complains of recurrent cough and hemoptysis. He has a history of recurrent pneumonias. He is a nonsmoker and has no occupational risk for pulmonary disease. Physical examination reveals decreased breath sounds in the right upper lobe. Chest x-ray reveals a small right upper quadrant mass. Bronchoscopy reveals an angioma. What is the most appropriate treatment for this patient?

a. Antibiotics
b. Corticosteroids
c. Left lobectomy
d. Right upper lobe lobectomy
e. Watchful waiting

88. A 55-year-old male presents to his primary care physician after noticing some blood-tinged urine 1 week ago. He denies any current pain and denies any fevers. His past medical history includes chronic obstructive pulmonary disease from many years of smoking cigarettes. CT scan reveals bilateral renal simple cysts, prostate enlargement, and an asymmetric thickening of the left side of the bladder. Left hydronephrosis is also present. His urinalysis is positive for microscopic hematuria. What is the most likely diagnosis?
a. Nephrolithiasis
b. Prostate cancer
c. Renal cell carcinoma
d. Transitional cell carcinoma of the bladder
e. Urinary tract infection

89. A 30-year-old man undergoes a CT scan of his abdomen after a motor vehicle accident. He was an unrestrained driver and was thrown from the vehicle. No acute abdominal injuries are found. The CT scan reveals bilateral enlarged kidneys with multiple cysts present in varying sizes. The right kidney is 15 cm and the left kidney is 16 cm in length. Physical examination of the heart, lungs, and abdomen are within normal limits, other than some mild tenderness to palpation in the right and left upper quadrants. Which of the following central nervous system pathologies are most strongly associated with this finding?
a. Circle of Willis aneurysm
b. Cysticercosis
c. Infarction
d. Glioma
e. Subdural hematoma

90. A 46-year-old female with polycystic kidney disease is receiving a kidney transplant. Within minutes of the anastomoses of the renal artery and vein to the respective external iliac artery and vein, the kidney rapidly regains a pink coloration and normal tissue turgor and begins excreting urine. The patient is discharged from the hospital and is seen at 1 month follow up. Serum creatinine is 4.2 mg/dL. Urine output is 20 mL/hour. Physical examination of the heart, lungs, and abdomen are within normal limits. The transplanted kidney is palpable in the right iliac fossa. Subsequent biopsy of the transplant shows extensive inflammation and edema. What is the most likely explanation for these findings?

a. Acute transplant rejection
b. Chronic transplant rejection
c. Graft-versus-host disease
d. Hyperacute transplant rejection
e. Normal posttransplant process

91. A 52-year-old man complains of chronic abdominal pain. He has been hospitalized seven times in the last 2 years for recurrent attacks of pain from chronic pancreatitis. He has been treated with analgesics and a partial distal pancreatectomy. His pain has still persisted. What is the next step in the treatment of this patient?
a. Continued use of oral analgesics
b. Corticosteroids
c. Splanchnicectomy
d. Total pancreatectomy
e. Watchful waiting

92. A 39-year-old man is evaluated by his physician for recurrent kidney stones. He has been treated in the past with extracorporeal shock wave lithotripsy, ureteroscopy, and a percutaneous nephrolithotripsy. Which of the following characteristics would suggest the diagnosis of primary hyperparathyroidism?
a. 1-mm stone on KUB x-ray
b. 2-mm stone on KUB x-ray
c. 1-mm and 2-mm right-sided stone on KUB x-ray
d. 1-mm, 2-mm, and 3-mm right- and left-sided stones on KUB x-ray
e. 4-mm right lower pole stone on CT scan

93. A physician wishes to deliver a local anesthetic subcutaneously to a patient with a suspicious lesion on his forehead. The lesion measures 1 cm and the surgeon plans an elliptical incision to remove it. Which of the following epidermal skin layers will the physician penetrate first with the local anesthetic needle?
a. Stratum basale
b. Stratum corneum
c. Stratum granulosum
d. Stratum lucidum
e. Stratum spinosum

94. A 35-year-old man with a history of Crohn's disease presents to his physician for a follow-up examination. He has diffuse ileocolonic disease on a recent CT scan. His current medications include sulfasalazine. Physical examination reveals right lower quadrant pain to deep palpation. Should antibiotic therapy be considered in this patient, which of the following organisms should be targeted?
a. *Mycobacterium species*
b. *Pseudomonas aeruginosa*
c. *Staphylococcus aureus*
d. *Streptococcus pneumoniae*
e. *Streptococcus pyogenes*

95. A 46-year-old woman presents to her physician with a history of progressive dysphagia. She has a history of a 15-lb weight loss in the last 6 months. Physical examination of the neck, heart, lungs, and abdomen are noncontributory. Laboratory testing reveals a hematocrit of 33% and a mean corpuscular volume of 70. Upper gastrointestinal endoscopy reveals an esophageal web. What is the most likely diagnosis?
   a. Carcinoid tumor
   b. Leukemia
   c. Lymphoma
   d. Plummer-Vinson syndrome
   e. Rheumatoid arthritis

96. A 47-year-old man is involved in a motor vehicle accident. He suffers fractures of ribs 9, 10, and 11 on the left side. He is hemodynamically unstable and has a blood pressure of 90/50 mm Hg and pulse of 120 beats/minute despite transfusion of 3 U of packed red blood cells. He is taken to the operating room for exploratory laparotomy. A ruptured spleen is identified and removed. In searching for a potential accessory spleen, which is the most likely location to encounter it?
   a. Greater omentum
   b. Right lower quadrant
   c. Right upper quadrant
   d. Splenic hilum
   e. Splenic ligaments

97. A 12-year-old boy is brought to his physician for evaluation of a neck mass. He has a history of recurrent sinusitis and tonsillar infections. Physical examination reveals a midline neck mass measuring 1.5 cm that moves with swallowing. There is no evidence of lymphadenopathy. What is the most likely diagnosis?
   a. Leukemia
   b. Lymphoma
   c. Thyroglossal duct cyst
   d. Thyroglossal fistula
   e. Thyroid carcinoma

98. During your Emergency Medicine rotation you are called to the emergency department to evaluate a patient with an ophthalmic injury. Which of the following ophthalmic trauma injuries requires immediate on-site management and referral to the ophthalmologist on call?
   a. Acid burn
   b. Corneal clouding
   c. Corneal laceration
   d. Hyphema
   e. Severe conjunctival chemosis

99. A patient presents to the emergency department after being slashed with a knife in the left leg. The wound appears clean and the edges are well opposed. Which of the following is the simplest method of wound closure for this injury?
   a. Delayed primary closure
   b. Graft
   c. Local flaps
   d. Primary closure
   e. Secondary intention

100. A 23-year-old female presents to her physician complaining of tenderness and pain in the right knee. The pain is constant throughout the day and has been present for approximately 3 weeks. Social history reveals that she is in a monogamous relationship. Physical examination reveals that her knee is slightly swollen and tender. A synovial aspiration is performed. Neither crystals nor bacteria are found. What is the most likely diagnosis?
   a. Bursitis
   b. Gonococcal arthritis
   c. Rheumatoid arthritis
   d. Septic bursitis
   e. Trauma

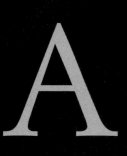

Answers

1. a (Chapter 2)

This patient likely has an abdominal aortic aneurysm. Ninety-five percent of aneurysms of the abdominal aorta are associated with atherosclerosis. This condition is responsible for approximately 15,000 deaths per year. Men are affected nearly 10 times more than women. Marfan syndrome can be associated with increased protease activity on histologic evaluation of the aneurysm wall. Syphilitic aneurysms occur in late-stage syphilis. Meningococcal infection is rarely associated with aneurysm formation. Trauma is a rare cause of abdominal aortic aneurysm.

2. e (Chapter 2)

This patient likely has acute mesenteric ischemia. Patients complain of sudden onset of abdominal pain with severe nausea, diarrhea, and/or vomiting. Pain is out of proportion to physical findings. Treatment involves surgical resection of infracted bowel as soon as possible. Aggressive surgical intervention should not be delayed because of the high index of suspicion of infracted bowel. Angiographic embolization may be diagnostic and therapeutic but is not considered a first-line therapy. Antibiotic therapy is considered an adjunctive therapy. Heparinization is not a first-line therapy for this condition.

3. c (Chapter 2)

A major portion of circulation for the lower extremity begins with the superficial femoral artery, which forms the popliteal artery passing behind the knee joint. This vessel then branches into the anterior tibial, posterior tibial, and peroneal arteries. There is no evidence to suggest rupture, hematoma, or spasm in these vessels. With knee injuries, the popliteal artery may go into spasm because of its location just posterior to the joint. It is important for practitioners to always palpate for a pulse in this artery in all patients with knee injuries. This vessel is also important, as it determines vascular supply to the distal leg.

4. d (Chapter 3)

Younger women have more fibrous tissue, which makes mammograms harder to interpret. Thus ultrasound is a useful testing modality. As women age, breast tissue transforms from fibrous tissue to adipose tissue. This change makes it easier for mammography to detect masses. Thus this modality is more useful in patients over the age of 35 years. Watchful waiting may be considered if the lesion is benign. Testing for the *BRCA* gene may be considered if the patient is suspect to a family history of breast cancer.

5. a (Chapter 3)

Women with mastitis need close follow-up for inflammatory breast disease. If a breast abscess developed, she would need antibiotics. If her breast abscesses were recurrent, the physician should consider resection of the involved ducts. If a patient with fibrocystic disease has straw-colored fluid on aspiration, she would need to be observed closely. If the patient had spontaneous galactorrhea, the physician would need to rule out a prolactinoma.

6. a (Chapter 3)

This patient should be treated with multiagent chemotherapy. This is the treatment of choice for a premenopausal patient with stage I or II breast cancer (size <1 cm), negative lymph nodes, and estrogen receptor—negative status. Watchful waiting may be appropriate for patients with small tumors and negative lymph nodes. External-beam radiotherapy is not indicated for this patient. High-energy focused ultrasound therapy is not indicated for the treatment of breast cancer. Tamoxifen is considered in patients who are estrogen receptor positive and have tumor size >1 cm.

7. b (Chapter 4)

This patient likely has ulcerative colitis. Colonoscopy may reveal thickened, friable mucosa. Fissures and pseudopolyps may also be present. This disease almost always involves the rectum and extends backward toward the cecum to varying degrees. Anoscopy is a limited procedure and will not allow visualization of the entire colon. Flexible or rigid sigmoidoscopy will allow visualization of the rectum and sigmoid colon but will miss higher levels of the colon. This patient requires further testing to establish a definitive diagnosis.

8. e (Chapter 4)

This patient has diverticulosis as a result of the presence of outpouchings in the wall of the colon that occur where the arterial supply penetrates the bowel wall. Patients who stop bleeding and are asymptomatic require no further treatment. Elective colectomy is not recommended at the first episode; thus right hemicolectomy, left hemicolectomy, or subtotal colectomy are not required. Intravenous antibiotic therapy is not required in this patient, because there is no evidence of infection.

9. d (Chapter 4)

This patient has sigmoid volvulus. This condition can be reduced with a rectal tube, which is the treatment of choice. In addition, one can consider decompression with enema. Cecal calculus is treated with surgical intervention. High-fiber diet has no role in the treatment of volvulus. Lactulose is unlikely to be of benefit in the management of this patient.

10. e (Chapter 5)

This patient likely has a prolactinoma, the most common type of pituitary neoplasm. Women may present with headaches, irregular menses, amenorrhea, or galactorrhea. A serum prolactin level of >300 μg/L suggests the diagnosis of pituitary adenoma. This can be confirmed with MRI. Ferritin levels would likely be normal in this patient. Hemoglobin and hematocrit levels should be normal in this patient. Iron levels should be normal in this patient.

11. c (Chapter 5)

This patient would be expected to have fibroblast dysfunction. Patients with inflammatory bowel disease may require treatment with exogenous corticosteroids. These agents suppress the immune system and impair inflammatory cell migration. Antibody production is impaired. This is appropriate in Crohn's disease. Other effects of corticosteroids include fibroblast dysfunction and impaired wound healing.

12. e (Chapter 5)

Renal failure is the most common cause of secondary hyperparathyroidism. This patient, who has had severe uncontrolled diabetes and lab values consistent in patients with diabetes, is most likely to have renal failure as the cause of his hypercalcemia. Whenever the kidney loses its ability to reabsorb calcium and hydroxylate vitamin D for calcium absorption from the gut, hypocalcemia triggers the parathyroid glands to increase their production of parathyroid hormone. Milk-alkali syndrome can cause hypercalcemia in patients who eat many antacids or drink an excessive amount of milk. This condition is more commonly found in patients who have gastric ulcers and frequently depend on milk and antacids for relief. Lithium can cause hypercalcemia by causing hyperparathyroidism. Parathyroid adenomas can cause hypercalcemia by increasing parathyroid hormone secretion.

13. a (Chapter 6)

The arcuate ligament does not inhibit gastroesophageal (GE) reflux and will not protect the esophageal mucosa from erosion. The esophagus limits its exposure to acid by several mechanisms, including salivation, gravity, gastric emptying, and the activity of peptic acid. Also important is the maintenance of a critical esophagogastric angle and appropriate diaphragmatic location of the GE junction.

14. b (Chapter 6)

This patient has diffuse esophageal spasm. Patients present with chest pain and dysphagia. Manometric studies reveal high-amplitude contractions and normal relaxation of the lower esophageal sphincter. Cricopharyngeal spasm occurs because of muscular dysfunction. Scleroderma is a collagen vascular disease that can affect the esophagus and cause motility dysfunction. Tuberculosis can be associated with esophageal diverticula of the traction type. This patient has no evidence to suggest a psychogenic swallowing disorder.

15. e (Chapter 6)

This child ingested a caustic alkaline substance. The child has difficulty breathing and has stridor. Airway edema is likely. Thus tracheostomy should be performed first. Antibiotics and corticosteroids are secondary to the important primary survey of airway, circulation, and breathing in this patient. Vomiting should not be induced for a patient with a caustic ingestion. Likewise, placement of a nasogastric tube should be deferred.

16. a (Chapter 7)

This patient likely has cancer of the gallbladder. Eighty percent of cases are due to adenocarcinoma. Approximately 10% are anaplastic carcinoma, whereas 5% are squamous cell carcinoma. A right upper quadrant mass may be palpable. Signs of jaundice are also possible. This lesion is unlikely to be a sarcoma. Transitional cell carcinoma occurs in the urinary tract. Tuberculosis granuloma is found in the lung.

17. e (Chapter 7)

This patient has a type II cholesterol stone. This is produced as a result of homogeneous nucleation and can produce large gallstones. This type of gallstone represents 5% to 20% of all

ANSWERS

gallstones. Type I cholesterol stones are small in size and often multiple. Calcium oxalate stones are often found in the kidney. Black and brown gallstones are smaller in size and multiple in number.

18. a (Chapter 7)

This patient has the Charcot triad of fever, jaundice, and upper quadrant pain. This triad is seen with acute cholangitis. Initial treatment consists of fluid resuscitation and antibiotics. Patients who do not respond to this therapy need to be decompressed with percutaneous transhepatic drainage. T-tube decompression can also be considered if there is failure to respond to antibiotics. Choledochojejunostomy is considered when the bile duct is dilated.

19. b (Chapter 8)

This patient has evidence of aortic stenosis. Progressive degeneration and calcification of the valve leaflets occur. Patients can complain of angina, syncope, and dyspnea. A crescendo-decrescendo murmur can be heard best in the second right intercostal space. Electrocardiogram reveals left ventricular hypertrophy. Bundle branch block is uncommon, as is T-wave inversion.

20. c (Chapter 8)

This patient has evidence of coronary artery disease that ultimately led to death. This is confirmed with the autopsy findings of myocardial necrosis and rupture of the left ventricle. Risk factors for coronary artery disease include hypertension, smoking, hypercholesterolemia, family history of heart disease, personal history of diabetes mellitus, and obesity. Atherosclerosis is the predominant pathogenic mechanism underlying obstructive disease of the coronary arteries.

21. c (Chapter 8)

This patient likely has a metastatic tumor to the heart. In this case, lymphoma is likely because of the following symptoms: fever, fatigue, weight loss, and an elevated white blood cell count beyond what would be expected with infection. Atrial myxoma would manifest as a mass lesion detectible with echocardiogram. Atrial fibrillation is unlikely given the findings presented. This patient has no colorectal symptoms; thus metastatic colorectal carcinoma is unlikely. Pericarditis is unlikely given the presenting findings in this patient.

22. c (Chapter 9)

This newborn has omphalocele, an opening in the abdominal wall at the umbilicus that is due to incomplete closure of the somatic folds of the anterior abdominal wall in the fetus. The omphalocele can be a part of the pentalogy of Cantrell, which is associated with a diaphragmatic hernia, cleft sternum, absent pericardium, intracardiac defects, and exstrophy of the bladder. Cleft lip and palate are not present in these patients.

23. e (Chapter 9)

The optimal time of convalescence after hernia repair is unknown. After traditional open surgery, patients have been asked to convalesce for 6 to 8 weeks. However, after laparoscopic mesh repair, patients may return to strenuous activity in 2 to 3 weeks. However, the true optimal time of convalescence is not known.

24. a (Chapter 9)

Femoral hernias are located in the femoral canal. The entrance to the canal is bounded superiorly and medially by the iliopubic tract, inferiorly by Cooper ligament, and laterally by the femoral vein. The inguinal ligament is more superficial. The ischial spine is not part of the femoral triangle. The lacunar ligament is not part of the femoral triangle. The femoral vein, not the femoral nerve, forms the lateral boundary of the triangle.

25. b (Chapter 10)

Although preservation of the bladder neck, nervi erigentes, and the size of the bladder neck have all been associated with continence, the only factor that is generally accepted as being related to urinary control after radical prostatectomy is preservation of the external sphincter.

26. c (Chapter 10)

This patient presents with a residual bulky mass after three courses of platinum-based chemotherapy. Although the chest x-ray and β-hCG are normal, the serum AFP remains slightly elevated. AFP production is usually attributed to yolk sac elements in a mixed germ cell tumor. It is also seen with a number of other conditions, such as hepatocellular carcinomas and benign hepatic disease, including alcohol hepatitis, as is probable in this case. Patients with persistent marker elevations after chemotherapy are usually considered very likely to harbor residual carcinoma and probably best managed by further chemotherapy. However, the AFP elevation seen in this case is more likely due to benign liver disease. Consequently, this patient would be best managed by retroperitoneal lymph node dissection instead. The most likely finding at retroperitoneal lymph node dissection would be either fibrosis or residual teratoma. CT scan–directed percutaneous needle biopsy would have considerable sampling error, and external-beam radiotherapy has no efficacy, particularly in the management of teratoma. Further observation is usually not warranted in patients who have residual retroperitoneal masses in excess of 2 to 3 cm.

27. a (Chapter 10)

The frequency of development of metachronous upper tract tumors in patients with superficial transitional cell carcinoma (TCC) of the bladder is not exactly known but has been estimated to be very low (1% to 3%). The incidence is higher in patients with higher stage (T2) primary lesions (2% to 8%).

Patients treated for high-risk superficial TCC with BCG demonstrate a higher rate (13% to 18%) of upper tract tumors over 3 years of follow-up. The best follow-up approach in patients treated with BCG is, therefore, the addition of upper tract imaging in the form of an intravenous pyelogram or CT urogram. Selective cytology as a routine practice is not recommended.

28. a (Chapter 11)

This patient likely has adenocarcinoma of the gallbladder, the most common pathology of gallbladder carcinoma. Ninety percent of patients have cholelithiasis. Metastases can occur to the lymph nodes and to the liver. Prognosis is poor and has a 5-year survival rate ranging from 0% to 10%. There are several rare benign tumors of the gallbladder, including fibroma, lipoma, myxoma, and myoma.

29. a (Chapter 11)

This patient has a congenital malformation of the pancreaticobiliary tree. Specifically, this is a type U choledochal cyst, which is a fusiform dilation of the common bile duct. The type II cyst is a diverticulum of the common bile duct. The type III cyst is a choledochocele involving the bile duct within the liver. The type IV cyst is a cystic celation of the intrahepatic ducts. The type V cyst does not exist.

30. d (Chapter 11)

This patient has sustained a penetrating injury. Gallbladder injuries are uncommon but are seen after such trauma, as in this patient. When the gallbladder is injured, one must search for other injuries. The most frequent associated injury, in 72% of cases, is to the liver. Aortic injuries are less common than are liver injuries. Colon injuries are less common than are liver injuries. Kidney injuries are commonly associated with penetrating trauma. Urinary bladder trauma is often associated with pelvic fractures.

31. e (Chapter 12)

The combination of cough, hemoptysis, wheezing, and smoking history suggests the diagnosis of lung cancer. Of the two lung cancers listed, squamous cell carcinoma is the one that may produce parathyroid hormone (PTH)–related peptide protein. PTH receptor leads to hypercalcemia. Small-cell carcinomas commonly produce antidiuretic hormone or adrenocorticotropin hormone. In a patient with Goodpasture, hemoptysis may present before hematuria, but because of the other symptoms, squamous cell carcinoma is the better choice. Renal cell carcinoma, not renal adenoma, may produce ectopic PTH-related protein, and smokers do have an increased risk, but these patients present with hematuria, a palpable mass, flank pain, and a fever. The lack of an immunoglobulin G or A spike on serum protein electrophoresis should rule out multiple myeloma.

32. b (Chapter 12)

Laryngeal papillomas are benign neoplasms usually located on the true vocal cords. In children, they present as multiple lesions and are usually caused by human papilloma virus. In adults, they occur as single lesions and sometimes undergo malignant change. A singer's nodule is a small benign laryngeal polyp associated with chronic irritation from excessive use or heavy cigarette smoking and is usually found on the true vocal cords. Thyroid carcinoma is unlikely in children.

33. e (Chapter 12)

Squamous cell carcinoma is the most common type of cancer of the larynx. Cigarette smoking is the most important risk factor. Laryngeal polyps are small and benign. They are usually associated with chronic irritation from excessive use or heavy cigarette smoking. Mucoepidermoid and adenocarcinoma of the larynx are not as common as squamous cell carcinoma and don't have dysplasia as a precursor. Laryngitis is acute inflammation of the larynx, trachea, and epiglottis and is most often caused by a viral infection.

34. e (Chapter 13)

Phimosis is an acquired or congenital condition in which the foreskin cannot be pulled back behind the glans penis. In acquired phimosis, there likely is a history of poor hygiene, chronic balanoposthitis, or forceful retraction of a congenital phimosis. Balanitis is inflammation of the glans of the penis. Hypospadias is an anomaly in which the urethral meatus opens on the ventral surface of the penis. Epispadias is an anomaly in which the urethral meatus opens on the dorsal surface of the penis. Paraphimosis is an emergency condition in which the foreskin, once pulled back behind the glans penis, cannot be brought down to its original position.

35. c (Chapter 13)

Dutasteride is 5-alpha reductase inhibitor used in the symptomatic treatment of benign prostatic hyperplasia that blocks the conversion of testosterone to dihydroxy testosterone (DHT) in target tissues. Because DHT is the major intracellular androgen in the prostate, dutasteride is effective in suppressing DHT and, subsequently, stimulation of prostatic growth and secretory function. Prostate size will decrease by approximately 25%. Ejaculatory dysfunction occurs in 5% to 8% of patients. Serum prostate-specific antigen will decrease by 50%. American Urological Association symptom scores typically improve by 5 to 7 points.

36. d (Chapter 13)

More than 90% of testicular tumors derive from germ cell tumors; the remainder are gonadal stromal tumors or metastatic from another site. The most common solid tumor

ANSWERS

in men between the ages of 15 and 40 is a seminoma. These tumors are typically confined to the testicle and associated with a hypoechoic area on ultrasound. This is an important feature, as most other testis tumors are associated with mixed echogenicity on ultrasound. Nonseminomatous germ cell tumors include embryonal carcinoma, choriocarcinoma, endodermal yolk sac tumor, and teratoma.

37. b (Chapter 14)

Arachnoid villi open at a pressure of 5 mm Hg. They act as one-way valves. Cerebrospinal fluid can be absorbed around the spinal nerve roots. Cerebrospinal fluid flows through the ventricles and exits by the foramen of Magendie. The total volume of cerebrospinal fluid is 150 mL.

38. c (Chapter 14)

Epidural hematoma results from hemorrhage into the potential space between the dura and the skull. The hemorrhage most likely results from rupture to a meningeal artery, which travels within this plane; the middle meningeal artery, which branches off the maxillary artery in the temporal area, is most common. Normally, the patient experiences a lucid interval, defined as an asymptomatic period of a few hours after the trauma. A Berry aneurysm results from a defect in the media of arteries and is usually located at bifurcation sites. Berry aneurysms are most commonly found in the circle of Willis. The source of bleeding due to subdural hematoma is from bridging veins; these often occur in older adults as a result of minor trauma, and symptoms usually occur slowly—days to weeks. Bacterial meningitis diagnosis is confirmed with lumbar puncture and demonstrates increased neutrophils/protein and decreased glucose in the cerebrospinal fluid.

39. d (Chapter 14)

This patient may have an acoustic neuroma. These lesions arise from the vestibular portion of cranial nerve VIII. MRI has now become the method of choice for evaluation of posterior fossa and cerebellopontine angle tumors, because they are better seen on MRI as compared with CT. Audiometric testing is useful for lesions of cranial nerve VIII. Brainstem-evoked potential testing is useful for lesions of cranial nerve VIII. Nystagmography is useful for evaluation of vestibular disorders.

40. b (Chapter 15)

The most appropriate incision for a single lung transplant is via lateral thoracotomy. Double lung transplants are usually performed through a transverse anterior thoracotomy incision. Chevron incisions are useful for renal surgery. Midline abdominal incisions are appropriate for abdominal surgeries, not thoracic surgeries. Pfannenstiel incisions are appropriate to approach the female genitourinary tract.

41. c (Chapter 15)

One thing to consider after lung transplantation is survival. It is similar when comparing single with double lung transplantation. It is also related to diagnosis. The best survival is with obstructive lung disease. This is followed by cystic fibrosis. The worst survival is associated with pulmonary hypertension. Bronchogenic carcinoma also has a poor survival rate. Patients with lung cancer are not considered candidates for lung transplantation.

42. a (Chapter 15)

Most candidates for liver transplantation have end-stage liver disease and are likely to die in 1 to 2 years. Children who require liver transplantation often have biliary atresia (in 50% of cases). In adults, postnecrotic cirrhosis accounts for 55% of cases, of which most are due to alcoholism or chronic hepatitis B. Approximately 15% of cases involve primary biliary cirrhosis and primary sclerosing cholangitis.

43. d (Chapter 16)

Pancreatic insufficiency, which is commonly seen in patients with cystic fibrosis, presents with malabsorptive issues and severe steatorrhea. Proper advice is to limit fat intake, as well as to increase ingestion of fat-soluble vitamins. Glucose malabsorption would not have such effects upon stooling. Menstrual loss could incur an anemic condition but not odorous stools. Bleeding ulcers can also cause anemia and black tarry stools, without the odor issues.

44. e (Chapter 16)

The exocrine pancreas is anastomosed to the bladder, and by measuring amylase, the exocrine product of the pancreas, one can monitor the functioning of the graft. Unless the patient had a pancreatectomy, the native pancreas may be making amylase. For the first several days postoperative, the serum glucose may not stabilize, and insulin may be required. The native pancreas may make a variably small amount of insulin, so direct measurement of the graft is not possible. The graft may have good blood flow but not be functioning well as a result of microvascular damage.

45. a (Chapter 16)

Ranson developed 11 criteria to determine the severity of pancreatitis. These factors are divided into admission criteria and initial 48 hours criteria. This patient's age of <55 years is reassuring. His blood glucose level is worrisome. His serum lactate dehydrogenase (LDH) level is worrisome. His serum calcium level is also worrisome. His serum calcium level is low and is also worrisome.

46. d (Chapter 17)

The superior parathyroid glands are located at the junction of the upper and middle third of the thyroid gland on the posteromedial aspect. The inferior parathyroids are located near the junction of the inferior thyroid and the recurrent laryngeal nerve. The carotid sinus is not near the location of the superior parathyroid glands.

47. e (Chapter 17)

Ultrasonography will define an enlarged parathyroid gland in 70% to 80% of cases. Dual tracer imaging can localize adenoma or hyperplasia in 70% of cases. Thyrocervical angiography is reserved for patients with recurrent hyperparathyroidism after surgical neck exploration. CT and MRI are helpful to locate enlarged parathyroid glands that are in the mediastinum.

48. c (Chapter 17)

This patient has tertiary hyperparathyroidism, which occurs in patients with chronic renal disease despite successful renal transplantation. Patients will have hypercalcuria (elevated urine calcium). There is no change in LDH levels. Serum phosphate levels are decreased. Serum and urine calcium levels are increased.

49. d (Chapter 18)

Melanocytes produce melanin and are chiefly responsible for pigmentation of the skin. They are of neural crest origin. One of the diseases associated with melanocytes is vitiligo, which is characterized by flat, well-demarcated zones of pigment loss. Keratinocytes produce keratin, which forms a waterproof layer. Langerhans cells are antigen-presenting cells. Merkel cells are epidermal cells that function in cutaneous sensation. Adipocytes are fat storage cells.

50. a (Chapter 18)

Basal cell carcinomas are the most common skin tumors. They tend to involve skin-exposed areas, most often in the head and neck. Grossly, they are characterized by a pearly papule with overlying telangiectatic vessels. The lower lip is actually the most common site for a tobacco user to develop squamous cell carcinoma. Malignant melanomas are the most likely primary skin tumors to metastasize systemically. Histiocytosis X (Langerhans cell histiocytosis) is caused by a proliferation of Langerhans cells, which are normally found in the epidermis. Seborrheic keratosis is a benign squamoproliferative neoplasm, associated with sunlight exposure. Fairskinned persons are at increased risk. Depth of tumor correlates with risk of metastases.

51. d (Chapter 18)

A keloid is an abnormal proliferation of connective tissue with an abnormal arrangement of collagen. This abnormal proliferation looks very similar to a tumorlike scar. Keloids are much more common in African American individuals and usually follow some sort of trauma—in this case, the ear piercing. The Spitz nevus can be confused with malignant melanoma.

However, the lack of color change or change in size would make melanoma a little less likely. Also, this patient is much younger than the average age of patients who present with melanomatous lesions. Spitz nevus is also known as juvenile melanoma; because of its benign nature, this name is falling out of use. It is important to always think of melanoma when this type of lesion is seen and to order appropriate tests to rule it out. Molluscum contagiosum is a viral disease caused by the DNA poxvirus. It is contracted via direct contact, and its lesions are characteristically pink, umbilicated, and dome-shaped.

52. d (Chapter 19)

Ovarian cancer is an associated risk for women with Peutz-Jegher's syndrome. Granulosa cell tumor is the most common. This condition is not associated with cervical carcinoma. Hereditary renal cell carcinoma can be associated with Von Hippel-Lindau disease. Hamartomas are not associated with liver carcinoma or pancreatic carcinoma.

53. d (Chapter 19)

This patient has carcinoid syndrome, which is caused by the release of substances from a carcinoid tumor. The medical treatment for carcinoid syndrome is octreotide, a somatostatin analog. Topical or intravenous corticosteroids are not beneficial for this patient. Furosemide is a loop diuretic used to treat fluid overload states. Tetracycline is an antibiotic and is not indicated in the treatment of carcinoid syndrome.

54. a (Chapter 19)

Appendicitis is predominantly seen in young adults. It causes right lower quadrant pain, nausea, vomiting, mild fever, and leukocytosis. The inflamed appendix may become gangrenous and perforate in 24 to 48 hours. Therefore, immediate appendectomy is standard treatment. Pancreatitis typically presents with epigastric pain radiating into the back, nausea, vomiting, and fever. Crohn's disease and ulcerative colitis are inflammatory bowel diseases that typically present with long-standing diarrhea. They do not typically present in an acute fashion, as in this patient. Diverticulitis is predominantly found in older adults and typically presents with left lower quadrant pain.

55. c (Chapter 20)

The left gastroepiploic artery runs through the gastrosplenic ligament to reach the greater omentum. The gastroduodenal artery and the right gastric artery branch off of the common hepatic artery. The gastroduodenal artery descends behind the first part of the duodenum. The right gastric artery runs to the pylorus and then along the lesser curvature of the stomach. The left gastric artery and the splenic artery arise from the celiac trunk. The left gastric artery runs upward and to the left toward the cardia, giving rise to esophageal and hepatic branches, and then turns right and runs along the lesser curvature within the lesser omentum to anastomose with the right gastric artery.

56. c (Chapter 20)

This child has a Meckel's diverticulum, which is a congenital anomaly resulting from an unobliterated yolk stalk. More specifically, it is a vestigial remnant of the omphalomesenteric duct. It presents as an ileal outpouching typically located close to the ileocecal valve. The presence of inflammation, ulceration, and gastrointestinal bleeding due to the presence of ectopic acid–secreting gastric epithelium is seen in approximately half of these patients. Remember the rule of 2s with Meckel's diverticulum: It occurs in approximately 2% of children, occurs within approximately 2 ft of the ileocecal valve, contains 2 types of ectopic mucosa (gastric and pancreatic), and its symptoms usually occur by age 2.

57. c (Chapter 20)

Because of the symptoms of decreased burning with food intake and weight gain, a preliminary differential diagnosis of *Helicobacter pylori* would be appropriate. Treatment with the triple therapy of bismuth salicylate, metronidazole, and an antibiotic such as amoxicillin would be in order. The presentation of *Escherichia coli* tends to be a more acute infection. *E. coli* is associated with bloody diarrhea, and *Shigella* with abdominal cramping and diarrhea.

58. e (Chapter 21)

Thrombocytopenia is not a complication of a splenectomy. Thrombocytosis is a possible complication postsplenectomy. Anemia is not a direct result of splenectomy. Patients are unlikely to have basophilia or eosinophilia. Subphrenic abscess, atelectasis, pancreatitis, gastric dilation, and sepsis are the possible complications of splenectomy.

59. c (Chapter 21)

The peripheral blood smear in a postsplenectomy patient will show Pappenheimer bodies, Howell-Jolly bodies, and Heinz bodies. Nucleated red blood cells are found in the blood of sickle cell patients. Basophilic stippling is found in the blood of patients with lead poisoning. Spherocytes are found in patients with hemolytic anemia. Blister cells are found in the blood of patients with glucose-6-phosphate deficiency.

60. d (Chapter 21)

Postsplenectomy patients should receive vaccinations against encapsulated organisms. The common encapsulated organisms are *Streptococcus pneumoniae, Neisseria meningitides,* and *Haemophilus influenzae.* The best time to vaccinate these patients is preoperatively.

61. b (Chapter 22)

This patient likely has Hashimoto thyroiditis. Patients have mild thyroid tenderness and fatigue. Laboratory features include the presence of thyroid autoantibodies. Frequently, no treatment is necessary for this condition. Acute thyroiditis is associated with fever, chills, and dysphagia. Papillary carcinoma is associated

with a palpable thyroid nodule. Riedel thyroiditis is associated with thyroid fibrosis. Symptoms of tracheal and esophageal compression are possible.

62. e (Chapter 22)

This patient has evidence of papillary carcinoma of the thyroid. Only 5% of patients with papillary carcinoma of the thyroid present with distant metastases. For tumors that are <1.5 cm and that are disease-confined to one lobe and no extracapsular extension, treatment with thyroid lobectomy is appropriate. External-beam radiotherapy is not required for this patient. Multiagent chemotherapy is not required for this patient. Subtotal and total thyroidectomy are not required for this patient.

63. a (Chapter 22)

Injury to the nerve causes bowing of the vocal cords during phonation. This can be a problem in singers who have difficulty reaching high-pitched notes. The nerve can be at risk during thyroid surgical procedures because of its proximity to the superior thyroid artery. The nerve is both sensory and motor to the larynx.

64. d (Chapter 23)

This patient is apneic. An airway must be established for this patient. However, he may also have fractures of the cervical spine. Thus the best treatment for this patient in terms of airway management is a tracheostomy. Nasotracheal intubation is inappropriate for a patient who is totally apneic. Oral intubation and oral intubation with head-chin lift is inappropriate because it requires some hyperextension of the neck. Intubation is necessary for a patient who is apneic.

65. b (Chapter 23)

It is unlikely that this patient has an open pneumothorax. Patients with pneumothorax are in obvious respiratory distress. They often have an obvious "sucking" chest wound. This patient has neither of the above findings. Left pneumothorax is possible in this patient and needs evaluation with a chest x-ray. Cardiac tamponade is possible in this patient, as is rupture of the main stem bronchus. Tension pneumothorax is also a consideration for this patient.

66. c (Chapter 23)

An amputated upper extremity body part can be replanted if properly recovered and transported with the patient. Cooling the body part in a chest filled with crushed ice and water may preserve the body part for up to 18 hours. The body part should not be placed in dry gauze or packed with dry ice. In addition, the body part should not be placed in warm water.

67. e (Chapter 23)

An ulcer will appear as a fluorescein-stained epithelial defect with a local corneal infiltrate. This patient appears to have no evidence of an ulcer. However, this form of testing does not rule out the presence of bacterial infection, iritis, trauma, or viral infection. This patient will benefit from treatment with quinolone eyedrops and avoidance of eye patching. Close follow-up with a physician is also recommended.

68. b (Chapter 23)

This patient has suffered a metallic foreign body to the eye with an epithelial rust ring. These should be removed immediately with an eye burr. Foreign bodies of the cornea can also be approached with a fine needle tip or an eye spud. Sterile water may be used, but alcohol exposure to the eye should be avoided. Cyanoacrylate glue adheres to the eyes and should also be avoided.

69. c (Chapter 23)

This patient has sustained a chemical burn to the eye. The eye should be immediately flushed at the scene with 1 to 2 L of normal saline, which should be continued in the emergency department. A topical anesthetic and a Morgan lens will facilitate flushing. Eye patch placement is not indicated. Placement of the eye under direct sunlight may damage the eye. Watchful waiting is not recommended; this patient needs eye lavage as soon as possible.

70. e (Chapter 25)

This patient likely has a compartment syndrome, which is caused by an increase in interstitial fluid pressure within an osteofascial compartment, leading to compromise of the microcirculation and myoneural necrosis. Diagnosis is confirmed by an intracompartmental pressure of 30 mm Hg or higher. Treatment of this condition is surgical fascial release.

71. a (Chapter 25)

Bursae are fluid-filled sacs that cushion areas of friction between tendon and bone or skin. Bursae are lined with special cells called synovial cells, which secrete a fluid rich in collagen and proteins. This synovial fluid acts as a lubricant when parts of the body move. When this fluid becomes irritated because of too much movement, the painful condition known as bursitis results. Rheumatoid arthritis is a multisystem disorder that results in symmetrical joint inflammation, articular erosions, and extra-articular complications. Infectious arthritis is unlikely in the absence of joint fluid aspiration that reveals an organism. Septic thrombophlebitis is unlikely given the history of this patient. Trauma is also unlikely given the history of this patient.

72. c (Chapter 25)

This patient may have suffered a tear of the rotator cuff. Most tears are small and may be treated symptomatically with rest, elevation, and anti-inflammatory agents. If the shoulder still

demonstrates pain after a trial of conservative therapy, surgical repair should be considered. Injection of corticosteroids or intravenous corticosteroids is not considered to be first-line therapy for this patient.

73. a (Chapter 26)

Multiple randomized controlled studies have demonstrated decreased mortality and morbidity with intraoperative beta blockade in high-risk patients. This is one of the few interventions that has been clearly shown to improve outcomes.

74. e (Chapter 26)

In the setting of a normal history and physical, it is not necessary to obtain preoperative labs for minor surgery, though many surgeons and institutions will do this.

75. d (Chapter 26)

Lactated Ringer's solution is a bicarbonate-rich solution with an electrolyte composition similar to stool output.

76. a (Chapter 1)

Although all of the options contain important principles of wound closure, the most relevant here is gentle handling of the tissue and closure without tension to prevent further damage that can result in poor healing, infection, or hypertrophic scar formation. Although debridement of devitalized tissue is important, in this type of injury, the surrounding tissue is generally healthy and well vascularized.

77. b (Chapter 16)

This patient has signs and symptoms of an abdominal aortic aneurysm. This is suggested by the mentioned risk factors and physical examination findings. CT scan will provide precise anatomical detail and location of the aneurysm. This is particularly important for consideration of stent graft repair. Aortogram may be useful as a secondary test to prepare for surgical resection. Ultrasound could be performed to determine the presence of clot in the aortic lumen. The ultrasound choices given in this question would be unlikely to determine clot in the lumen because they are focusing on the upper quadrants and not the midline.

78. d (Chapter 14)

Younger women have more fibrous tissue, which makes mammograms harder to interpret. Thus ultrasound is a useful testing modality. This patient has a family history of breast cancer. Therefore, ultrasound and consideration for breast biopsy would be most prudent. As women age, breast tissue transforms from fibrous tissue to adipose tissue. This change makes it easier for mammography to detect masses. Thus this modality is more useful in patients older than 35 years. Watchful waiting may be considered if the lesion is benign. Testing for the *BRCA* gene may be considered if the patient is suspect to a family history of breast cancer.

79. e (Chapter 5)

This patient likely has ulcerative colitis. Patients complain of bloody diarrhea, fever, and weight loss and have frequent attacks of symptoms. Colonoscopy often reveals thickened, friable mucosa. Fissures and pseudopolyps are also common. Diverticulosis is rare in a patient younger than 30 years. Although internal hemorrhoids are a possible cause of bleeding in this patient, they do not present with the associated findings of abdominal pain and weight loss.

80. c (Chapter 15)

This patient has a glucagonoma, a tumor produced by pancreatic alpha cells that increases glycogenolysis and gluconeogenesis and leads to increased blood glucose levels. Glucagonomas are associated with necrolytic migratory erythema, a characteristically red, scaly rash usually located on the face but also occurring in other locations. Typical patients are thin and have an insidious onset of symptoms. Insulinoma would produce dizziness, diaphoresis, anxiety, and tremor because of the increased production of insulin and resulting hypoglycemia. Patients with type II diabetes mellitus are often obese and have a gradual onset of symptoms. Patients with Verner Morrison disease often complain of watery diarrhea, hypokalemia, and achlorhydria.

81. c (Chapter 19)

This patient likely has esophageal cancer by history. Any older patient with dysphagia should be assumed to have esophageal cancer until proven otherwise. This patient is a smoker with progressive dysphagia and lymphadenopathy, placing him at high risk. Definitive diagnosis requires biopsy at the time of esophagogastroscopy. CT and MRI may evaluate the presence of regional lymphatic spread. Barium study will detect lesions in more than 90% of patients but will not provide tissue for pathologic examination.

82. d (Chapter 7)

This patient likely has sickle cell anemia. Calcium bilirubinate stones are found in association with the following conditions: chronic biliary infection, cirrhosis, and hemolytic processes such as sickle cell anemia. A high-cholesterol diet has a role in the pathogenesis of cholesterol stones.

83. b (Chapter 17)

Atrial septal defects are often mild until later in life. As a result of the low pressures of both atria, only a small left-to-right shunt will occur. Over time, this increase in blood return to the right heart leads to pulmonary hypertension and right ventricular hypertrophy. Ventricular septal defect is associated with late cyanosis because of the left to right shunt. Patent ductus arteriosis is also associated with a left-to-right shunt and late cyanosis. The posterior descending artery can close with indomethacin treatment. Tetralogy of Fallot is the most common cause of early cyanosis. It is the result of a right-to-left shunt and results in early cyanosis.

84. c (Chapter 11)

Umbilical hernias are the result of a patent umbilical ring at birth. Some of the other choices in this question, such as patent omphalomesenteric duct, are seen in association with umbilical hernias, but this is likely coincidence as opposed to causality. Most of these hernias will resolve without the need for operation.

85. e (Chapter 21)

This patient has a uric acid stone. These stones are visible on CT scan but not on KUB x-rays. Calcium and struvite stones, on the other hand, are visible on both CT scan and on KUB x-rays. Knowing the visibility of stones on imaging modalities assists with treatment decisions.

86. b (Chapter 6)

Recurrent pancreatitis occurs within 6 weeks in nearly 50% of patients. When this occurs, complications of pancreatitis can be severe. Although the other choices are possible, they are not nearly as common.

87. e (Chapter 18)

Angioma is a benign tumor that frequently regresses, and simple observation (watchful waiting) with serial examinations and imagines studies is recommended. There is no need for other treatments such as corticosteroids, antibiotics, or lobectomy.

88. d (Chapter 22)

This patient likely has transitional cell carcinoma of the bladder. This is a common cause of painless gross hematuria in patients older than 50 years. This consideration is strengthened by the CT scan findings in this question (hydronephrosis and bladder mass). Both renal cell carcinoma and advanced prostate cancer can present with hematuria, but it is less likely. Urinary tract infections are also a cause of hematuria, but are not common in men. Nephrolithiasis can cause hematuria, but are more likely to cause flank pain.

89. a (Chapter 20)

This man most likely has adult polycystic kidney disease, an autosomal dominant disease. It is the most common inherited disorder of the kidney. Adult polycystic kidney disease is often associated with berry aneurysm in the circle of Willis. These aneurysms are prone to rupture, leading to subarachnoid hemorrhage. Cerebellar hemangioma is associated with von Hippel-Lindau disease, an autosomal dominant disease of chromosome 3.

90. a (Chapter 26)

Acute rejection typically occurs days to months after transplantation and is characterized by significant inflammation. Acute rejection is primarily T-cell mediated. These patients typically present with symptoms of acute renal failure. Hyperacute rejection occurs within minutes or hours of the transplantation and is due to preformed antibodies against the donor. In a hyperacute kidney rejection, the graft would rapidly become cyanotic, mottled, and flaccid and does not produce urine. Chronic rejection is probably more correctly termed chronic allograft nephropathy and presents years after transplantation with chronic changes on biopsy. Patients typically present clinically with a progressive increase in serum creatinine levels over a 4-to 6-month period.

91. c (Chapter 9)

This patient has suffered from chronic pain which is presumed to be of pancreatic origin. This can initially be treated with oral analgesics. For patients for whom this treatment fails, operative drainage is considered next. All of the above steps have failed, and therefore, this patient would best benefit from interruption of sympathetic nerve fibers (splanchnicectomy).

92. d (Chapter 13)

Patients with primary hyperparathyroidism can have renal stones. Typically, patients have multiple and bilateral stones. Thus a patient with 1-mm, 2-mm, and 3-mm stones bilaterally and visible on KUB suggests calcium stones.

93. b (Chapter 23)

Histologically, the epidermis has five layers, which are demarcated on the basis of microscopic morphology. The most superficial layer, the stratum corneum, is characterized by anucleate cells filled with keratin filaments. Beneath the stratum corneum is the stratum lucidum, which is only seen well in thick skin and is considered to actually be a subdivision of the stratum corneum. The stratum granulosum is beneath the stratum lucidum and contains keratohyalin granule-containing cells. The stratum spinosum, beneath the stratum granulosum, is composed of spiny-looking cells. Finally, the stratum basale, the deepest layer of the epidermis, is composed of a single layer of stem cells from which keratinocytes arise.

94. a (Chapter 4)

Because of the presence of granulomas in the colon, mycobacterial infection is thought to be the causative agent. Thus if one were to consider antibiotic therapy in such a patient, it should be directed toward this agent. However, no specific immunologic disturbance has been described for this disease.

95. d (Chapter 3)

This patient has postcricoid carcinoma, which is associated with Plummer-Vinson syndrome. Dysphagia is nearly always a symptom of organic disease rather than a functional complaint. Lymphoma and leukemia are rarely associated with iron deficiency anemia. Rheumatoid arthritis is associated with arthralgias of joints of the hands. Iron deficiency anemia is uncommon with this condition.

96. d (Chapter 8)

Accessory spleens are present in approximately 25% of patients. They are most often found in the splenic hilum. The second most common location is the splenic ligaments and greater omentum. Accessory spleens are almost never found in the right upper or lower quadrants.

97. c (Chapter 12)

This patient has a thyroglossal duct cyst. These are most commonly seen in children and appear as a single painless lump in the midline that moves with swallowing. Thyroid carcinoma is rare in children. Leukemia and lymphoma would be associated with palpable lymphadenopathy in the neck.

98. a (Chapter 27)

There are two ophthalmic injuries that require immediate treatment: acid/alkali burns and an unremovable corneal or conjunctival foreign body. The other choices should be referred immediately and do not require immediate on site treatment.

99. d (Chapter 24)

Primary closure is the simplest and most common method of wound closure. Surgical wounds created during a procedure are typically closed in this fashion. Delayed primary closure is considered if the wound is contaminated or requires debridement.

100. a (Chapter 25)

Bursae are fluid-filled sacs that cushion areas of friction between tendon and bone or skin. Bursae are lined with special cells called synovial cells, which secrete a fluid rich in collagen and proteins. This synovial fluid acts as a lubricant when parts of the body move. When this fluid becomes irritated because of too much movement, the painful condition known as bursitis results. Rheumatoid arthritis is a multisystem disorder that

ANSWERS

results in symmetrical joint inflammation, articular erosions, and extra-articular complications. Gonococcal arthritis is unlikely in the absence of joint fluid aspiration that reveals Gram-negative diplococci. Rheumatoid arthritis is an autoimmune disease that affects the synovial joints, with pannus formation in the joints (metacarpophalangeal, proximal interphalangeal), subcutaneous rheumatoid nodules, ulnar deviation, and subluxation. Septic bursitis is unlikely in the absence of a joint fluid aspiration that reveals organisms on Gram stain. Trauma is unlikely given the history in this patient.

Index

Note: Page numbers referencing figures are italicized and followed by an "*f*". Page numbers referencing tables are italicized and followed by a "*t*".